Case Studies in Neurology

Editor

RANDOLPH W. EVANS

NEUROLOGIC CLINICS

www.neurologic.theclinics.com

Consulting Editor
RANDOLPH W. EVANS

August 2016 • Volume 34 • Number 3

ELSEVIER

1600 John F. Kennedy Boulevard • Suite 1800 • Philadelphia, Pennsylvania, 19103-2899

http://www.theclinics.com

NEUROLOGIC CLINICS Volume 34, Number 3
August 2016 ISSN 0733-8619, ISBN-13: 978-0-323-45979-2

Editor: Lauren Boyle
Developmental editor: Donald Mumford

Neurologic Clinics (ISSN 0733-8619) is published quarterly by Elsevier Inc., 360 Park Avenue South, New York, NY 10010–1710. Months of issue are February, May, August, and November. Periodicals postage paid at New York, NY, and additional mailing offices. Subscription prices are $300.00 per year for US individuals, $578.00 per year for US institutions, $100.00 per year for US students, $375.00 per year for Canadian individuals, $701.00 per year for Canadian institutions, $415.00 per year for international individuals, $701.00 per year for international institutions, and $210.00 for Canadian and foreign students/residents. To receive student/resident rate, orders must be accompanied by name of affiliated institution, date of term, and the *signature* of program/residency coordinator on institution letterhead. Orders will be billed at individual rate until proof of status is received. Foreign air speed delivery is included in all *Clinics* subscription prices. All prices are subject to change without notice. **POSTMASTER:** Send address changes to *Neurologic Clinics*, Elsevier Health Sciences Division, Subscription Customer Service, 3251 Riverport Lane, Maryland Heights, MO 63043. **Customer Service: Telephone: 1-800-654-2452 (U.S. and Canada); 314-447-8871 (outside U.S. and Canada). Fax: 314-447-8029. E-mail: journalscustomerservice-usa@elsevier.com (for print support); journalsonlinesupport-usa@elsevier.com (for online support).**

Reprints. For copies of 100 or more of articles in this publication, please contact the Commercial Reprints Department, Elsevier Inc., 360 Park Avenue South, New York, New York, 10010-1710; Tel.: +1-212-633-3874; Fax: +1-212-633-3820, and E-mail: reprints@elsevier.com.

Neurologic Clinics is also published in Spanish by Nueva Editorial Interamericana S.A., Mexico City, Mexico.

Neurologic Clinics is covered in *Current Contents/Clinical Medicine, MEDLINE/PubMed (Index Medicus), EMBASE/Excerpta Medica, and PsycINFO, and ISI/BIOMED.*

Contributors

CONSULTING EDITOR

RANDOLPH W. EVANS, MD
Clinical Professor, Department of Neurology, Baylor College of Medicine, Houston, Texas

EDITOR

RANDOLPH W. EVANS, MD
Clinical Professor, Department of Neurology, Baylor College of Medicine, Houston, Texas

AUTHORS

ALEC L. AMRAM, MD
Department of Ophthalmology, University of Texas Medical Branch, Galveston, Texas

ALON Y. AVIDAN, MD, MPH
Professor, Department of Neurology, Director, UCLA Sleep Disorders Center, Director, UCLA Neurology Clinic, David Geffen School of Medicine at UCLA, Los Angeles, California

SHIN C. BEH, MD
Department of Neurology and Neurotherapeutics, University of Texas Southwestern Medical Center, Dallas, Texas

GAMZE BALCI CAMSARI, MD
Fellow of Behavioral Neurology, Department of Neurology, Mayo Clinic, Jacksonville, Florida

ALAN CARSON, MB ChB, MD, FRCP, FRCPsych
Consultant Neuropsychiatrist and Honorary Reader in Neuropsychiatry, Departments of Clinical Neurosciences and Psychological Medicine, Western General Hospital, University of Edinburgh, Edinburgh, United Kingdom

RANDOLPH W. EVANS, MD
Clinical Professor, Department of Neurology, Baylor College of Medicine, Houston, Texas

MUHAMMAD U. FAROOQ, MD, FACP, FAHA
Division of Stroke and Vascular Neurology, Mercy Health Hauenstein Neurosciences, Grand Rapids, Michigan

ELLIOT M. FROHMAN, MD, PhD, FAAN, FANA
Departments of Neurology and Neurotherapeutics, Ophthalmology, University of Texas Southwestern Medical Center, Dallas, Texas

TERESA C. FROHMAN, PA-C, MPAS
Department of Neurology and Neurotherapeutics, University of Texas Southwestern Medical Center, Dallas, Texas; Department of BioEngineering, University of Texas at Dallas, Richardson, Texas

PAULA GARDINER, MSc, Dip CBT
NeuroSpecialist Physiotherapist/CBT Therapist, Department of Clinical Neurosciences, Western General Hospital, University of Edinburgh, Edinburgh, United Kingdom

JEANNETTE GELAUFF, MD
PhD-Student, Department of Neurology, University Medical Center Groningen, University of Groningen, Groningen, Netherlands

PHILIP B. GORELICK, MD, MPH, FACP, FAAN, FANA, FAHA
Professor, Department of Translational Science and Molecular Medicine, Medical Director, Mercy Health Hauenstein Neurosciences, Michigan State University College of Human Medicine, Grand Rapids, Michigan

NEILL R. GRAFF-RADFORD, MBBCh, FRCP (UK)
David Eisenberg Professor, Department of Neurology, Mayo College of Medicine, Mayo Clinic, Jacksonville, Florida

BENJAMIN GREENBERG, MD, MHS
Department of Neurology and Neurotherapeutics, University of Texas Southwestern Medical Center, Dallas, Texas

INGRID HOERITZAUER, MB ChB, BSc, MRCP
Research Fellow in Neurology, Department of Clinical Neurosciences, Western General Hospital, University of Edinburgh, Edinburgh, United Kingdom

EMILY L. JOHNSON, MD
Epilepsy Fellow, Department of Neurology, Johns Hopkins School of Medicine, Baltimore, Maryland

JAMES C. JOHNSTON, MD, JD
Legal Medicine Consultants, San Antonio, Texas

ERIC J. KILDEBECK, MD, PhD
Department of Neurology and Neurotherapeutics, University of Texas Southwestern Medical Center, Dallas, Texas; Center for Engineering Innovation, University of Texas at Dallas, Richardson, Texas

INNA KLEYMAN, MD
Assistant Professor, Department of Neurology, Columbia University College of Physicians and Surgeons; The Neurological Institute of New York, New York, New York

GREGORY L. KRAUSS, MD
Professor, Department of Neurology, Johns Hopkins School of Medicine, Baltimore, Maryland

ANDREW G. LEE, MD
Department of Ophthalmology, Blanton Eye Institute, Houston Methodist Hospital, Houston, Texas; Department of Ophthalmology, University of Texas Medical Branch, Galveston, Texas; Department of Ophthalmology, Baylor College of Medicine, Houston, Texas; Departments of Ophthalmology, Neurology, and Neurosurgery, Weill Cornell Medicine, New York, New York; Section of Ophthalmology, UT MD Anderson Cancer Center, Houston, Texas

ALEX LEHN, MD, FRACP
Consultant Neurologist, Mater Centre for Neurosciences; School of Medicine, University of Queensland, Queensland, Australia

MELISSA E. MURRAY, PhD
Assistant Professor, Department of Neuroscience, Mayo Clinic, Jacksonville, Florida

RAM NARAYAN, MD
Department of Neurology and Neurotherapeutics, University of Texas Southwestern Medical Center, Dallas, Texas

MARY ANGELA O'NEAL, MD
Director of Women's Neurology, Brigham and Women's Hospital; Instructor of Neurology, Harvard Medical School, Boston, Massachusetts

LORI ANI PANOSSIAN, MD
Medical Director, Sleep Laboratory, East Bay Division, Department of Neurology, Veterans Affairs Northern California Health Care System, Martinez, California

ALEJANDRO A. RABINSTEIN, MD
Professor, Department of Neurology, Mayo Clinic, Rochester, Minnesota

ELSA M. RODARTE, MD
Department of Neurobiology and Anatomy, University of Texas Health Science Center at Houston, Houston, Texas

AMRA SAKUSIC, MD
Research Fellow, Department of Critical Care, Mayo Clinic, Rochester, Minnesota; Departments of Internal Medicine and Pulmonary Medicine, Tuzla University Medical Center, Tuzla, Bosnia and Herzegovina

THOMAS P. SARTWELLE, BBA, LLB
Deans and Lyons, LLP, Houston, Texas

TAD SEIFERT, MD
Director, Sports Concussion Program, Norton Healthcare; Head, NCAA Headache Task Force, Louisville, Kentucky

AZIZ SHAIBANI, MD, FAAN, FACP, FANA
Director, Nerve and Muscle Center of Texas, Clinical Professor of Medicine, Baylor College of Medicine, Houston, Texas

VICKI L. SHANKER, MD
Assistant Professor of Neurology, Icahn School of Medicine at Mount Sinai, New York, New York

STACY V. SMITH, MD
Department of Ophthalmology, Blanton Eye Institute, Houston Methodist Hospital, Houston, Texas

JON STONE, MB ChB, PhD, FRCP
Consultant Neurologist and Honorary Reader in Neurology, Department of Clinical Neurosciences, Western General Hospital, University of Edinburgh, Edinburgh, United Kingdom

KATHERINE TREADAWAY, LCSW, ACP
Department of Neurology and Neurotherapeutics, University of Texas Southwestern Medical Center, Dallas, Texas

ANNE VAN GILS, MD
Specialty Registrar in Psychiatry, University Medical Center Groningen, Interdisciplinary Center Psychopathology and Emotion Regulation, University of Groningen, Groningen, Netherlands

LOUIS H. WEIMER, MD
Professor, Department of Neurology, Columbia University College of Physicians and Surgeons; The Neurological Institute of New York, New York, New York

KNUT WESTER, MD, PhD
Department of Clinical Medicine K1, University of Bergen; Department of Neurosurgery, Haukeland University Hospital, Bergen, Norway

Contents

favors a myopathic cause for distal weakness. Electromyogram confirms this diagnosis. Profuse spontaneous discharges are common in inflammatory, metabolic, and myofibrillar myopathy (MFM). If the clinical picture indicates a specific disease such as facioscapulohumeral muscular dystrophy (FSHD), genetic testing provides the quickest diagnosis. Otherwise, muscle biopsy can distinguish specific features. The common causes of myopathic distal weakness are FSHD, myotonic dystrophy, and inclusion body myositis. Other causes include MFM, distal muscular dystrophies, metabolic myopathies, and congenital myopathies.

challenges facing the neurointensivist. Life-threatening medical complications after severe acute ischemic stroke, seizures and extreme agitation from autoimmune encephalitis, refractory seizures after subdural hemorrhage, neurologic and systemic complications related to aneurysmal sub arachnoid hemorrhage, and status epilepticus after cardiac arrest are discussed in this article.

Many dementia subtypes have more shared signs and symptoms than defining ones. We review 8 cases with 4 overlapping syndromes and demonstrate how to distinguish the cases. These include focal cortical presentations of Alzheimer's disease (AD; posterior cortical atrophy and corticobasal syndrome [CBS]), fluent aphasia (semantic dementia and logopenic aphasia), late-onset slowly progressive dementia (hippocampal sclerosis and limbic predominant AD) and rapidly progressive dementia (Creutzfeldt–Jakob disease and limbic encephalitis). Recognizing the different syndromes can help the clinician to improve their diagnostic skills, leading to improved patient outcomes by early and accurate diagnosis, prompt treatment, and appropriate counseling and guidance.

The anatomic and physiologic changes that occur during pregnancy are unique. A neurologist needs to be aware of normal pregnancy-induced physiologic changes in the cardiovascular, renal, hematologic, and autoimmune systems, and the local anatomic changes, which include alteration of body habitus and pelvic ligaments. These changes are clearly advantageous, but in certain circumstances may predispose to pathology. In addition, pregnancy effects treatment of chronic neurologic conditions as regards medication safety and metabolism. This case-oriented review discusses the important aspects of pregnancy physiology and an approach to treatment of common disorders encountered during pregnancy including stroke, multiple sclerosis, epilepsy, and compression neuropathies.

With regard to persistent posttraumatic headache, there is legitimate concern that duration of symptoms may have an impact on the efficacy of future treatment attempts. Without neuropathologic confirmation, a clinical diagnosis of chronic traumatic encephalopathy cannot be made with a high degree of confidence. Sport-related headaches are challenging in a return-to-play context, because it is often unclear whether an athlete has an exacerbation of a primary headache disorder, has new-onset headache unrelated to trauma, or is in the recovery phase after concussion. Regular physical exercise may prove beneficial to multiple neurologic disease states.

A young woman presents with an intracranial arachnoid cyst. Another is diagnosed with migraine headache. An elderly man awakens with a stroke. And a baby delivered vaginally after 2 hours of questionable electronic fetal monitoring patterns grows up to have cerebral palsy. These seemingly disparate cases share a common underlying theme: medical myths. Myths that may lead not only to misdiagnosis and treatment harms but to seemingly never-ending medical malpractice lawsuits, potentially culminating in a settlement or judgment against an unsuspecting neurologist. This article provides a case studies approach exposing the fallacies and highlighting proper management of these common neurologic presentations.

NEUROLOGIC CLINICS

RELATED INTEREST

Psychiatric Clinics, December 2015 (Vol. 38, Issue 4)
Sleep Disorders and Mental Health
Andrew Winokur and Jayesh Kamath, *Editors*

THE CLINICS ARE AVAILABLE ONLINE!
Access your subscription at:
www.theclinics.com

Preface

Case Studies in Neurology

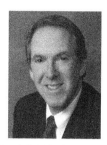

Randolph W. Evans, MD
Editor

n = 1. That's the formula for the clinical interactions of neurologists, diagnosing and treating patients one by one, with their unique genomics, demographics, comorbidities, and clinical presentations. As we all know too well, evidence-based medicine is sometimes helpful, often not. Perhaps 40% of medical practice is either not effective or harmful, and often we don't know.[1] The art of medicine is flourishing in clinical neurology.

The May 2006 issue, "Neurology Case Studies," was very well received. We are again providing you with another case-based issue, which is an excellent exercise in active learning where you can consider each case, come to your own conclusions, and then compare them to the subspecialty experts who review the latest evidence and give their opinions.

This issue of the *Neurologic Clinics* reviews cases and topics in cerebrovascular disease, multiple sclerosis, syncope, neuromuscular disease, sleep disorders, epilepsy, neuro-ophthalmology, headache, tremor, functional neurologic disorders, neurocritical care, dementia, neurology of pregnancy, sports neurology, and neurologic malpractice. The disorders range from the rare to the commonplace, and the issues range from the most controversial to those widely accepted. We hope you find this issue as educational and stimulating to read as we did to write.

I thank our distinguished contributors for their outstanding articles. I also thank Lauren Elise Boyle, *Clinics* editor, Donald Mumford, senior developmental editor, and the Elsevier production team for an excellent job. Finally, I am grateful for the support of my wife, Marilyn, and our children, Elliott, Rochelle, son-in-law, Corry, and Jonathan.

Randolph W. Evans, MD
Baylor College of Medicine
1200 Binz #1370
Houston, TX 77004, USA

E-mail address:
revansmd@gmail.com

Neurol Clin 34 (2016) xiii–xiv
http://dx.doi.org/10.1016/j.ncl.2016.05.002
0733-8619/16/$ – see front matter © 2016 Published by Elsevier Inc.

neurologic.theclinics.com

REFERENCE

1. Prasad VK, Cifu AS. Ending medical reversal: improving outcomes, saving lives. Baltimore (MD): Johns Hopkins, 2015.

Neurology Case Studies
Cerebrovascular Disease

Muhammad U. Farooq, MD[a],*, Philip B. Gorelick, MD, MPH[b]

KEYWORDS

- Intracranial stenosis • Intracranial occlusive disease • Migrainous stroke
- Susac syndrome • Cerebral autosomal dominant arteriopathy with subcortical infarcts and leukoencephalopathy • Posterior reversible encephalopathy syndrome
- Eclampsia

KEY POINTS

- This article provides a series of interesting neurologic cases practice and discusses diagnosis and treatment.
- Because several of the cases are uncommon causes of stroke, there is no high-level evidence base to guide the clinician in relation to diagnosis and treatment.
- One must recognize the pattern of clinical features to arrive at the proper diagnostic workup and diagnosis and exercise good clinical judgment in relation to reasonable treatment.
- Careful neurologic history and examination remain paramount to determining the correct diagnosis and subsequent treatment.

CASE 1: MANAGEMENT OF SYMPTOMATIC INTRACRANIAL ARTERY STENOSIS
Case Presentation

A 79-year-old man with a medical history of hypertension, type-2 diabetes mellitus, hyperlipidemia, and coronary artery disease presented with spells of intermittent left hand grip weakness and left hand numbness. His wife observed facial asymmetry and speech impairment with some of the episodes. The duration of the spells was up to 1 hour, and they occurred over a 2- to 3-week period. In the emergency department (ED), the National Institutes of Health Stroke Scale (NIHSS) score was 1 (left upper extremity sensory impairment). The patient did not receive intravenous (IV) thrombolytic therapy because of delay in presentation to the ED. He had no history of cardiac

Conflict of Interest: None.
[a] Division of Stroke and Vascular Neurology, Mercy Health Hauenstein Neurosciences, 200 Jefferson Street Southeast, Grand Rapids, MI 49503, USA; [b] Department Translational Science & Molecular Medicine, Mercy Health Hauenstein Neurosciences, Michigan State University College of Human Medicine, 220 Cherry Street Southeast, Room H 3037, Grand Rapids, MI 49503, USA
* Corresponding author.
E-mail address: farooqmu@mercyhealth.com

Neurol Clin 34 (2016) 467–482
http://dx.doi.org/10.1016/j.ncl.2016.04.001
0733-8619/16/$ – see front matter © 2016 Elsevier Inc. All rights reserved.

neurologic.theclinics.com

arrhythmia such as atrial fibrillation. His low-density lipoprotein cholesterol level was 111 mg/dL, and HbA1c was 7.4%. The patient had computerized axial tomography (CT) and MRI of the brain. Brain CT was unremarkable, but brain MRI showed areas of restricted diffusion (Fig. 1A, B). The areas of restricted diffusion were interpreted as being consistent with embolic stroke. There was no evidence of hemodynamically significant stenosis of the carotid arteries. Magnetic resonance angiography (MRA) of the brain without contrast was limited by motion artifact. CT angiography (CTA) was not obtained, as there was renal impairment caused by diabetes. Echocardiography with bubble study did not show evidence of a cardiac source of stroke. The patient was discharged to home on aspirin, 81 mg daily, and atorvastatin, 40 mg at bed time. He underwent cardiac event monitoring for 28 days, and there was no evidence of atrial fibrillation.

The patient was readmitted to the hospital almost 4 weeks later with left arm and leg weakness, decrease sensation of the left arm, dysarthria, and left facial droop. His symptoms improved, and in the ED his NIHSS score was 3 (left arm and leg drift and left arm sensory loss). In spite of previous stroke education, there was a delay in the patient's presentation to the ED, and he did not receive IV tissue plasminogen activator therapy. Brain CT in the ED did not show an acute intracranial process. Brain MRI again showed multiple new areas of restricted diffusion consistent with embolic strokes (Fig. 1C, D). The patient had conventional cerebral angiography, which showed hemodynamically significant stenosis of the right M1 segment of the middle cerebral artery (MCA) (Fig. 2A, B).

Despite intensive medical management with clopidogrel, 75 mg/d, aspirin, 81 mg/d, and atorvastatin, 80 mg/d, the patient had fluctuations of neurologic symptoms and signs that were blood pressure (BP) dependent and required IV fluids and vasopressors for 2 days. His examination findings remained stable after 2 days, and he was discharged to an acute rehabilitation hospital with an intensive risk factor control regimen. The BP target for this patient was 130/80 mm Hg.

The patient had a third hospital admission for worsening neurologic symptoms about 4 weeks later. He had pronounced left-sided weakness. His NIHSS score was 8. Brain CT did not show an acute process. Brain MRI showed multiple new areas of restricted diffusion (Fig. 1E, F). With a relative decrease in BP, the patient had significant fluctuation and worsening of focal neurologic deficits during hospitalization. His BP ranged from 160/84 mm Hg to 126/68 mm Hg.

Clinical Questions

1. What is the diagnosis in this patient?
2. What is the significance of BP variability and BP augmentation in this patient?
3. According to current American Heart Association/American Stroke association guidelines, how should this patient be treated?

Discussion

Recurrent cerebral ischemic symptoms in a single vascular territory, such as in this patient, suggest a high-grade focal large artery stenosis. The symptoms can be caused by cerebral hypoperfusion or artery-to-artery embolism. In this patient, there was no evidence of a high-risk source of cardiac embolism. Given the constellation of symptoms and neuroradiologic findings, we believe that intracranial occlusive disease with artery-to-artery embolism was the most likely cause of stroke.

Intracranial occlusive disease is common in many Asian countries where transcranial Doppler may be used for detection of microembolic signals.[1–5] Therefore, noninvasive imaging by means of CTA, MRA, or transcranial Doppler of the intracranial vasculature is recommended to exclude the presence of proximal intracranial stenosis or occlusion (class I; level of evidence A).[6]

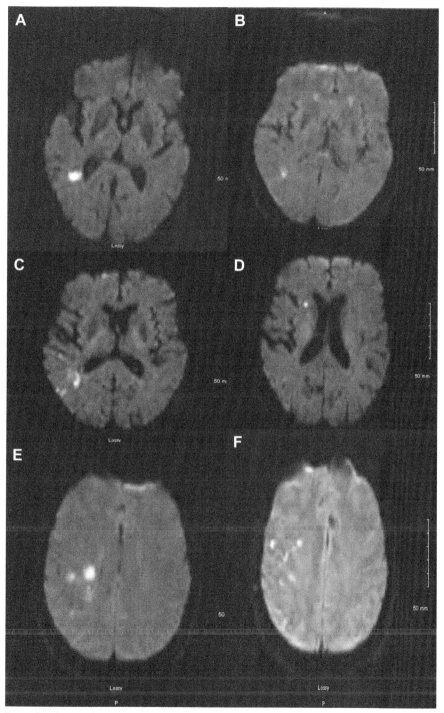

Fig. 1. (*A–F*) MRI of the brain (axial sequence) DWIs show multiple areas of restricted diffusion in the brain in the right MCA territory at different time points according to the patient's symptom course over an approximately 8-week period.

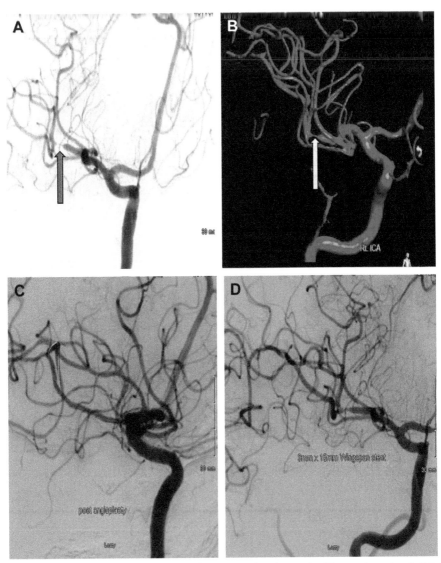

Fig. 2. (*A* and *B*) Conventional cerebral angiography shows significant stenosis of distal right MCA M1 segment. (*C*) Conventional cerebral angiography shows improvement in right MCA stenosis after angioplasty. (*D*) Conventional cerebral angiography shows patency of right MCA after Wingspan stent placement. An *arrow* delineates the key neuroradiological feature referred to in the respective figure segment.

Blood pressure variability in acute stroke patients with intracranial atherosclerotic occlusive disease may be associated with neurologic deterioration and poor neurologic outcome.[7] Therefore, augmentation of BP and reduction of BP fluctuations in the acute setting may be useful, especially when auto-regulatory mechanisms are compromised in the area of cerebral infarction and the surrounding penumbra. The penumbra may be thought of as a shadow zone of compromised cerebral blood flow or perfusion in which brain tissue is rendered ischemic and dysfunctions, but frank infarction has not occurred. The rationale to augment BP is to salvage the ischemic penumbra. Elevation of BP may augment collateral blood flow.[8,9]

Our patient was treated with intravenous fluids and required vasopressors to elevate the BP and to avoid further fluctuations in neurologic status. Systolic BP was then maintained at greater than 150 mm Hg, and worsening of neurologic status ceased. However, with attempted weaning of vasopressors, there was recurrence of neurologic signs and symptoms.

For patients with recent stroke or transient ischemic attack (ie, within 30 days) attributable to severe stenosis (70%–99%) of a major intracranial artery, the addition of clopidogrel, 75 mg/d, to aspirin therapy for 90 days may be reasonable (class IIb; level of evidence B).[10] Our patient was on dual antiplatelet and statin therapy at the time of his third admission to the hospital. Aggressive medical management is found to be efficacious when there is high-grade (70%–99%) symptomatic intracranial large artery occlusive disease according to findings from the SAMMPRIS trial.[11] However, the Wingspan stent system is not recommended as an initial treatment (class III; level of evidence B).[10] Because of hemodynamic compromise, our patient underwent angioplasty and stenting of the right MCA stenosis. The procedure was successful, and there were no complications (**Fig. 2**C, D). Thus, although angioplasty and stenting of major intracranial arteries is not generally recommended in practice, when there is a high-grade stenosis and inability to wean a patient from vasopressors because of hemodynamic compromise, intracranial angioplasty and stenting may be indicated.

CASE 2: AN INTERESTING CASE OF MIGRAINE HEADACHE AND STROKE
Case Presentation

A 27-year-old woman presented to the ED with left temporal throbbing headache, left facial and left arm numbness, and left arm weakness. She had intractable headaches with some fluctuation for the past 3 to 4 weeks. The focal neurologic symptoms lasted for 30 minutes and then completely resolved. Her BP was 120/70 mm Hg. She had a history of migraine headache but never had focal neurologic symptoms. The patient was not pregnant and had never taken birth control pills. There was no history of cigarette smoking. Brain MRI did not show an acute intracranial process. The diffusion-weighted images (DWI) were unremarkable. In the ED the patient was treated with sumatriptan injection, and dihydroergotamine mesylate (DHE) was administered during acute hospitalization over a 12-hour period. Her symptoms completely resolved within 24 hours of hospitalization.

However, the next day she woke up and could not see off to the left side. There was a left visual field defect but no other focal neurologic impairment. The patient had a repeat brain MRI and MRA. MRI brain showed findings consistent with right occipital ischemic stroke, and brain MRA showed narrowing of the right posterior cerebral artery (PCA) (**Fig. 3**A, B). Diagnostic studies for blood markers of inflammation, hypercoagulable testing, and cerebrospinal fluid (CSF) analysis were unremarkable. Her BP was not elevated at any time during hospitalization or stay in the ED. She was headache free at the time of discharge but had a visual field defect. Repeat brain MRA after 3 months was unremarkable, and there were no findings suggestive of vasculitis. A clinically significant visual field deficit was still present 1 year later.

Clinical Questions

1. What is the diagnosis in this case?
2. What is the mechanism of stroke?
3. Is it safe to administer sumatriptan and DHE concurrently in a migraine patient to abort an acute headache?

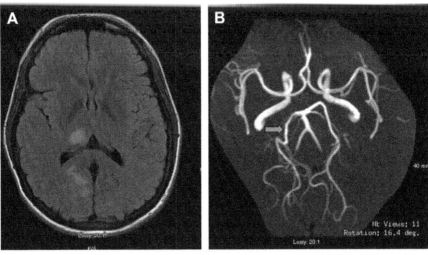

Fig. 3. (*A*) MRI of the brain (axial sequence) FLAIR image shows multiple hyperintensities in the right PCA distribution involving occipital lobe and thalamus. (*B*) MRA of the brain shows irregularity of right PCA concerning for possible vasculitis or other vasculopathy. An *arrow* delineates the key neuroradiological feature referred to in the respective figure segment.

Discussion

The differential diagnosis in this case includes migrainous infarction, vasculitis, hypercoagulable condition, posterior reversible encephalopathy syndrome (PRES), and a complication related to medications administered during hospitalization to treat the headache. The diagnostic workup, including laboratory studies and CSF analysis, was not suggestive of vasculitis or a hypercoagulable condition. Moreover, repeat brain MRA after 3 months was essentially unremarkable. The patient declined to have a conventional cerebral angiography study. PRES was unlikely, as BP was normal throughout the hospital stay. Therefore, it is thought that the patient may have had stroke related to sumatriptan and DHE, used to treat the headache, although the mechanisms underlying cerebral ischemia associated with migraine are many (eg, vasospasm, endothelial injury, platelet aggregation, prothrombotic state, cortical spreading depression, cerebral arterial dissection, genetic variants, and traditional vascular risk factors).[12]

One should be cautious when using vasoconstrictive medications in patients with migraine cephalalgia. Triptans may be safe if used to treat migraine even with associated neurologic symptoms.[13,14] However, these medications should be used with caution, especially in combination with other drugs that can cause vasoconstriction such as DHE. This may deserve additional emphasis if the patient has an underlying disorder predisposing to stroke such as vasculitis or hypercoagulable condition. DHE is an ergot alkaloid and has potential for vasoconstriction; therefore, it may be preferred not to use multiple medications concurrently (eg, at least within 24 hours) that have such properties.[15] However, there are no clear guidelines to support the latter timeframe.

CASE 3: A PATIENT WITH RETINAL ARTERY OCCLUSIONS AND OTITIC NERVOUS SYSTEM INVOLVEMENT
Case Presentation

A 34-year-old woman presented with visual disturbance, headaches, intermittent vertiginous feeling, and behavioral changes for almost 2 years. She had progressive worsening of visual acuity and blurry vision but never had complete or sudden visual loss. The patient described a vertiginous feeling as being lightheaded or as a spinning sensation.

She was initially diagnosed with amaurosis fugax at an outside hospital because of visual impairment. However, she never had sudden monocular visual loss but rather had progressive visual impairment over time. She was treated with aspirin, 81 mg/d, and had stroke diagnostic studies before being examined in our clinic. The diagnostic studies including those of the cervical and intracranial vasculature were unremarkable. Transesophageal echocardiography found a patent foramen ovale. Her patent foramen ovale was closed at an outside hospital at the recommendation of other consultants.

Her family reported a few episodes of acute confusion in the last year. They also reported that her interpersonal interactions were abnormal. The patient stopped working and driving because of her episodic confusion, behavior change, and difficulty with balance and hearing.

Brain MRI was done at an outside hospital and showed multiple hyperintensities on T2 fluid-attenuated inversion recovery (FLAIR) images involving the corpus callosum (**Fig. 4**). The patient was referred for an ophthalmologic evaluation, which found bilateral and multiple branch retinal artery occlusions on fluorescein angiography. Later she had an otolaryngology evaluation, which confirmed bilateral sensorineural hearing loss.

Clinical Questions

1. What is the diagnosis in this case?
2. What is the cause of visual symptoms in this patient, and why was a careful neurologic history so important in this case?
3. Was there any indication for oral anticoagulation therapy in this patient?

Discussion

The differential diagnosis in this case includes a demyelinating disorder such as multiple sclerosis, vasculitis, ischemic stroke, and an endotheliopathy such as Susac syndrome. Lesions predominantly of the corpus callosum are not common and are not pathognomonic of multiple sclerosis, vasculitis, or stroke. Based on the neuroradiologic findings,

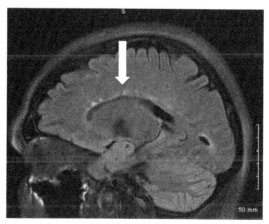

Fig. 4. MRI of the brain (sagittal sequence) T2 (FLAIR) image shows multiple hyperintensities involving the central fibers of the corpus callosum and typical of a neuroradiologic diagnosis of Susac syndrome. An *arrow* delineates the key neuroradiological feature referred to in the respective figure segment.

one should consider a diagnosis of Susac syndrome, as lesions involve the central fibers of the corpus callosum, sparing the more peripheral ones.[16] Patients with Susac syndrome have associated visual and hearing impairment as seen in our patient.

Susac syndrome is an immune modulated endotheliopathy. It is characterized by the triad of encephalopathy, cochlear hearing loss, and retinal artery occlusions. The clinical course of Susac syndrome is usually self-limited and fluctuating and lasts from 2 to 4 years, but duration varies. Some patients recover with little or no residual issues, but others can be profoundly impaired. Options for therapy include corticosteroids, intravenous immunoglobulin, and other immunosuppressant drugs.[17,18]

This patient had visual symptoms caused by the involvement of retinal arterial occlusions and not by amaurosis fugax. A careful neurologic history is important when making a diagnosis of amaurosis fugax. Patients with amaurosis fugax usually have sudden loss of vision in one eye that may be described as a shade coming over the eye or from the side and as a blackening, greying, or clouding of vision. Visual loss is not progressive over weeks or months but rather typically occurs over seconds to minutes or longer.

In this patient, the clinicians stopped antiplatelet therapy and administered oral anticoagulation. Use of oral anticoagulation is generally reserved for patients with certain types of cardiac source embolism (eg, atrial fibrillation), certain hypercoagulable states (eg, antiphospholipid antibody syndrome), and deep vein thrombosis or pulmonary embolism who have stroke.[10]

CASE 4: INTRACRANIAL OCCLUSIVE DISEASE
Case Presentation

A 49-year-old woman with a medical history of bipolar disorder had an episode of lightheadedness, dizziness, visual disturbance, confusion, and impaired level of consciousness during a trip to Paris. The episode lasted for 10 to 15 minutes with complete resolution of symptoms except for a mild headache, which lasted for 1 to 2 hours. The patient had no medical history of headache or similar symptoms in the past. She underwent brain MRI and MRA of the head and neck in Paris and was informed that all of the imaging findings were unremarkable. She underwent hypercoagulable workup, echocardiography, and electroencephalography on her return to the United States and was told that all diagnostic findings were unremarkable.

She had 2 more episodes of similar symptoms within 1 month of her return to the United States. The spells lasted longer than her first episode. She also had associated difficulty with speech and mild left temporal headache. The patient had vascular migraine headache diagnosed and was advised to take topiramate. Topiramate was administered for several months at a dose of 100 mg twice a day, but the patient continued to have 1 to 2 episodes of focal symptoms every month. She was referred to our vascular neurology clinic for a second opinion. Brain MRI findings were normal, but MRA of the head and neck carried out in Paris showed significant vascular abnormalities. She underwent CTA of the head and neck and conventional cerebral angiography. These studies showed complete occlusion of the internal carotid arteries on both sides and a vascular network of collateral circulation at the base of the brain (**Fig. 5**).

Clinical Questions

1. What is the diagnosis in this case?
2. Does this disease entity occur worldwide and in adults preferentially?
3. What are the surgical options for these patients?

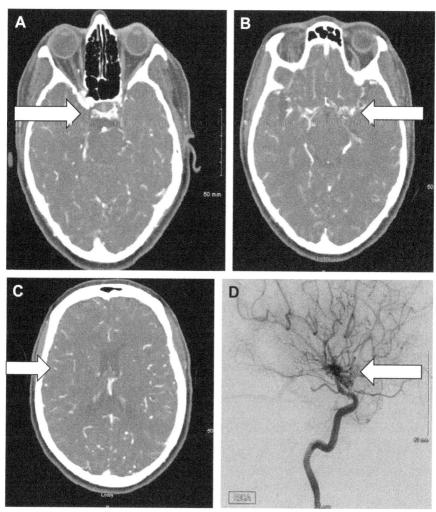

Fig. 5. (*A*) CTA of the brain shows complete occlusion of both internal carotid arteries. (*B*) CTA of the brain shows abnormal vascular network at the base of the brain. (*C*) CTA of the brain shows dilated collateral blood vessels close to the brain surface that are normally not seen in healthy individuals. (*D*) Conventional cerebral angiography of the brain shows abnormal vascular network known as *puff of smoke* (moyamoya). An *arrow* delineates the key neuroradiological feature referred to in the respective figure segment.

Discussion

The differential diagnosis in this case includes cerebral ischemia, vascular migraine, seizure disorder, autonomic instability, and cardiac arrhythmia. In retrospect, the initial neuroimages from France were not normal, emphasizing the potential importance of personally reviewing neuroimages or reviewing them with a neuroradiologist when possible. Based on the neurologic and neuroradiologic findings, a diagnosis of Moyamoya syndrome was made. If a patient with vascular migraine continues to have focal symptoms in spite of taking prophylactic medication, consider ordering imaging of the cervical and intracranial vasculature to rule out vascular pathology.

There is some misconception about the prevalence of Moyamoya disease. Although Moyamoya syndrome is common in some persons of Asian heritage, it can be seen in whites.[19] It is a chronic, occlusive cerebrovascular disease of unknown etiology. It is characterized by bilateral steno-occlusive changes at the terminal portion of the internal carotid arteries. These patients also develop an abnormal vascular network at the base of the brain with extensive collaterals to compensate for main vessel occlusion. The collateral circulation at the base of the brain may look like a puff of smoke or what is referred to as *moyamoya* in Japanese. The disease primarily affects children, but it can also occur in adults. Children may present with cerebral ischemic symptoms after crying, as hyperventilation may cause cerebral artery constriction and trigger a reduction of cerebral blood flow given tenuous collateral blood flow.

Moyamoya syndrome can lead to ischemic or hemorrhagic strokes. Surgical revascularization procedures may help prevent ischemic vascular complications in these patients. These procedures include direct revascularization—superficial temporal artery middle cerebral artery bypass—and indirect revascularization—encephalo-duro-arterio-synangiosis and encephalo-myo-synangiosis. Our patient underwent encephalo-duro-arterio-synangiosis on the right side and had the same procedure on the left side after 3 months. She tolerated these procedures well and is symptom free for the last 1 year and has been free of disability.[20]

CASE 5: AN IMPORTANT HERITABLE CAUSE OF STROKE AND VASCULAR DEMENTIA
Case Presentation

A 41-year-old woman with a history of traumatic brain injury, tinnitus, chronic daily headaches, and seizure disorder was evaluated for worsening memory, mood disorder, unsteady gait, and balance problems. She had no history of vascular risk factors such as hypertension, hyperlipidemia, or diabetes mellitus. MRI of the brain showed multiple hyperintensities on T2 FLAIR images with involvement of the tips of temporal lobes (**Fig. 6**).

She underwent extensive diagnostic workup for markers of inflammation and demyelination. Study findings were normal, including CSF analysis, with the exception of syphilis antibody titer, which was elevated, and Treponema pallidum antibodies, which were reactive. Her CTA scans of the head and neck were unremarkable. She was evaluated by an infectious disease consultant, and meningovascular syphilis was diagnosed, which was treated with intravenous penicillin therapy. The patient did not have improvement in her symptoms over time and continued to have headaches, memory and mood disorder, and intermittent focal neurologic symptoms. Based on MRI brain findings, especially involvement of the tips of the temporal lobes, and clinical features, genetic testing was obtained. The results showed the presence of a NOTCH 3 gene mutation on chromosome 19.

Clinical Questions

1. What is the diagnosis in this case?
2. Is there curative or high-level evidence-based preventive therapy for this disorder?
3. Can these patients be treated with thrombolytic therapy if they have an acute ischemic stroke?

Discussion

The differential diagnosis in this case includes stroke, vasculitis, a demyelinating disorder such as multiple sclerosis, neurosyphilis, and cerebral autosomal dominant arteriopathy with subcortical infarcts and leukoencephalopathy (CADASIL). One should consider a diagnosis of CADASIL when there is a history of migraine headache, absent

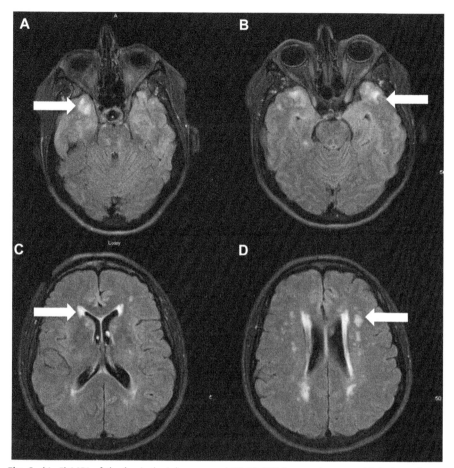

Fig. 6. (*A, B*) MRI of the brain (axial sequence) T2 (FLAIR) image shows multiple hyperintensities involving the white matter of the tips of temporal lobes. (*C*) MRI of the brain (axial sequence) T2 (FLAIR) image shows multiple hyperintensities involving the periventricular white matter. (*D*) MRI of the brain (axial sequence) T2 (FLAIR) image shows multiple hyperintensities involving the subcortical white matter. An *arrow* delineates the key neuroradiological feature referred to in the respective figure segment.

or few vascular risk factors (eg, cigarette smoking may be present), mood disorder, and neurologic symptoms and signs. Characteristically, there is involvement of the white matter of the tips of temporal lobes on brain MRI. This patient underwent genetic testing and had a NOTCH 3 gene mutation confirming the diagnosis of CADASIL. This mutation is expressed predominantly in vascular smooth muscle. There is progressive degeneration of the smooth muscle cells in blood vessels, and the vasculopathy is generalized. Mutations in the NOTCH 3 gene cause abnormal accumulation of protein in vascular smooth muscle cells in the cerebral and extracerebral vessels including the skin. On microscopic examination there are osmophilic granules in the blood vessel wall.

Clinically, CADASIL is characterized by history of migraine headache, recurrent ischemic strokes, cognitive decline, and psychiatric affective symptoms. CADASIL begins with migraine with aura in almost one-third of patients. It is the most common heritable cause of stroke and vascular dementia in adults. These patients have transient

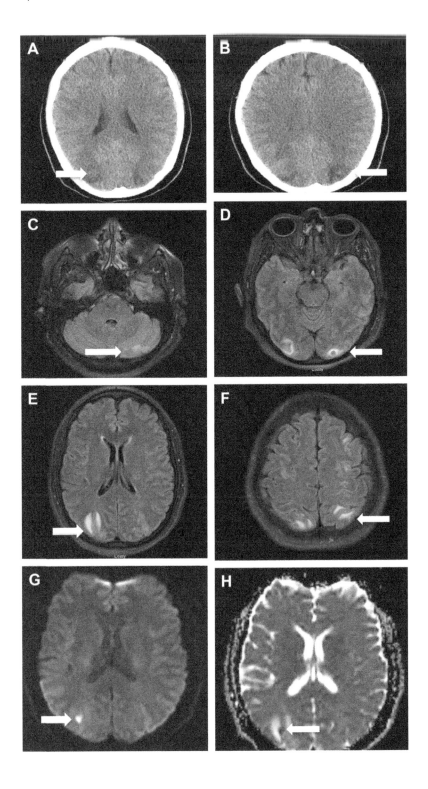

ischemic attacks and strokes between the ages of 30 and 50 years. There are multiple, small, deep cerebral infarcts, and neuroimaging findings are consistent with leukoence-phalopathy. During the time course of CADASIL, women earlier on may have fewer small deep infarcts compared with men. Frank dementia is usually a late complication. Diagnostic studies include MRI of the brain and skin biopsy or genetic testing. The NOTCH 3 gene mutation test is the favored means to establish a diagnosis.[21–24]

There is no definitive prevention or treatment for CADASIL. However, antiplatelet drugs rather than anticoagulants are often administered. The role of calcium channel-blocking agents and other BP-lowering medications with vessel wall–protective properties are often used though remain to be formally tested in a large-scale clinical trial.[23]

If a CADSIL patient has an acute ischemic stroke, thrombolytic therapy may be administered. However, safety of tissue plasminogen activator in patients with CADASIL is not well characterized, and there is no definite recommendation about CADASIL patients and administration of acute thrombolytic therapy for ischemic stroke in current American Heart Association/American Stroke guidelines.

CASE 6: AN INTERESTING CLINICO-NEURORADIOLOGIC ENTITY IN PREGNANCY
Case Presentation

A 35-year-old woman, gravida 2, para 2, aborta 0, 5 days postpartum after an uncom-plicated vaginal delivery presented to the ED after multiple seizure spells. She had 2 wit-nessed tonic-clonic seizure spells at home and one more spell en route to the hospital and a prolonged postictal state. The patient had a mild continuous retro-orbital head-ache since delivery and had blurry vision with worsening of headache. Her BP in the ED was 187/119 mm Hg. She was started on IV nicardipine and magnesium sulfate.

CT of the brain showed areas of hypodensities involving the occipital lobes (**Fig. 7**A, B), and brain MRI showed multiple hyperintensities on T2 FLAIR images, which were mainly located posteriorly (**Fig. 7**C–F). The DWI images showed areas of hyperintensities and corresponding areas on apparent diffusion coefficient study consistent with ischemic injury (**Fig. 7**G, H). CT angiography and MR venography of the brain were unremarkable. Transesophageal echocardiography did not show any high-risk cardiac source of embolic stroke.

Clinical Questions

1. What is the diagnosis in this case?
2. What is the underlying pathophysiology and etiology of this clinicoradiologic syndrome?
3. How should you treat a patient with this disorder?

Discussion

The differential diagnosis in this case includes ischemic stroke, cerebral venous thrombosis, hypertensive encephalopathy, PRES/reversible cerebral vasoconstrictive syndrome and eclampsia, and neoplasm. Taking into account the clinical presentation

◀

Fig. 7. (A, B) CT scan of the brain (axial sequence) shows multiple hypodensities involving the occipital lobes bilaterally. (C–F) MRIs of the brain (axial sequence) T2 (FLAIR) image show mul-tiple hyperintensities involving the left cerebellar hemisphere (C), occipital lobes (D–F), and part of the frontoparietal lobes (F). (G, H) MRIs of the brain (axial sequence) DWI image (G) show an area of hyperintensity close to the parieto-occipital lobe on the right side and a cor-responding area of low signal on apparent diffusion coefficient sequence (H). An *arrow* delin-eates the key neuroradiological feature referred to in the respective figure segment.

and imaging studies, the most likely diagnosis is PRES associated with eclampsia. The clinical features of PRES include headache, seizure, encephalopathy, and visual disturbance.

The neuroradiologic findings include focal reversible vasogenic edema that is best seen on brain MRI. However, PRES is a misnomer, as there can be involvement of the anterior circulation of the brain and gray matter. In addition, the neuroradiologic findings may be irreversible.

The precise underlying pathophysiology is not well defined. Rapidly developing hypertension leads to a breakdown in cerebral autoregulation. It is more pronounced in the posterior circulation of the brain, where there is a relative lack of a protective sympathetic innervation compared with the anterior brain circulation. Hyperperfusion leads to protein and fluid extravasation, which results in focal vasogenic edema. There is endothelial dysfunction in PRES patients with associated preeclampsia, eclampsia, and those who are treated with chemotherapeutic agents.[21,25] PRES has been reported in patients with hypertensive encephalopathy, eclampsia, renal impairment, and toxicity related to various chemotherapeutic and immunosuppressive agents (eg, gemcitabine, carboplatin, ciclosporin), especially in patients with hematopoietic malignancies in whom high-dose chemotherapeutic agents are used.[25]

Moreover, a strong association between eclampsia and the characteristic neuroradiologic findings of PRES have been reported. Furthermore, the symptoms of PRES in nonpregnant patients are similar to the prodromal symptoms of eclampsia. In one study, the incidence of PRES was more common among cases of postpartum eclampsias compared with antepartum eclampsias. Also, it was noted that PRES was more common in primigravidas and younger age group patients.[26] Furthermore, PRES and the seizures of eclampsia seem to be pathophysiologically related.[27]

Early recognition of PRES is important for proper management and avoidance of complications.[28] In patients with PRES, immediate withdrawal of triggers, such as chemotherapeutic agents and rapid control of BP are recommended.[25] We are not aware of any large-scale clinical trials that address precise BP-lowering targets and time to reach the BP-lowering target in PRES. Based on one source, we believe that it is reasonable to decrease the mean arterial pressure by 20% to 25% within the first 2 hours and to bring the BP down to a target of 160/100 mm Hg within the first 6 hours. Furthermore, too rapid BP reduction is not recommended, as it might decrease the cerebral perfusion pressure resulting in cerebral hypoperfusion and ischemia.[27] In addition, a sudden decrease in BP may adversely affect uteroplacental blood flow; therefore, close maternal BP and fetal monitoring are recommended.[29,30]

Prognosis is good in most of the cases of PRES; however, secondary complications, such as status epilepticus, intracranial hemorrhage, and large ischemic stroke can cause significant morbidity and mortality.[28,29,31] Our patient did not have any long-term complications. She had complete recovery of focal deficits at the time of her 6-month follow-up visit.

SUMMARY

We provide a series of interesting neurologic cases from our practice and discuss diagnosis and treatment. As a number of the cases are uncommon causes of stroke, there is no high-level evidence base to guide the clinician in relation to diagnosis and treatment. Therefore, one must recognize the pattern of clinical features to arrive at the proper diagnostic workup and diagnosis and exercise good clinical judgment in relation to reasonable treatment. Careful neurologic history and examination remain paramount to determining the correct diagnosis and subsequent treatment.

REFERENCES

1. Gorelick PB, Wong KS, Bae HJ, et al. Large artery intracranial occlusive disease: a large worldwide burden but a relatively neglected frontier. Stroke 2008;39(8): 2396–9.
2. Qureshi AI, Caplan LR. Intracranial atherosclerosis. Lancet 2014;383(9921):984–98.
3. Kim JS, Nah HW, Park SM, et al. Risk factors and stroke mechanisms in atherosclerotic stroke: intracranial compared with extracranial and anterior compared with posterior circulation disease. Stroke 2012;43(12):3313–8.
4. Wang Y, Zhao X, Liu L, et al. Prevalence and outcomes of symptomatic intracranial large artery stenoses and occlusions in China: the Chinese Intracranial Atherosclerosis (CICAS) Study. Stroke 2014;45(3):663–9.
5. Kim JM, Jung KH, Sohn CH, et al. Middle cerebral artery plaque and prediction of the infarction pattern. Arch Neurol 2012;69(11):1470–5.
6. Jauch EC, Saver JL, Adams HP Jr, et al. Guidelines for the early management of patients with acute ischemic stroke: a guideline for healthcare professionals from the American Heart Association/American Stroke Association. Stroke 2013;44(3): 870–947.
7. Chung JW, Kim N, Kang J, et al. Blood pressure variability and the development of early neurological deterioration following acute ischemic stroke. J Hypertens 2015;33(10):2099–106.
8. Aiyagari V, Gorelick PB. Management of blood pressure for acute and recurrent stroke. Stroke 2009;40(6):2251–6.
9. Singh V, Edwards NJ. Advances in the critical care management of ischemic stroke. Stroke Res Treat 2013;2013:510481.
10. Kernan WN, Ovbiagele B, Black HR, et al. Guidelines for the prevention of stroke in patients with stroke and transient ischemic attack: a guideline for healthcare professionals from the American Heart Association/American Stroke Association. Stroke 2014;45(7):2160–236.
11. Chimowitz MI, Lynn MJ, Derdeyn CP, et al. Stenting versus aggressive medical therapy for intracranial arterial stenosis. N Engl J Med 2011;365(11):993–1003.
12. Harriott AM, Barrett KM. Dissecting the association between migraine and stroke. Curr Neurol Neurosci Rep 2015;15(3):5.
13. Jamieson DG. The safety of triptans in the treatment of patients with migraine. Am J Med 2002;112(2):135–40.
14. Artto V, Nissila M, Wessman M, et al. Treatment of hemiplegic migraine with triptans. Eur J Neurol 2007;14(9):1053–6.
15. Farooq MU, Naravetla B, Bhatt A, et al. Possible iatrogenic bilateral cerebral ischemic infarcts in a woman with vasculitis. J Headache Pain 2008;9(3):189–90.
16. Susac JO. Susac's syndrome. AJNR Am J Neuroradiol 2004;25(3):351–2.
17. Kleffner I, Duning T, Lohmann H, et al. A brief review of Susac syndrome. J Neurol Sci 2012;322(1–2):35–40.
18. Grygiel-Gorniak B, Puszczewicz M, Czaplicka E. Susac syndrome - clinical insight and strategies of therapy. Eur Rev Med Pharmacol Sci 2015;19(9):1729–35.
19. Kraemer M, Heinemann FM, Horn PA, et al. Inheritance of moyamoya disease in a Caucasian family. Eur J Neurol 2012;19(3):438–42.
20. Fujimura M, Tominaga T. Diagnosis of moyamoya disease: international standard and regional differences. Neurol Med Chir (Tokyo) 2015;55(3):189–93.
21. Guidetti D, Casali B, Mazzei RL, et al. Cerebral autosomal dominant arteriopathy with subcortical infarcts and leukoencephalopathy. Clin Exp Hypertens 2006; 28(3–4):271–7.

22. Kalimo H, Ruchoux MM, Viitanen M, et al. CADASIL: a common form of hereditary arteriopathy causing brain infarcts and dementia. Brain Pathol 2002;12(3):371–84.

23. Gorelick PB. CADASIL: do the clinical and MRI profiles differ for women and men? Stroke 2012;43(1):8–10.

24. Choi JC. Cerebral autosomal dominant arteriopathy with subcortical infarcts and leukoencephalopathy: a genetic cause of cerebral small vessel disease. J Clin Neurol 2010;6(1):1–9.

25. Bhatt A, Farooq MU, Majid A, et al. Chemotherapy-related posterior reversible leukoencephalopathy syndrome. Nat Clin Pract Neurol 2009;5(3):163–9.

26. Bembalgi S, Kamate V, Shruthi KR. A study of eclampsia cases associated with posterior reversible encephalopathy syndrome. J Clin Diagn Res 2015;9(7):QC05–7.

27. Legriel S, Pico F, Azoulay E. Understanding posterior reversible encephalopathy syndrome. In: Vincent J-L, editor. Annual update in intensive care and emergency medicin. Berlin; Heidelberg (Germany): Springer; 2011. p. 631–53.

28. Roth C, Ferbert A. The posterior reversible encephalopathy syndrome: what's certain, what's new? Pract Neurol 2011;11(3):136–44.

29. Wagner SJ, Acquah LA, Lindell EP, et al. Posterior reversible encephalopathy syndrome and eclampsia: pressing the case for more aggressive blood pressure control. Mayo Clin Proc 2011;86(9):851–6.

30. Hobson EV, Craven I, Blank SC. Posterior reversible encephalopathy syndrome: a truly treatable neurologic illness. Perit Dial Int 2012;32(6):590–4.

31. Kutlesic MS, Kutlesic RM, Koratevic GP. Posterior reversible encephalopathy syndrome in eclamptic patients: neuroradiological manifestation, pathogenesis and management. Med Pregl 2015;68(1–2):53–8.

Neurotherapeutic Strategies for Multiple Sclerosis

Teresa C. Frohman, PA-C, MPAS[a,b],*, Shin C. Beh, MD[a],
Eric J. Kildebeck, MD, PhD[a,c], Ram Narayan, MD[a],
Katherine Treadaway, LCSW, ACP[a], Benjamin Greenberg, MD, MHS[a],
Elliot M. Frohman, MD, PhD[a,d],*

KEYWORDS

- Multiple sclerosis • Exacerbation • Corticosteroids • Adrenocorticotrophic hormone
- Disease-modifying therapy • MS • Pregnancy

KEY POINTS

- Multiple sclerosis is the most common disabling neurologic disease of young adults.
- There are now 16 US Food and Drug Administration–approved disease-modifying therapies for multiple sclerosis as well as a cohort of other agents commonly used in practice when conventional therapies prove inadequate.
- Pregnancy is a state of immunomodulation associated with an antiinflammatory milieu that leads to a reduction in disease activity. The postpartum period has been associated with a resurgence of disease activity.
- An MS exacerbation can be defined as a neurologic event lasting more than 24 hours in the absence of increased body temperature or infection. A Psudo-exacerbation is when the patient experiences a reemergence or deterioration of neurologic deficits, lasting less than 24 hours, and/or occurring in the presence of increased body infection with or without infection (also known as Uhthoffs Phenomenon).

[a] Department of Neurology and Neurotherapeutics, University of Texas Southwestern Medical Center, 5323 Harry Hines Boulevard, Dallas, TX 75390, USA; [b] Department of BioEngineering, University of Texas at Dallas, 800 West Campbell Road, Richardson, TX 75080, USA; [c] Center for Engineering Innovation, University of Texas at Dallas, Institute for Innovation and Entrepreneurship, 800 West Campbell Road, Richardson, TX 75080, USA; [d] Department of Ophthalmology, University of Texas Southwestern Medical Center, 5323 Harry Hines Boulevard, Dallas, TX 75390, USA
* Corresponding author. Department of Neurology and Neurotherapeutics, University of Texas Southwestern School of Medicine, 5323 Harry Hines Boulevard, Dallas, TX 75235.
E-mail addresses: teresa.frohman@utsouthwestern.edu; elliot.frohman@utsouthwestern.edu

Neurol Clin 34 (2016) 483–523
http://dx.doi.org/10.1016/j.ncl.2016.05.001
0733-8619/16/$ – see front matter © 2016 Elsevier Inc. All rights reserved.

neurologic.theclinics.com

INTRODUCTION

The inception of an organization solely dedicated to the investigation and ultimate cure of multiple sclerosis (MS) was set in motion in 1946, when Silvia Lowry established the National Multiple Sclerosis Society after publishing an advertisement she took out in the New York Times, inquiring to the world whether anyone had identified a potential treatment that might be used for her brother, who had a particularly aggressive and accelerated course of the disease.

No affirmative replies were forthcoming in time to shift Sylvia's brother's disease trajectory, and he ultimately succumbed to the disease. As if establishing the National MS Society (which continues to be the most important advocacy organization for the research and treatment of MS worldwide) was not a sufficient individual contribution to the world, Sylvia lobbied Congress in 1950, arguing that the time had come for the government to play a leading role in advancing the understanding of the pathobiological underpinnings of neurodegenerative disorders in general, and for MS in particular.

Through her efforts, the government established the National Institute of Neurological Disorders and Stroke, with the government contributing a mere $14,000 for the investigation of MS before the founding of the institute, whereas since that time Congress has appropriated in excess of $1.5 billion dollars for the investigation of a landscape of neurologic disorders, and in excess of $110 million dollars has been dedicated to MS. The reason for opening this article with this preamble is that it powerfully underscores what is possible, when confronted by one of the most challenging neurologic disorders, before the advent of disease-modifying therapies. Further, this story also emphasizes the impact that even a single individual can have on the process of patient care, education, and discovery. The remainder of this article provides the details on an expanding repertoire of innovative neurotherapeutic capabilities, all of which are derivatives of the scaffolding assembled by Sylvia Lowry.

UNITED STATES FOOD AND DRUG ADMINISTRATION–APPROVED MULTIPLE SCLEROSIS THERAPIES

Table 1 provides a list of common side effects and adverse effects.

Injectables

Interferon-beta
Several clinical trials for interferon-beta (IFNB) have shown significant reductions in clinical and radiologic measures of disease activity and severity; in general, IFNB reduces Annualized relapse rate (ARR) by about one-third and radiologic activity by two-thirds to 90%.[1–10] Intramuscular interferon (IFN)-1a (Avonex) is administered once weekly, subcutaneous IFN-1a (Plegridy) is given every other week, subcutaneous IFNB-1a thrice weekly (Rebif), and subcutaneous IFNB-1b every other day (in our center, we recommend dosing of Betaseron/Betaferon and Extavia 3 times weekly, as with Rebif administration).

Most studies show no significant differences in efficacy among these IFNB products.[11–17] By contrast, the INCOMIN and EVIDENCE trials suggested that high-dose IFNB-1b and high-dose subcutaneous IFNB-1a were slightly superior to low-dose intramuscular IFNB-1a, respectively.[18,19] Despite slightly greater efficacy, higher dose IFNB carries the increased risk of neutralizing antibodies (NABs) and side effects (flulike symptoms, injection site reactions, transaminitis, dysthyroidism, anemia, leukopenia, alopecia, and depression).[11,15–17]

Table 1
Summary of common side effects and adverse reactions as well as monitoring recommendations for some common disease-modifying agents in MS

	Side Effects and Adverse Reactions	Comments	Monitoring
Interferon-beta	Flulike symptoms Injection site reactions Alopecia Depression Leukopenia Dysthyroidism Increased transaminase level NABs	For injection site reactions, consider using topical ethyl chloride (100%) or Cetacaine, topical diphenhydramine, and rotate injection sites Naprelan with or without a triptan 1 hour before injection to prevent headaches and flulike symptoms	CBC; LFT; TFT at months 1, 2, and 3, then quarterly NAB levels annually
Glatiramer acetate	Isolated postinjection reaction Lipoatrophy Injection site reactions	Injection site reactions can be managed as for interferon-beta	—
Natalizumab	Infusion reaction NABs Lymphocytosis Eosinophilia Increased transaminase level PML Increase in minor infections	IVMP 250 mg with the first 3 infusions may reduce infusion reactions and the risk of NAB development In patients at increased risk of PML, consider switching to natalizumab infusions every 8 wk	NAB levels (at months 6 and 12, then annually) CBC, LFTs (at months 1, 2, 3, and then every 6 mo) JCV antibodies (every 6 mo)
Teriflunomide	Alopecia GI upset Oral herpetic infections Nasopharyngitis Leukopenia Increased transaminase level Teratogenicity	—	CBC and LFT (baseline, at 2 wk; months 1, 3, 6; and then every 6 mo)
DMF	Flushing GI upset Pruritus Asymptomatic proteinuria Lymphopenia Increased transaminase level	Premedication with glycopyrrolate 0.5–1 mg, aspirin 81 mg, and cetirizine 10 mg about 30–60 min before taking DMF, and then take DMF with apple sauce or peanut butter	CBC with differential and LFT (baseline, months 3 and 6, and then every 6 mo)

(continued on next page)

Table 1
(continued)

	Side Effects and Adverse Reactions	Comments	Monitoring
MMF	GI upset Alopecia Upper respiratory infections Urinary tract infections Headaches Asthenia Lymphopenia Anemia Thrombocytopenia Eosinophilia Increased transaminase level	Start MMF at 250 mg twice daily for 1 wk and then increase by 250 mg twice daily per week until a target dose of 1000 mg twice daily is achieved Take MMF on an empty stomach (either 1 h before or 2 h following a meal)	CBC with differential and LFT (baseline, weekly for the first month, biweekly for the second and third months, monthly up to the sixth month, then quarterly)

Abbreviations: CBC, complete blood count; DMF, dimethyl fumarate; GI, gastrointestinal; JCV, John Cunningham virus; LFT, liver function test; MMF, mycophenolate mofetil; NAB, neutralizing-antibody; PML, progressive multifocal leukoencephalopathy; TFT, thyroid function test.

Monitoring interferons

Because of the potential for transaminitis, hematologic abnormalities, and thyroid abnormalities, the authors recommend checking complete blood count (CBC), liver function test (LFT), and thyroid function tests at months 1, 2, 3, and then annually. Asymptomatic transiently increased transaminase levels in the first months after starting therapy are common; IFNB discontinuation should be considered only if liver enzyme levels remain persistently increased, or if there is other evidence of liver damage.

Adverse reactions

To minimize injection site reactions, the authors advise patients to allow the drug to warm to room temperature before injection, apply topical diphenhydramine, and rotate injection sites. Spraying ethyl chloride (100%), or Cetacaine, on the skin before injection helps reduce pain. Taking a nonsteroidal antiinflammatory drug (NSAID) 1 hour before injection often helps mitigate these symptoms. Although generic naproxen, ibuprofen, or even acetaminophen may be helpful,[18] most of our patients report significant benefit with controlled-release naproxen (Naprelan). Should Naprelan fail or if headache is a major complaint, the addition of a triptan (or using a drug that combines both; eg, Treximet) often provides significant relief.

Neutralizing antibodies

In general, NABs may develop as early as 4 to 6 months after commencing therapy. Patients who develop seropositivity (defined as 2 consecutive positive titers of at least 20 neutralizing units per milliliter 3 months apart) most often do so within the first 2 years of treatment.[20–22] However, it has been our experience that a cohort of patients who had been on Avonex for up to 10 years, and who were NAB free for the first several years, seroconverted to being positive for NABs when tested because of disease breakthrough. As discussed previously, the incidence of NABs is greatest with high-frequency, high-dose IFNB therapy.[21]

Glatiramer acetate

Glatiramer acetate (GA) is a random polymer of 4 amino acids found in myelin basic protein (glutamic acid, lysine, alanine, and tyrosine). US Food and Drug Administration (FDA)–approved formulations include Copaxone (injected subcutaneously at 20 mg daily, or 40 mg 3 times weekly) and Glatopa (injected subcutaneously daily). Clinical trials have shown that GA is effective in reducing clinical and radiologic activity in patients with MS.[23–25] Comparisons between GA and IFNB suggest similar levels of efficacy.[26–28]

Adverse reactions

Isolated postinjection reaction About 10% to 15% of patients experience an idiosyncratic, transient (15–20 minutes) reaction, characterized by dyspnea, chest tightness, palpitations, anxiety, and flushing.[29] In our experience, this distressing reaction may develop at any time during the course of treatment with GA, and not necessarily with the first dose.

Injection site reactions The authors advise patients to allow GA to warm to room temperature before injection, and to rotate injection sites (each site at least 5 cm [2 inches] away from the previous one). The application of a cold compress or spraying ethyl chloride (100%) or Cetacaine before injection may mitigate injection-related pain.

Lipoatrophy GA-associated lipoatrophy, attributed to localized inflammation (leading to panniculitis), is a significant and extremely common cosmetic problem; it is reported in as many as 45% of patients with MS on long-term GA. The application of ice 5 minutes before and after the injection and topical diphenhydramine may help reduce this complication.[29–33]

Orals

Fingolimod

The first FDA-approved oral disease modifying therapy (DMT) for MS, fingolimod, is phosphorylated by sphingosine kinase into its active form, fingolimod phosphate, which binds to the lymphocyte sphingosine 1-phosphate type-1 (S1P1) receptor and leads to receptor internalization and degradation. This process results in functional antagonism of lymphocyte egress from secondary lymphoid tissue, leading to reversible sequestration of lymphocytes in lymph nodes.[34,35] Fingolimod is administered at a dosage of 0.5 mg orally once a day.

Two large, phase III, double-blind, randomized trials (FREEDOMS and TRANS-FORMS) showed the impact of fingolimod on relapsing remitting multiple sclerosis (RRMS). Compared with placebo, it decreased the ARR by 54%, the risk of disability progression by 37% at 6 months, T2 lesion load by 74%, and the number of gadolinium-enhancing lesions by 82%. Compared with IFNB-1a, fingolimod reduced the ARR by a relapse rate (RR) of 52%, T2 lesion load by 35%, and the number of gadolinium-enhancing lesions by 55%.[36–39]

Adverse effects

Laboratory derangements Lymphopenia, with absolute CD4 counts comparable with those in human immunodeficiency virus (HIV) infection or myelotoxic chemotherapy, is common.[35] Within a month, lymphocyte counts typically decrease by about 75%; as such, lymphopenia can be considered a laboratory marker of therapy complaince.[40,41] The lymphopenia is almost always reversible but may persist for weeks after discontinuation.[36–38] Another common finding is reversible increased alanine aminotransferase level; other liver enzyme levels are typically normal.[40,41]

Cardiac effects S1P1 receptors are present in cardiac myocytes. A transient, dose-dependent decrease in heart rate, developing within an hour of administration and reaching its nadir 3 to 5 hours later, is common. In most patients, this effect is asymptomatic, improves after 8 hours, and resolves within 24 hours.[42,43] However, severe, prolonged bradycardia, asystole, and cardiac-related death have been reported.[44–46]

Ophthalmic complications The risk of macular edema is 0.2% to 0.4% and it usually occurs within 4 months of starting therapy. Diabetes mellitus and prior uveitis increase this risk, and, in general, fingolimod is contraindicated in patients with a history of either disorder.[47]

Infections Fingolimod-induced lymphopenia is a result of lymphocyte sequestration, not depletion. Further, peripheral effector memory T cells are spared, and as such recall antigen immune responses are preserved (eg, polio, measles).[48] Serious infections caused by herpesviruses, including herpes simplex virus (HSV) encephalitis, have been reported, as well as slightly more localized numbers of dermatologic malignancies. Rates of cough, dyspnea, and reversible changes in pulmonary function tests were slightly increased in patients taking fingolimod compared with controls.[49–51]

In the FREEDOMS study, the proportion of patients with herpesvirus infections was 7.9% on placebo, 8.7% on 0.5 mg, and 5.8% on 1.25 mg of fingolimod; the proportions of serious herpes infections were 0%, 0.2%, and 0.2%, respectively.[37] A total of 48 patients had serious infections (from among 2315 patients in a phase 2 and 2 phase 3 trials); 12 of these cases were caused by herpesviruses, including HSV encephalitis.[36–38] Other cases of severe herpesvirus infections in fingolimod-treated patients have been reported.[49–51]

Neoplasms Slightly more localized dermatologic malignancies (especially basal cell carcinoma) and breast cancer were diagnosed in the fingolimod group. These numbers are insufficient to determine causality. Although fingolimod may increase the risk of certain malignancies, S1P1 inhibition apparently suppresses other cancers.[52,53]

Pulmonary complications Rates of cough, dyspnea, and reversible changes in pulmonary function tests were slightly increased in patients taking fingolimod compared with controls.[36,37]

Worsening of disease activity Several reports describe a paradoxic worsening of disease activity (even resulting in tumefactive lesions) after starting fingolimod.[54,55] The immunoetiologic underpinnings of this phenomenon remain unclear. Fingolimod discontinuation may result in a resurgence of disease activity, possibly the consequence of massive egress of previously sequestered lymphocytes.[56–60]

Monitoring Please refer to Box 1 for further details.

Teriflunomide

After it is hepatically metabolized into its active form (leflunomide), teriflunomide inhibits mitochondrial dihydroorotate dehydrogenase, disrupting pyrimidine synthesis and impairing lymphocyte proliferation. Additional favorable immunologic effects include inhibition of proinflammatory cytokine (IFNγ, interleukin [IL]-2) secretion, nuclear factor kappa-B, astrocytic inducible nitric oxide synthase, and cyclooxygenase-2, as well as shifting the immune profile toward a Th2 bias.[61–63]

A phase III study (TEMSO) comparing teriflunomide with placebo in patients with RRMS showed an RR of ARR of just more than 30%, diminished 12-week disability

Box 1
Monitoring for fingolimod therapy

In view of the adverse effects and based on current FDA recommendations, the authors propose the following:

Contraindications:

• Diabetes mellitus.

• Existing, or a history of, uveitis, macular disease, or retinal vascular disease.

• Recent (within 6 months) myocardial infarction, unstable angina, stroke, transient ischemic attack, class III/IV congestive heart failure, decompensated congestive heart failure requiring hospitalization.

• Existing, or a history of, Mobitz type II second-degree or third-degree atrioventricular block or sick sinus syndrome (unless the patient has a pacemaker).

• Baseline corrected QT (QTc) greater than 500 milliseconds.

• Current use of class 1a (quinidine, procainamide) and class III (amiodarone) antiarrhythmic drugs.

Evaluations before therapy:

• Laboratory tests: complete blood count (CBC), liver function test (LFT), varicella-zoster antibodies (if no immunity, administer varicella vaccination and delay fingolimod for 1 month), pregnancy test.

• Electrocardiogram (ECG; refer to a cardiologist if abnormal before starting therapy).

• Ophthalmic examination (including optical coherence tomography [OCT]).

• Pulmonologist referral in patients with asthma, chronic obstructive pulmonary disease, smoking, or other pulmonologic disorders.

First-dose monitoring:

• ECG before administration of fingolimod.

• Observe patient with hourly vital signs for at least 6 hours for any sign of bradycardia or hypotension.

• ECG 6 hours after the administration of fingolimod.

• Overnight observation with continuous telemetric monitoring is required if:
  ○ Lowest heart rate develops 6 hours after administration
  ○ Symptomatic bradycardia
  ○ Heart rate less than 45 beats/min
  ○ New-onset second-degree heart block or higher
  ○ Prolonged QTc interval (baseline or after administration)
  ○ Other risk factors for QT prolongation (eg, antipsychotics, calcium-channel blockers, β-blockers)
  ○ Pharmacologic intervention required to treat bradycardia
  ○ Patients expected to be less tolerant of first-dose bradycardia, or those on concomitant negative chronotropic medications

• First-dose monitoring is needed in patients reinitiating therapy if:
  ○ Interrupted more than 1 day during weeks 1 to 2 of therapy
  ○ Interrupted more than 7 days during weeks 3 to 4 of therapy
  ○ Interrupted more than 14 days after a month of therapy

Long-term monitoring:

• Laboratory tests (CBC, LFTs) at 3, 6, and 12 months. If stable, every 6 months .

• OCT at 3, 6, and 12 months. If stable, every 12 months.

• Home weekly visual self-examination with an Amsler grid. Urgent ophthalmologic referral is recommended if the patient loses visual acuity or develops metamorphopsia.

• Annual dermatologic evaluation.

progression, as well as significant reductions in radiologic markers of disease activity. The second phase III study (TOWER) comparing teriflunomide 14 mg with placebo showed an RR in ARR of 36.3% and a 31.5% reduction in the risk of 12-week sustained disability accumulation.[64,65]

Adverse effects

Teriflunomide has generally been shown to be safe and tolerable. Side effects include nasopharyngitis, gastrointestinal (GI) upset, alopecia, nausea, and increased oral herpetic infections. Laboratory abnormalities include leukopenia (usually transient) and increased liver transaminase levels (particularly alanine transaminase [ALT]).Because leflunomide is the active metabolite, leflunomide's long-term safety data may also apply to teriflunomide. Most of leflunomide's adverse effects are similar to those of teriflunomide; however, there have been reports of hepatotoxicity, hypertension, pneumonitis, pancytopenia, and peripheral neuropathy.[62–64] Two cases of progressive multifocal leukoencephalopathy (PML) have been reported with leflunomide since it received FDA approval in 1998 but both patients had prior exposure to immunosuppressants.[66,67]

Teriflunomide is potentially teratogenic; while on treatment, strict contraception is recommended for women of reproductive age, and men because teriflunomide is secreted in seminal fluid.[62] Patients who become pregnant while on teriflunomide should undergo a cholestyramine-based or activated charcoal–based washout procedure after treatment discontinuation, and a plasma level less than 0.02 g/L should be confirmed to minimize risk to the pregnancy. Without the washout procedure, systemic clearance of teriflunomide may take up to 2 years.[67] **Table 2** provides details of the washout of teriflunomide.

VIGNETTE 1: CHILDBEARING-AGED WOMAN ON TERIFLUNOMIDE WHO WANTS TO BECOME PREGNANT

A 30-year-old woman with stable relapsing-remitting MS has been on teriflunomide for 3 years. She got married recently and wants to discuss family planning.

Should the clinician stop or continue the DMT? Should the clinician withdraw the DMT entirely? Should the clinician withdraw and bridge with monthly steroids? Should the clinician switch the DMT and, if so, to what?

In general, the failure rates of various contraceptive methods are the same in patients with MS as in the general population. With regard to the effects of oral contraceptives in MS, the limited data available suggest no negative effect and seem to suggest that there may be delayed onset of MS and mitigation of symptoms in patients who have MS.

If the patient is not currently planning a pregnancy (with good reliability), teriflunomide can be continued. A pregnancy test should be checked in all women of child-bearing age who are started on this medication. If the patient is planning on pregnancy or if the reliability of contraceptive methods is not good, it is recommended that this patient comes off teriflunomide therapy and washout protocol is initiated (see **Box 2**). During the washout period, she must be kept on folic acid. If her disease is stable (as with this patient) then it may be recommended that she stays off DMTs when she is trying to get pregnant. If her disease is active/aggressive, she might need to be bridged with safer DMTs like GA or IFN-beta during the periconceptional period. Alternatively, she can be put on monthly pulse steroids until she gets pregnant. Steroids are not advisable during the first trimester. With regard to the use of other DMTs in the periconceptional period, refer to the previous vignette.

Dosing and monitoring

Patients should be screened for latent tuberculosis, using a tuberculin skin test or the QuantiFERON-TB Gold In-Tube test; positive cases should be treated before starting

Table 2
Use of disease-modifying therapies for MS in pregnancy

Medication	FDA Pregnancy Category	Comments
Glatiramer acetate	B	Most favorable pregnancy rating. May be safe during breast feeding as well
Interferon beta	C	No major effects on infants after 6 mo of exclusive breast feeding
Fingolimod	C	Increased risk for fetal malformations in animal models. Takes 2 mo to be eliminated after discontinuation. Excreted into breast milk
BG-12/dimethyl fumarate	C	Embryotoxicity, testicular toxicity, and neurobehavioral adverse effects in animal models. Unclear if excreted into breast milk
Natalizumab	C	Reversible hematological abnormalities on human studies. Excreted in low levels in breast milk. Takes 3 mo to be eliminated after discontinuation; this can be expedited with a 3–5 cycles of plasma exchange
Mitoxantrone	D	Low birth weight, increased risk for prematurity. Pregnancy not advised for 6 mo after discontinuing therapy. Significant excretion in breast milk
Teriflunomide	X	Fetal malformations and intrauterine death. Only DMT that needs consideration for men who are planning to have children because it is secreted into the semen. Pregnancy test is recommended before starting therapy. Can persist for up to 24 mo and so a washout is required (protocol listed in **Box 2**)
Anti-CD20s (rituximab)	C	Reduced B-cell lymphoid tissue in newborns for 6 mo, increased risk for infections
Alemtuzumab	C	No data available
Daclizumab	C	Early prenatal loss in animal models
Laquinimod	Unknown	No data available

treatment. Teriflunomide in our center is started at a dosage of 7 mg orally once daily, which can be increased to 14 mg after 2 to 4 weeks. CBC and LFTs should be checked before starting therapy, at 2 weeks, month 1, month 3, month 6, and then every 6 months.

Dimethyl fumarate

Fumaric acid esters have been used since the 1990s for the treatment of psoriasis in a proprietary formulation called Fumaderm. In 2000, a neurologist noticed that patients with MS had disease stabilization after starting Fumaderm. This finding eventually led to research into the effect of dimethyl fumarate (DMF) on MS, eventually culminating in FDA approval in early 2013.[68]

DMF immunomodulatory effects are mediated via activation of the nuclear factor (erythroid-derived 2)–related factor-2 antioxidant pathway, the main cellular defense line against oxidative damage, as well as by shifting dendritic cell differentiation, suppressing proinflammatory cytokine secretion, and increasing antiinflammatory Th2 cytokine production.[68–70] The antioxidant properties make DMF a novel and particularly attractive DMT, because it may confer neuroprotection and hence delay or even prevent the inevitable march to the progressive, neurodegenerative phase of MS.

DMF's efficacy was shown in 2 randomized, double-blind, placebo-controlled, multicenter, phase III studies. In the DEFINE study, DMF 240 mg twice daily reduced ARR by 53%, the risk of relapse by 50%, disability progression by 38%, enhancing lesions by 68%, and new/enlarging T2 lesions by 85%.[69] In the CONFIRM study, DMF 240 mg twice daily reduced ARR by 44%, risk of relapse by 34%, risk of disability progression by 21%, new/enlarging T2-lesions by 71%, and T1 black holes by 57%.[70]

Adverse effects

Flushing and GI upset are common side effects and tend to abate after the first month, but may be severe enough to compromise treatment adherence, or prompt discontinuation. Flushing is a result of activation of the G protein–coupled receptor hydroxycarboxylic acid receptor 2 (GPR109A) in epidermal cells.[69–71]

One method of reducing the flushing and abdominal complaints in our experience has been to premedicate with glycopyrrolate 0.5 to 1 mg, aspirin 81 mg, and cetirizine 10 mg about 30 to 60 minutes before taking DMF, and then take DMF with apple sauce or peanut butter. The authors have also prescribed montelukast 10 mg once daily to help mitigate the GI effects of DMF. Precooling (eg, ingestion of ice-cold liquids, use of cold towels) may mitigate Uhthoff phenomenon in those susceptible to heat intolerance.

Other common side effects include pruritus and asymptomatic proteinuria unrelated to renal failure.[69] The incidence of mild infections was marginally higher in DMF-treated patients compared with placebo.[70] However, several cases of PML have been reported in patients who had received fumaric acids and DMF.[72–74]

Lymphopenia is a common laboratory finding. Lymphocyte counts typically diminish (by approximately 30%) in the first year and then plateau, usually in the lower end of the normal range. Lymphopenia less than 0.5×10^9/L was observed in 4% to 5% of patients. Increased liver transaminase (usually ALT) levels may be observed between months 1 and 6 but no cases of hepatotoxicity were reported.[69,70]

Dosing and monitoring

It is recommended that patients start at 120 mg twice daily orally for 7 days before increasing it to the full dose of 240 mg twice daily. Patients should have a CBC and LFT checked before treatment, at month 3, at month 6, and every 6 months thereafter. More recently, for those intolerant to dose escalation after only 1 week of 120 mg twice a day, the authors extend the use of the lower dose regimen to 4 weeks before commencing the maintenance dose regimen of 240 mg twice a day.

VIGNETTE 2: ORAL THERAPIES

A series of problems starting with Gilenya, then problems with Tecfidera, and then transitioning to Aubagio. The patient is keen to try Aubagio, but is preoccupied with the issue of hair thinning. A discussion ensues, and some additional recommendations are made (eg, biotin, multiminerals, and spironolactone).

Darrell is a 32-year-old white man with celiac disease who was diagnosed with MS at the age of 22 years in February of 2010, before the oral disease-modifying agents. After diagnosis, he was originally started on Copaxone because he was already being treated for major depressive disorder and was concerned that the interferons may exacerbate that problem. When the new formulation of 40 μg given 3 times a week was approved he switched to that formulation. He remained fairly stable from a clinical and radiographic standpoint but after 6 years his MRI showed 2 enhancing lesions in noneloquent sites, so they were not accompanied by any clinical changes that were visible or perceptible to the patient or the provider. When visiting with his MS provider to discuss the MRI results, Darrell admitted that he was nonadherent to the 3-times-a-week regimen and was "probably getting on average 2 shots per week in." This adherence was a patient who did not have issues with injection site reactions or lipoatrophy but was experiencing so-called needle fatigue. After further discussion, the patient decided that he wanted to try one of the 3 available oral therapies: Gilenya, Tecfidera, or Aubagio.

On discussion with the health care provider, it was decided not to start with Tecfidera because it has a high incidence of GI symptoms when initially starting therapy (this tends to lessen or resolve completely within a few months) and he was hesitant because of his already present GI issues with celiac disease. He and his wife were going to be starting a family soon, so this removed Aubagio as an option because it is classified as teratogenic to the unborn fetus. There was no history of heart disease, retinal disease, or diabetes within the immediate family, and all the initial testing (optical coherence tomography [OCT], electrocardiogram [ECG], dermatologic examination, and serology testing) was within normal limits, so Darrell decided to start Gilenya. He was informed that the first dose would be given in a monitored setting because approximately a quarter of patients experience a 13 to 20 beats/min decrease in pulse rate at some point during the 6-hour monitoring after the first dose of Gilenya. He completed the first-dose monitoring without incident. He was informed that if his therapeutic dosing was to be interrupted by 2 weeks or more, then he would need to undergo the first dosing regimen again.

Infusions

Natalizumab
Natalizumab is a recombinant, humanized immunoglobulin (Ig) G4κ monoclonal antibody that targets the $\alpha 4\beta 1$ (adhesion molecule VLA-4) and $\alpha 4\beta 7$ integrins on lymphocyte membranes, blocking them from binding to VCAM-1 (present on activated cerebrovascular endothelial cells), thus preventing lymphocyte egress across the blood-brain barrier into the central nervous system (CNS).[75,76] Compared with placebo in the AFFIRM trial, natalizumab reduced ARR by 68%, 3-month disability progression by 42%, new/enlarging T2 lesions by 83%, T1-hypointense lesions by 76%, and enhancing lesions by 92%.[77,78] Compared with IFNB-1a monotherapy in the SENTINEL trial, natalizumab combined with IFNB-1a reduced the ARR by 55%, 3-month disability progression by 24%, new/enlarging T2 lesions by 83%, enhancing lesions by 89%, and the rate of brain atrophy.[77–79]

Natalizumab has several notable benefits. It effectively controls MS disease activity shortly after initiation and is thus useful in patients who need rapid control of highly active disease. Natalizumab is also effective in patients of African descent (who tend to have more aggressive disease activity) and in pediatric MS.[80–82] In addition, natalizumab reduces cortical lesion accumulation and accrual of cortical atrophy, as well as decreasing cerebrospinal fluid (CSF) markers of axonal injury and neurodegeneration.[83]

Infusion-related reactions
Less than 10% of patients have infusion-related reactions.[77,78] These reactions are typically minor and include headache, dizziness, and nausea; pretreatment with antihistamines and acetaminophen is typically effective. Severe reactions, including anaphylactoid reactions, are rare and typically occur with the second infusion; treatment with corticosteroids and/or antihistamines is effective.

Antinatalizumab antibodies
Hypersensitivity reactions typically coincide with antinatalizumab antibodies (ANT-ZAbs). About 4.5% to 15.7% of natalizumab-treated patients develop antibodies against the drug; although some are transiently positive, 3.5% to 8.2% remain persistently positive (ie, detectable at 2 or more time points at least 6 weeks apart). Persistent seropositivity is associated with a reduction in treatment efficacy.[84–89]

To mitigate infusion reactions and ANTZAbs development, the authors give intravenous methylprednisilone (IVMP) 250 mg with the first 3 infusions when initiating therapy, as well as when reinitiating therapy after an interruption longer than 3 months (eg, discontinuation during pregnancy). The authors recommend checking for ANTZAbs annually as long as patients remain on therapy; 1 of our patients developed ANTZAbs after her 40th infusion, which was associated with a disease relapse (unpublished data).

Laboratory abnormalities

Increased lymphocyte and eosinophil count may occur in some patients. Transaminitis and hepatitis have been reported. Our surveillance laboratory plan includes monthly CBC, and LFT after treatment initiation for 3 months, then every 6 months.[90,91]

Infections

Pharyngitis and herpes virus infections are most common in natalizumab-treated patients.[92–94] In our experience, some patients experience an increase in cellulitis, urinary tract infections, and vaginal yeast infections.

Progressive multifocal leukoencephalopathy

In 2005, natalizumab was briefly withdrawn from the market after 3 cases of PML were identified in the clinical trials; in July 2006, after establishment of a global risk-management program, it was reintroduced to the market with a warning about the possibility of developing PML.

PML is a rare, often-fatal, lytic infection of oligodendrocytes caused by the pathogenic form of the John Cunningham virus (JCV), a ubiquitous neurotropic virus that rarely causes disease in immunocompetent hosts.[95] From 50% to 90% of healthy adults have been exposed to this virus, with 19% to 27% of them shedding JCV (most typically the nonpathogenic form) in their urine[96,97]; the primary infection is asymptomatic and the latent virus resides in the kidneys, bone marrow, and lymphoid tissue. The JCV noncoding control region (NCCR) is hypervariable; NCCR rearrangement during periods of immunosuppression determines neurotropism and neurovirulence. The archetype NCCR is not associated with PML. Prototype NCCRs are the pathogenic variants of JCV isolated from tissues of patients with PML.[98–102]

Natalizumab-associated PML carries a mortality of 22%; among survivors, 40% are left with severe disability. Clinical manifestations of PML include subacute, progressive visual disturbances (typically retrochiasmal, cortical, or subcortical), aphasia, behavioral abnormalities, and hemiparesis. In contrast with MS, optic nerve and spinal cord involvement is rare, and seizures are more common. Characteristic MRI lesions include large, bilateral but asymmetric, multifocal (which later become confluent), T2/fluid-attenuated inversion recovery (FLAIR)–hyperintense, T1-hypointense, diffusion-hyperintense subcortical lesions typically affecting the parietal or frontal lobes; these lesions are often described as scalloped with a sharp border facing the gray matter but an ill-defined border toward the white matter. These lesions may involve the thalami and basal ganglia. Unlike HIV-related PML, natalizumab-associated PML often shows gadolinium enhancement (punctate or rimlike).[103]

As of 2015, the overall PML risk incidence in natalizumab-treated patients with MS is 3.96 per 1000 patients. Three risk factors predispose natalizumab-treated patients to PML: anti–JCV-antibody seropositivity (and recently further risk stratification has been achieved through the operationalization of the antibody index), prior exposure to immunosuppressants, and increased duration of treatment with natalizumab (>24 consecutive monthly infusions). A 2-step assay, using a detection enzyme-linked immunosorbent assay (ELISA) and a confirmation assay, was developed to detect and confirm the presence of anti-JCV antibodies to stratify the risk of PML for patients. This risk is less than 1 in 1000 for patients who are JCV-antibody seronegative (regardless of other risk factors). Approximately 50% to 60% of patients with MS are seropositive, and about 2% to 3% seroconvert annually. Seropositivity increases PML risk to 1 in 300; this risk is low in the first 2 years of treatment (0.7 per 1000 patient years), but increases to 5.3 per 1000 patient years after 2 to 4 years, and 6.1 per 1000 patient years after 4 to 6 years.[104–109]

Although this assay was reported to have a false-negative rate of 2.5% to 2.7%, false-negative rates as high as 37% have been observed. Therefore, a single assessment of JCV activity may not be enough to stratify PML risk in patients taking natalizumab. It is important to realize that JCV antibody–seronegative natalizumab-treated patients may have JC viremia and viruria. Furthermore, PML has been reported in JCV antibody–negative patients, underscoring the importance of clinical vigilance for this serious complication in natalizumab-treated patients.[74,105,110–112]

Prior immunosuppressant use (irrespective of type, duration of exposure, or intervening period between its use and natalizumab) increases the risk of PML. In JCV antibody–seropositive patients, this increases the risk of PML to 1.8 per 1000 patient years for the first 2 years of therapy, and 11.2 per 1000 patient years in the subsequent 2 years.[113–115]

There is currently no specific prophylaxis for PML, or effective anti-JCV treatment. The diagnosis of PML should be considered in patients with the appropriate clinical and radiologic data, and confirmed by the presence of CSF JCV DNA by high-precision polymerase chain reaction techniques. Most patients have a low viral load at the onset (<500 copies/mL), and therefore a high-sensitivity assay (capable of detecting <50 copies/mL) is important.[104] A single negative test does not immediately rule out PML; it should be repeated in those with suggestive clinical and/or radiologic features.

The main goal of managing natalizumab-associated PML is to allow a buffered immune reconstitution; in essence, the return of competent immune surveillance to clear the virus, while avoiding the collateral and potentially cataclysmic phenomenon widely recognized as the immune reconstitution inflammatory syndrome (IRIS). Our therapeutic approach has been to immediately commence plasmapheresis to remove circulating natalizumab, thereby permitting lymphocytes to once again enter the CNS compartment to battle the infection. Further, we immediately start weekly high-dose corticosteroids (IVMP 1 g) for a total of 12 consecutive weeks, then reducing to every other week for 6 doses, and then monthly for 3 months. Following plasmapheresis, we treat with intravenous immunoglobulin (IVIg) at 0.4g/kg/d for 5 consecutive days. This therapy provides some additional capability to block the action of natalizumab, and simultaneously confers antiinflammatory properties to help mitigate IRIS.

Other DMTs implicated in PML include fingolimod, DMF, rituximab, and mycophenolate mofetil (MMF), but the risk is lower than for natalizumab.[113–117]

Cessation of natalizumab therapy

Concerns about PML led some clinicians to explore treatment interruptions (so-called drug holidays), which led to resurgent disease activity. This recrudescence typically occurs 4 to 7 months (but sometimes as early as 3 months) after stopping natalizumab, which is unsurprising because it takes about 3 months for complete natalizumab clearance. The risk of rebound disease may be higher in patients with shorter natalizumab treatment duration; post-hoc analyses of natalizumab trials and phase 2b studies show that, although MS disease activity returns after treatment discontinuation, the risk of rebound disease is very low for those treated for the duration of the trials. On discontinuation of natalizumab, recrudescence of disease activity usually mirrors prenatalizumab levels of disease activity.[118–125]

De-escalation of treatment from natalizumab to less efficacious agents has also been associated with resurgent clinical and radiologic disease activity, and may even result in tumefactive lesions. For example, when switching from natalizumab to fingolimod, more than 50% of patients experience recrudescent disease activity. However, cessation of natalizumab without any immunomodulatory drugs results in more severe disease, compared with when patients are put on a less efficacious DMT. Furthermore, the nonscientific, unsubstantiated practice of a washout period when switching from natalizumab to another DMT does more harm than good.[125–127]

Our approach to de-escalation from natalizumab has involved the use of high-dose corticosteroid bridging; we administer IVMP 1 g (or equivalent) daily for 5 days for the first month after treatment cessation; 3 days for the second month; and 1 day for the third and final month. This regimen has been almost uniformly effective, irrespective of which DMT the patient is converting to. Therefore, unless the patient develops persistent ANTZAbs, the authors recommend against abruptly stopping natalizumab without a carefully formulated bridging strategy.[126]

Extended-interval dosing of natalizumab

After natalizumab was reintroduced in 2006, several of our patients complained of an increase in the incidence of mild but bothersome infections. Based on data showing that disease activity returned as early as 12 weeks after natalizumab discontinuation, the authors decided to offer a modified dosing regimen of intravenous (IV) natalizumab 300 mg every 8 weeks. This modified regimen resulted in complete resolution of our patients' infections, without any return of disease activity (either clinical or on serial MRI performed at 3-month intervals for the first year after this transition). As such, in natalizumab-treated patients with any of the 3 PML risk factors, the authors have offered a similar dosing schedule. Based on retrospective review of 905 patients on extended-dosing-interval natalizumab therapy from 9 MS centers, we found that extended dosing was similar in efficacy to standard dosing; furthermore, no cases of PML were found in this cohort (compared with 4 in the standard monthly natalizumab dosing group).[127]

VIGNETTE 3: TYSABRI 4-WEEK VERSUS 8-WEEK DOSING

Janet is a 40-year-old woman with an 8-year history of MS. She has 3 children aged 12, 10, and 8 years. Janet works part time as a financial consultant. Janet originally was diagnosed at the age of 29 years, 3 months after the birth of her first child. At that time, she presented with cerebellar symptoms and mild sensory changes in her upper extremities. She was treated with IV Solu-Medrol 1 g for 5 days and then started on Avonex. Eight months later she had a severe exacerbation with enhancing lesions in the cervical and thoracic cord and CellCept 1000 mg twice a day was added to her Avonex regimen. Two years later she presented with profound optic neuritis in the left eye. She was found to have interferon antibodies (clinicians must test for interferon antibodies even if the patient has been on interferon for >2 years if a new exacerbation occurs). She again was treated with IV Solu-Medrol 1 g for 5 days and symptoms resolved. She was taken off Avonex and CellCept and was started on natalizumab every 4 weeks. At the time she tested JCV antibody negative. Janet continued to do well with no new exacerbations or evidence. Because of the chance of seroconversion, she continued to be tested for the JCV antibody every 3 months. At month 18 she seroconverted to JCV antibody positive with an index titer of 1.65. She was reluctant to change disease-modifying therapies because she had been stable on the natalizumab and felt better on it than she had since she had been diagnosed. At that time, her infusion regimen was changed to every other month (8 weeks), with clinical monitoring visits every 3 months and MRI every 6 months. She has remained stable with no symptomatic or radiographic progression for the past 5 years.

Discussion: natalizumab (Tysabri; Biogen, Cambridge, MA) is a humanized monoclonal antibody that inhibits α4 integrin, a transmembrane leukocyte receptor. It prevents leukocyte adhesion to vessel walls and subsequent migration across the blood-brain barrier. It is administered via IV infusion once every 4 weeks. The AFFIRM and SENTINEL trials effectually established natalizumab as one of the most efficacious of the approved agents in terms of relapse prevention.

The primary safety concern with natalizumab is the associated risk of PML; a serious, potentially fatal brain infection caused by the John Cunningham polyoma virus. Approximately 50% to 60% of the population have been exposed to the virus as shown by positive antibodies.

Before starting therapy with natalizumab, patients must be risk stratified for the presence of serum JCV antibodies. In JCV antibody–negative patients, the authors think that natalizumab can be safely used as an initial therapy. The risk/benefit ratio is favorable in patients with aggressive disease onset but also reasonable for those with seemingly mild disease onset who are JCV antibody negative. After starting therapy, it is recommended that JCV antibody status is checked at least every 6 months but preferably every 3 months because patients can be subsequently exposed to the virus. There is a negative to positive seroconversion rate of the 2-step ELISA assay of 1% to 2% per year.[104]

There are 3 major risk factors for the development of PML: presence of serum antibodies to JCV, history of prior immunosuppression, and length of natalizumab exposure greater than 2 years. Rates of PML are estimated to increase from less than 0.1 per 1000 in patients who are seronegative for JCV antibodies, to 0.5 per 1000 for JCV-positive patients without prior immunosuppressants in the first 2 years, to 4.6 per 1000 for JCV antibody–positive patients without prior immunosuppressants after 2 years, to 11.1 per 1000 for JCV antibody–positive patients with a history of immunosuppression who have been exposed to natalizumab for more than 2 years.[95]

It is the author's experience that, for those patients who are JCV antibody positive or seroconvert to JCV antibody positive, the strategy is to change infusions to every 8 weeks. From previous clinical trials when patients who were on natalizumab were discontinued from therapy and not put on another disease-modifying therapies, patients generally did well (clinically and radiographically) for 8 to 10 weeks but by 12 weeks the immune system was able to reconstitute and a recrudescence of MS activity resumed.

Ongoing studies of extended-interval dosing of natalizumab (every 8 weeks) are ongoing and preliminary results indicate a significantly reduced risk of PML for those patients who are JCV antibody positive and receiving doses every 8 weeks.[127]

Alemtuzumab

Alemtuzumab is a humanized monoclonal antibody against CD52, a receptor highly expressed on T and B cells, and at lower levels on monocytes, macrophages, and eosinophils; very little CD52 is expressed on neutrophils, natural killer cells, and hematopoietic stem cells. Peripheral lymphocytes are depleted within minutes of a single infusion of alemtuzumab. Its success in treating MS is caused by alteration of the immune repertoire via homeostatic lymphocyte reconstitution. Although T-cell populations reconstituted slowly, reaching normal baseline levels in about a year, B-cell numbers returned to normal within 6 months.[128–132]

Alemtuzumab is infused intravenously (12 mg/d) for 5 consecutive days in the first cycle, and for 3 consecutive days in the second cycle. Extension of the phase II trials showed that efficacy from 2 cycles endured to 5 years of follow-up. Both the CARE-MSI and CARE-MSII showed that alemtuzumab is more effective than IFNB-1a in reducing the ARR (RR of approximately 55%), radiologic markers of disease activity (new/enlarging T2 lesions and number of gadolinium-enhancing lesions), and the degree of brain volume loss; alemtuzumab is effective in treatment-naive patients and in those whose disease was inadequately controlled with prior therapy. Another remarkable observation was a sustained reduction in mean disability compared with IFNB-1a.[129,130]

Adverse effects
Infusion-related reactions Infusion-related reactions are almost universal; most were considered mild (pyrexia, headache, rash, urticaria, flushing, and chills) but some serious events were reported (cardiac dysrhythmias, hypotension, pleurisy, angioedema, and anaphylaxis).[128–130]

De novo autoimmunity The most salient adverse effect of alemtuzumab is the induction of novel autoimmunity, the likely consequence of reconstitution of the lymphocyte population.[128] The greatest risk of developing alemtuzumab-induced autoimmune disease is in the 12 to 36 months following the initial infusion.[133] The most common autoimmune disorder is thyroiditis (usually Graves disease), which occurs in about a quarter of treated patients[129–131]; the risk is higher in smokers and those with a family history of autoimmune disease.[133]

Other autoimmune conditions include idiopathic thrombocytopenic purpura and Goodpasture syndrome. Single cases of autoimmune neutropenia and autoimmune hemolytic anemia have been reported as well. The development of autoimmunity does not depend on the total dose, treatment frequency, or treatment interval with alemtuzumab.[129,130,134,135]

Although T-cell populations reconstitute slowly and reach normal baseline levels in about a year, B-cell numbers return to normal within 3 to 6 months. The authors hypothesize that this earlier reconstitution of the B-cell population (without the modulating effect of the Th2 cells) may be responsible for inducing de novo autoimmunity.

Infections Mild to moderate infections (mucocutaneous herpetic, respiratory, and urinary tract) are more frequent in patients treated with alemtuzumab, and peak during the first month after the first treatment course. More serious infections like herpes zoster and pulmonary tuberculosis were also observed. Surprisingly, PML has not been reported in alemtuzumab-treated patients with MS, but has occurred in patients with chronic lymphocytic leukemia who received alemtuzumab.[128–130]

Malignancy Three cases of papillary thyroid carcinoma (possibly related to Graves disease) and a case of non-EBV Burkitt lymphoma were reported.[130]

Role in multiple sclerosis therapy
Alemtuzumab is infused intravenously (12 mg/d) for 5 consecutive days in the first cycle, and 3 consecutive days in the second cycle. Extension of the phase II trials showed that efficacy from 2 cycles endured to 5 years of follow-up.[136] Some clinicians have suggested waiting for a return of disease activity after the second cycle of alemtuzumab before proceeding with further infusions. This wait-and-watch approach carries the risk of a debilitating relapse, but the adverse effects and risk of developing NABs mitigates against a routine annual administration of alemtuzumab. In a long-term open-label study of 87 patients with MS, additional courses of alemtuzumab were given 12 months after the second cycle for relapses. Additional cycles of treatment resulted in improved or unchanged disability; the incidence of de novo autoimmunity was also higher, but could be attributed to the longer follow-up.[137] The authors suggest that alemtuzumab should be used to stabilize highly active disease activity before the patient is put on a less toxic DMT.

The premedication, as well as screening and monitoring requirements for patients treated with alemtuzumab, are extensive and laborious, in view of the adverse effects and safety risks of the drug. A detailed discussion of these procedures is beyond the scope of this article.

Rituximab

Rituximab, a chimeric monoclonal antibody against CD20, specifically lyses circulating B cells while sparing stem cells, pro-B cells, and mature plasma cells. It is FDA approved for non-Hodgkin lymphoma, chronic lymphocytic leukemia, rheumatoid arthritis, Wegener granulomatosis, and microscopic polyangiitis.[138,139] It is highly effective for treating MS, even though it has not received explicit FDA approval for this purpose.

Two published studies clearly support the efficacy of rituximab monotherapy in treating RRMS, without any serious events.[139,140] Both studies showed a reduction of gadolinium-enhancing lesions exceeding 90%. A similar rate was found when a 4-week course of rituximab was added to the therapeutic regimen of patients with MS with breakthrough disease on IFNB and GA.[141,142] In the OLYMPUS study, although it failed to meet its primary end point, rituximab reduced T2-lesion volume and slowed progression in the subgroup with gadolinium-enhancing lesions.[143]

Rituximab is a reasonable treatment of choice when diagnostic confusion between MS and neuromyelitis optica exists, because it effectively treats both. Further, because its efficacy is comparable with natalizumab, it is therefore a good option for patients who develop ANTZAbs that result in breakthrough disease activity.

Dosage and monitoring

The authors recommend IV administration of rituximab 1 g together with IVMP 250 mg, acetaminophen, and diphenhydramine hydrochloride to minimize infusion reactions. Complete depletion of CD20+ peripheral B cells (as measured by CD19+ expression) should be expected. Lymphocyte counts should be checked monthly and when CD19+ cell counts begin increasing another 1-g dose of rituximab should be administered.

Adverse reactions

All 3 studies[139–141] report infusion-related reactions (eg, pruritus, dyspnea, rash, asthenia, fatigue, headaches) that are most pronounced with the first infusion and are most likely a consequence of B-cell lysis. Although PML risk is much lower compared with natalizumab, the mortality in rituximab-associated PML is far higher; however, rituximab-related PML has almost always occurred in hematologic malignancies that already predispose to PML.[144,145]

Azathioprine

A purine analogue that disrupts B-cell and T-cell proliferation, azathioprine is not FDA approved for the treatment of MS but has been used off label for this purpose nonetheless.[146]

Azathioprine seems to be as effective as IFNB in reducing ARR and disability progression[147] but has been associated with GI symptoms, myelosuppression, and hepatotoxicity.[146] As such, careful dose adjustment and regular surveillance laboratory tests (CBC and LFT) are mandatory. Before starting therapy, patients should be screened for thiopurine-S-methyltransferase deficiency, an autosomal recessive trait resulting in excessive thioguanine nucleotide accumulation in hematopoietic tissues, which causes severe myelosuppression.[148,149] In addition, azathioprine has been associated with a cumulative (>600 g) dose risk of malignancies (typically after 5–10 years of use).[150,151]

Methotrexate

Methotrexate, an antimetabolite that inhibits dihydrofolic acid reductase, interferes with DNA synthesis and repair. There is no significant benefit of adding low-dose mothotroxato to pationts with MO on IFNB-1a with evidence of active disease. Long-term use carries the risk of myelosuppression, hepatic fibrosis, hepatotoxicity, opportunistic infections, nephrotoxicity, and potentially fatal GI toxicity.[152,153] As such, the authors do not recommend methotrexate as a long-term DMT in MS.

Mycophenolate mofetil

MMF is an oral immunosuppressant that interrupts lymphocyte DNA synthesis (by selectively inhibiting inosine 5'-monophosphate dehydrogenase type II, responsible for de novo synthesis of the purine nucleotide guanine), thereby inhibiting lymphocyte proliferation, IFNγ release, IL-6 secretion, and blood-brain barrier egress. MMF disrupts the same general pathways as azathioprine but is more selective, accounting for its more favorable safety and side effect profiles.[154–158]

Several small, prospective studies have supported the efficacy of MMF as an add-on therapy for IFNB and GA. MMF is also an effective monotherapy for MS.[159–164]

Adverse effects In general, MMF is well tolerated and safe. Side effects (usually transient) include GI upset, an increase in mild infections (predominantly upper respiratory and urinary), headache, and asthenia. Rare side effects include oral ulcerations, GI hemorrhage, esophagitis, gastritis, duodenitis, ischemic colitis, urticaria, dyshidrotic eczema, blistering hand dermatitis, and onycholysis. Potential laboratory abnormalities include lymphopenia, anemia, thrombocytopenia, eosinophilia, and increased hepatic transaminase levels.[159–164] MMF is classified as FDA pregnancy category D.

Dosing and monitoring The authors recommend starting MMF at 250 mg twice daily for 1 week and then escalated by 250 mg twice daily per week until a target dose of 1000 mg twice daily is achieved. Patients should be instructed to take MMF on an empty stomach (either 1 hour before or 2 hours following a meal). CBC and LFT should be checked before therapy commences, weekly for the first month, biweekly for the second and third months, monthly up to the sixth month, and then 3 monthly.

Advantages of using MMF include its oral formulation, generic availability, as well as efficacy. Drawbacks include the need for regular surveillance laboratory studies, and having to take MMF on an empty stomach twice daily (which may affect compliance).

Mitoxantrone

Mitoxantrone is a cytotoxic chemotherapeutic agent that intercalates with DNA and inhibits topoisomerase II; it is the only FDA-approved drug for secondary progressive multiple sclerosis (SPMS). In vitro, it inhibits B-cell, T-cell, and macrophage proliferation; it also disrupts antigen presentation as well as secretion of IFN, tumor necrosis factor-alpha, and IL-2. Its efficacy in treating MS is well documented[165–169] but mitoxantrone carries significant risks, including cardiotoxicity, leukemia, myelosuppression, and teratogenecity.[169,170]

Both cardiotoxicity and leukemia may occur acutely or years after cessation of treatment. In view of the adverse effects mentioned earlier, patients who receive mitoxantrone should have an annual echocardiogram (or multigated acquisition scan) and CBC for life. The current repertoire of DMTs and the safety risks of mitoxantrone restrict its use as a last-resort drug to be used in patients with aggressive disease activity refractory to other therapies.

Choosing a DMT

Although it is tempting to categorize drugs as first-line agents, second-line agents, and so on, this simplistic approach is not appropriate if there is disease and individual heterogeneity. Each patient with MS is an individual and thus deserves a personalized treatment plan.

The first step is to stratify patients into low-risk or high-risk categories. The low-risk category encompasses patients with clinically isolated syndrome (CIS), minimal disability, low MRI lesion load, as well as favorable prognostic indicators (being young, white, female, and experiencing sensory attacks). High-risk patients include those with moderate to severe disability, highly active disease, high radiologic lesion load, and those with poor prognostic factors (being older, male, nonwhite, and experiencing cerebellar or motor attacks).

Patients in the low-risk category may be candidates for IFNB or GA, because many patients respond to them with minimal side effects. Those who prefer oral therapy, or who cannot tolerate IFNB side effects, may consider teriflunomide, fingolimod, or DMF. The decision to initiate fingolimod therapy should be weighed carefully in view of its potential adverse effects, and the requirement for close monitoring. Patients in the high-risk category should be considered candidates for fingolimod, DMF, or natalizumab. PML risk factors may favor the use of fingolimod, DMF, or 8-weekly natalizumab infusions. Monthly natalizumab may be used in those without such risk factors. If a patient develops NABs against natalizumab with breakthrough disease, rituximab should be considered.

Patients who relapse on IFNB but remain in the low-risk category may be switched to GA, or vice versa. Those who fail both agents may be switched to fingolimod, teriflunomide, or DMF. Alternatively, clinicians may consider adding either MMF or monthly steroid therapy to those already on IFNB or GA. Again, if they transition to the high-risk category, escalating to natalizumab or DMF should be considered.

The presence of other risk factors should also be weighed against a DMT's side effect profile before starting any DMT.

Fertility and pregnancy

Pregnancy is a state of immunomodulation associated with an antiinflammatory milieu that leads to a reduction in disease activity. The postpartum period has been associated with a resurgence of disease activity (**Box 2**).

GA, IFNB, fingolimod, and natalizumab have not been shown to affect human fertility.[171] However, mitoxantrone and cyclophosphamide have been associated with both female and male gonadal toxicity.[172–175]

Although women are often advised to discontinue immunomodulatory therapy before conceiving, prenatal exposure to these agents still occurs because about half of pregnancies are unplanned. GA is the only DMT considered pregnancy category B (ie, no controlled human studies are available but either no or minimal risk to the fetus in animal studies). No negative side effects have been reported with GA use during pregnancy and breastfeeding. IFNB (pregnancy class C) was associated with lower mean birth weight, shorter mean birth length, and preterm birth (<37 weeks); no serious teratogenic effects have been observed to date. No negative side effects

---

Box 2
Washout protocol for teriflunomide

1. Oral cholestyramine 8 g every 8 hours for 11 days, reduce to 4 g every 8 hours if not tolerating well or oral activated charcoal 50 g every 12 hours for 11 days

2. Get teriflunomide level at day 12, goal less than 0.02 mg/L

3. Supplement folic acid during washout period during pregnancy or during the periconceptional period

4. Washout days do not have to be consecutive

have been reported with natalizumab (pregnancy class C) use in pregnancy to date.[171,176–179]

Although there is a lack of data regarding fingolimod (pregnancy class C), the authors advise against its use in pregnant and breastfeeding women because it may interfere with critical S1P1 signaling pathways that contribute to various cellular processes and embryogenesis. Anti-DNA agents (eg, mitoxantrone, MMF, azathioprine, teriflunomide, and cyclophosphamide) are contraindicated in pregnancy and breastfeeding; patients on these agents should be advised to use contraception.

Patients on DMTs other than GA should be advised to discontinue therapy when they plan to become, or find out that they are, pregnant. Patients who discontinue a DMT while trying to become pregnant, or who are pregnant, can be on pulsed corticosteroid therapy. Corticosteroids are generally safe for use in pregnancy and are used by obstetricians to promote lung maturity in preterm births.[171] It may be preferable to use prednisone, prednisolone, and methylprednisolone because these are inactivated by 11β-hydroxysteroid dehydrogenase in the placenta, thus minimizing fetal exposure. In contrast, dexamethasone can cross the placenta.[171] Patients with a history of difficult-to-control disease may need monthly IVMP or IVIg throughout gestation and until 12 weeks postpartum.

VIGNETTE 4: DMTs DURING PREGNANCY

A 25-year-old right-handed, recently married nulliparous woman was diagnosed with relapsing MS after she developed acute optic neuritis of the right eye with T2/FLAIR and gadolinium-enhancing lesions of the brain and cervical spine. Her CSF analysis corroborated this diagnosis. She had received a 3-day course of high-dose steroids (1g/d of IV methylprednisolone) with almost complete resolution of her symptoms. Three weeks later she presents to the neurologist's office for follow-up. She expresses a desire to have children. However, she is also concerned about the effects of MS disease–modifying therapies during pregnancy and about the risk of having a relapse if she was off disease-modifying therapy during pregnancy.

The prototypical patient with MS is a woman in the child-bearing age group and so this clinical scenario is common in MS clinics. First, the timing of pregnancy could be made based on personal decisions made between the couple rather than based on the disease activity because there is enough evidence that the MS disease process and pregnancy do not adversely affect each other for the most part, with rare exceptions (that are not discussed in this vignette).

First the patient must be counseled on the topics listed in **Table 1**.

Treatment concerns in MS during pregnancy can be divided into 3 parts: (1) use of DMTs, (2) treatment of relapses, (3) use of symptomatic therapies.

Use of DMTs DURING PREGNANCY

The National MS Society consensus statement states that, as far as possible, DMTs should not be used in patients with MS who are pregnant, trying to become pregnant, or breast feeding. Most pregnancy registries for any of the DMTs have not clearly shown teratogenic effects. **Table 2** shows the effects of the currently used DMTs in pregnancy. For the most part, only a minority of pregnant patients with MS (especially those with severe or highly active MS) might have to remain on therapy. Although there is no clear consensus regarding when to stop a DMT before trying to become pregnant, the following recommendations are widely agreed on. One month is reasonable for the interferon-βs, GA, and dimethyl fumarate (BG-12)/DMF, and 2 months for fingolimod. Although 3 months have been recommended with natalizumab, it may be that 1 month is sufficient, and the antibody does not need to be totally gone from the system before a patient tries to become pregnant; the level is much lower at 1 month, longer washout is associated with risk of activity, the patient is not likely to get pregnant immediately, and no negative pregnancy effect has been documented. Teriflunomide should always be washed out (discussed later).

Management of acute relapses during pregnancy

In general, when there is a concern for relapse, there is a tendency to obtain MRI of the brain and/or spinal cord. MRI is considered safe during pregnancy; however, guidelines recommend MRI only if essential. Contrast is contraindicated in pregnancy because gadolinium crosses the placenta and its effects on the fetus are not clearly known.

With regard to treatment, a short course of high-dose steroids is the standard symptomatic treatment to speed up recovery from an acute attack of MS during pregnancy. Typically, the equivalent of 1 g of methylprednisolone (IV or oral) is given daily for 3 to 7 days, depending on the severity of the attack. No oral taper is recommended. It is advisable to avoid steroids during the first trimester to avoid the increased risk of cleft palate and reduce birth weight. However, steroids can be used fairly safely in the second and third trimesters. In general, dexamethasone and betamethasone are avoided in pregnancy because they cross the placenta readily compared with prednisone, prednisolone, or methylprednisolone, which are preferred to minimize adverse effects on the fetus.

It should be remembered that patients who relapse during pregnancy are at an increased risk of relapse postpartum and a plan for postpartum relapse management should be formulated early during pregnancy.

Use of symptomatic therapies

Clinicians should attempt nonpharmacologic strategies for symptom management related to MS during pregnancy and breast feeding. Symptomatic therapies should be minimized as much as possibly during pregnancy. If deemed essential, a minimum effective dose may be used.

IVIg (which is safe in pregnant and lactating women) has been shown to mitigate against postpartum resurgence in MS disease activity.[180–183] The authors use the same protocol as Achiron and colleagues,[182] as shown in **Box 3**.

Multiple Sclerosis Exacerbation and its Management

An acute MS exacerbation can be defined as a neurologic event lasting more than 24 hours, in the absence of increased body temperature or infection. Pseudoexacerbation should be suspected if the patient experiences a reemergence or deterioration of previously sustained neurologic deficits, lasting less than 24 hours, and/or occur in the presence of an increased body temperature, with or without infection. Pseudoexacerbations caused by Uhthoff phenomenon may be treated with antipyretic therapy and/or cooling techniques.

VIGNETTE 5: A PATIENT WITH MS WITH ACUTE OPTIC NEURITIS AND UHTHOFF PHENOMENON

A 27-year-old woman with optic neuritis OS (oculus sinister [left eye]), who is a nationally ranked tennis player, awoke 1 week ago with severe eye pain and light flashes when moving her eyes in darkness, and now describes brightness sensitivity, color desaturation, and the illusion of the tennis ball moving in an elliptical trajectory across the court. She also describes the even more conspicuous change in visual-motor function, in which she is overhitting the ball in one direction, and underhitting in the other. She describes eye strain headache (ie, asthenopia from visual corrective disparity). Examination shows that high-contrast letter acuity (ie, 100%) is 70 out of 70 letters identified OD, and 68 OS. On low-contrast letter acuity at 2.5%, she correctly identifies 40 letters OD, and 5 letters OS; 48 letters OU (consistent with the principle of binocular summation; parallax effect), large left RAPD, a cecocentral field suppression OS on Humphrey 30 to 2 fields, prolongation in the P100 VEP latency and amplitude on the left, and a loss of the melanopsin-mediated pupillary light reflex on the left (which she wants to know whether this could be affecting her change in sleep and waking, mood regulation, and change in her menstrual cycle). Fundus examination is normal. OCT reveals an RNFL thickness on the right of 100 μm and 125 μm on the left. However, GCL + IPL is essentially equivalent OU.

Notwithstanding the administration of 1g of IVMP/d/3 d, starting on the day of symptom onset, the patient describes minimal improvements. What should be done?

Answer: admit to hospital and initiate another round of IVMP, while placing a central line (given that she has poor peripheral venous access), and commence plasma exchange (at 1 volume/d × 5 treatments; this ultimately takes 8 days because of the fibrinogen levels). Before starting she is given supplemental iron plus vitamin C to avoid PLEX-related iron deficiency. She is discharged on the day of her last PLEX, and within 1 to 2 weeks she notes near-complete resolution of her attack-related deficits. Examination shows recovery of low-contrast letter acuity to 42 letters OD, 30 letters OS, and 45 letters OU. The field defect and color desaturation has resolved. The large left RAPD is now trace, and the fundus examination reveals very mild pallor OS, in a temporal quadrant distribution. VEP reveals improvement of the prolonged P100 latency and amplitude (from 125 milliseconds on the left to 113 milliseconds; whereas on the right the P100 latency was originally 98 milliseconds, and is now 100 milliseconds), whereas the OCT now reveals RNFL thicknesses of 101μm OD, and 90 μm OS. The GCL + IPL thickness measures are only modestly reduced on the left versus the right. There is no significant macular quadrant thinning. All pupillary responses are improved, including the melanopsin-mediated pupillary light reflex, in conjunction with resynchronization of her sleep-wake cycle, improved mood, and normalization of the menses. However, she continues to have the visual illusory movements of the tennis ball on the court, but only after playing for about 30 minutes (a time she describes as occurring conspicuously when feeling warmer than usual). When asked, she acknowledges that, for many years, she has been a poor sweater. These features are in keeping with the Uhthoff phenomenon, prompting us to recommend the following:

1. Use of the Frog Tog Chilly pad wrapped around her neck while playing.

2. Liberal ingestion of ice-cold liquids before starting play.

3. Given that the above were only modestly, albeit objectively, helpful, we then recommended that she start Ampyra, a long-acting formulation of 4-aminopyridine (4-AP) that serves as a general potassium channel antagonist, thereby prolonging action potential duration, and FDA approved to help patients with MS with walking. Our patient starts with 10 mg in the early morning, and takes the second dose about 9 hours later (rather than 12 hours in order to avoid insomnia, which is well known to occur with this agent when the second dose is taken close to bedtime, while the drug's concentration is increasing over 3–4 hours to achieve its maximum level).

Abbreviations: GCL, ganglion cell layer; IPL, inner plexiform layer; OD, oculus dextres (right eye); OU, oculus uterque (both eyes); PLEX, plasmapheresis or plasma exchange; RAPD, relative afferent pupillary deficit; RNFL, retinal nerve fiber layer; VEP, visual evoked potential.

Acute exacerbations are usually managed with corticosteroids, whereas steroid-refractory relapses should be considered for treatment with plasmapheresis or IVIg. Occasional circumstances arise in which a serious and treatment-resistant exacerbation evolves, usually with a limited window of opportunity to rescue the target tissue. In this context the authors often use parenterally administered chemotherapeutic options such as cyclophosphamide, high-dose methotrexate with leucovorin rescue, or mitoxantrone.

Box 3
Treatment protocol for IVIg in pregnancy, the postpartum, and in breastfeeding mothers

- Give 0.4 g/kg/d for 5 consecutive days within the first week after delivery.
- Give additional booster doses of 0.4 g/kg/d at 6 and 12 weeks postpartum.

In patients with a history of aggressive disease, 0.4 g/kg body weight/d for 5 consecutive days within the 6 to 8 weeks of gestation with additional booster doses of 0.4 g/kg body weight/d once every 6 weeks until 12 weeks postpartum.

Corticosteroid therapy
Both corticosteroids and adrenocorticotrophic hormone have been used to treat MS exacerbations since the 1950s.[184] Corticosteroids play an important role in the treatment of acute exacerbations and also may be part of the long-term immunomodulatory strategy.

Corticosteroid therapy for acute exacerbations
Pulse corticosteroid therapy for acute exacerbations has also been shown to result in short-term immunologic and electrophysiologic improvement, hastening time to recovery but not affecting long-term disability. However for first-time acute optic neuritis (AON) high-dose corticosteroid therapy accelerates recovery and decreases the rate of conversion to clinically definite MS, for up to 2 years following the inception point of treatment intervention.[184–190] Most MS relapses are treated for 3 to 5 days with oral high-dose corticosteroids (IVMP 1 g daily or equivalent); a subsequent steroid taper is optional. High-dose oral steroids are now recognized as bioequivalent and equally efficacious as IV steroids.[191–196] Furthermore, oral corticosteroids are less costly, and place less demand on health care resources and work productivity.

Pulsed corticosteroid therapy
Although pulsed corticosteroid therapy is an established method for controlling disease activity in MS,[197–200] published trials use different dosing regimens. Most give high-dose corticosteroids on a monthly basis, as monotherapy or as adjuncts to patients' DMT regimens. Various studies have shown that pulsed corticosteroid therapy can delay progression of disability of SPMS, reduce postpartum relapse rate, and reduce the development of T1 black holes and brain atrophy.[200] An added dividend of adjunctive pulsed corticosteroid therapy, when added to IFNB treatment, is the lower risk of developing NABs.[201,202]

Adverse effects
Steroids have been associated with GI upset, dysgeusia, insomnia, mood disturbances (typically euphoria and irritability), tremor, weight gain, edema, hypertension, and hyperglycemia. As such, antacids and sleep aids may be required. Patients with hypertension or diabetes may need closer blood pressure and glycemic monitoring, respectively. Long-term monthly pulsed steroid therapy has been associated with osteoporosis and avascular necrosis.[184,203]

Plasmapheresis
Plasmapheresis involves the nonselective separation of the entire plasma volume from the corpuscular blood components either by centrifugation or membrane filtration. Mechanistically, the efficacy achieved with this technique it is thought to be associated with the depletion of pathogenic humoral factors, which in turn restrains the cellular immune response, and has been used to treat various autoimmune disorders.[203] Steroid-refractory MS relapses have been shown to respond favorably to plasmapheresis.[204,205] In contrast, plasmapheresis does not seem to improve progressive MS.[206–209] An important point to remember is that steroid-refractory MS relapses may still derive benefit from plasmapheresis, even 6 or more months after the relapse. Most patients experience improvement in their symptoms within 3 to 5 exchanges.[210]

A typical regimen is exchanges of 1 to 1.5 plasma volumes for 3 to 5 treatments over 10 days.

Adverse effects
Although plasmapheresis is usually well tolerated; typical side effects include anemia, hypotension, and hypocalcemia. Heparin-induced thrombocytopenia and iron

deficiency anemia, if used as a maintenance therapy, may develop in patients who are predisposed (because heparin is used to maintain the fluidity of extravascular blood on the apheresis circuit). The citrate used in plasmapheresis may cause complications related to hypocalcemia.[211] If a central IV catheter is required, central line–related complications may arise. The sequence of the exchanges is at least in part influenced by changes in coagulation parameters in order to avoid bleeding diatheses. The authors have observed that a significant proportion of patients develop iron deficiency anemia, particularly if plasmapheresis is used as a maintenance therapy.

Dose A typical regimen is exchanges of 1 to 1.5 plasma volumes for 3 to 5 treatments over 10 days.[211]

Intravenous immunoglobulin
IVIg is the pooled, polyvalent IgG extracted from the plasma of multiple donors. Its precise mechanism of action is unclear but it is used to treat a variety of dysimmune conditions. IVIg has been shown in a few small studies to be as efficacious as corticosteroid therapy.[212,213] Of note, IVIg may benefit corticosteroid-refractory MS AON. Administration of IVIg monthly up to 3 months, but not more than 6 months, after the onset of the relapse may be beneficial.[214,215]

Intravenous immunoglobulin for long-term immunomodulation Monthly IVIg reduced the ARR in 4 randomized, double-blind studies but 1 trial failed to replicate these results.[180,216–220]

Intravenous immunoglobulin for pregnancy and lactation IVIg is also effective in preventing MS relapses in the postpartum period, and is the only immunomodulating medication that is safe for lactating mothers.[181,221–223]

Dosing For steroid-refractory MS relapses in patients unable or unwilling to undergo plasmapheresis, IVIg may be given at a dose of 400 mg/kg/d for 5 days. For long-term immunomodulation, a monthly (or every 2 months, or quarterly) infusion of 400 mg/kg/d may be given.

Adverse reactions Although most patients experience infusion-related reactions, including headaches, nausea, and chills, these are easily remedied by reducing the rate of infusion, in addition to treatment with NSAIDs. Fluctuations in blood pressure may also be managed by adjusting the rate of infusion. More serious, albeit infrequent, adverse effects have been reported.

Cyclophosphamide
Cyclophosphamide is a nonspecific, alkylating immunosuppressant that is metabolized hepatically to yield cytotoxic metabolites. Its effect on MS is thought to be mediated by its lymphotoxic effects, and by shifting the immune system toward an antiinflammatory Th2 response.[224] Pulse or high-dose cyclophosphamide therapy is effective in patients with active, inflammatory disease, particularly those refractory to standard therapy.

Cyclophosphamide's pharmacology is responsible for its highly immunosuppressive, but not myeloablative, effects.[224]

Cyclophosphamide pulse therapy
Cyclophosphamide pulse therapy has been used in treatment of MS for many years. Induction therapy with IV cyclophosphamide is effective at stabilizing disease and inducing temporary remission; however, recrudescence of disease activity usually begins in the second year in the absence of concomitant or subsequent application of

disease-modifying therapy.[224–226] The Northeast Cooperative MS Treatment Group study supported the benefit of cyclophosphamide induction therapy but also showed that bimonthly IV cyclophosphamide pulses significantly prolonged the time to treatment failure.[226] The most marked benefits of cyclophosphamide pulse therapy are seen in younger patients with active, relapsing disease; it does not seem to benefit progressive MS that lacks a concomitant relapsing component.[227,228]

Cyclophosphamide pulses may also be added to standard DMT regimens to induce clinical stability. Multiple studies have shown that IFNB with adjunctive cyclophosphamide pulse therapy is more effective than IFNB alone.[229–233]

How and when to use pulse cyclophosphamide therapy Cyclophosphamide may be used to treat acute exacerbations refractory to steroids and plasmapheresis, as well as induction or adjunctive therapy in rapidly progressive MS (2 or more relapses in a year, or rapid progression of disability) before transitioning to a less toxic DMT. **Box 4** provides a summary of the treatment protocol.

Box 4

Protocols for administration of cyclophosphamide in MS

For steroid-refractory and plasmapheresis-refractory exacerbations:

- Cyclophosphamide 1000 mg IV given as a single infusion. For induction or adjunctive therapy.

For induction or adjunctive therapy:

- Monthly IV cyclophosphamide infusions (1000 mg) for 6 months to 1 year before transitioning to a more standard DMT monotherapy.

Precautions and monitoring during cyclophosphamide infusions:

- IV mesna (which binds to acrolein, the urotoxic metabolite of cyclophosphamide) at a dose 20% of the total cyclophosphamide dose should be given as 3 equal doses: 30 minutes before, then 4 and 8 hours after the cyclophosphamide infusion to prevent hemorrhagic cystitis.

- Urinalysis should be performed before and 12 hours after the infusion to screen for hematuria, which would necessitate further monitoring.

- IV hydration should begin just before, and continue for several hours after, the cyclophosphamide infusion.

- Patients should be encouraged to drink plenty of fluid (at least 3.8 L [1 gallon]) daily for the 2 days following therapy.

High-dose cyclophosphamide therapy treatment protocol:

- Cyclophosphamide 50 mg/kg (based on ideal body weight) is infused intravenously over an hour via a central venous catheter on 4 consecutive days.

- IV mesna (10 mg/kg) is administered 30 minutes before, and at 3, 6, and 8 hours after, cyclophosphamide to prevent hemorrhagic cystitis.

- Pancytopenia almost always occurs following treatment; platelet or pure red blood cell (leukocyte-poor) infusions may be required.

- Beginning 6 days after the last infusion of cyclophosphamide, the patient should be given granulocyte colony-stimulating factor (5 μg/kg/d) until the absolute neutrophil count (ANC) is greater than 1.0×10^9/L.
  Prophylactic antimicrobials (fluconazole 400 mg/d; norfloxacin 400 mg/d; and valacyclovir 500 mg twice daily) can be given on the last day of cyclophosphamide until the ANC exceeds 0.5×10^9/L. Pneumocystis prophylaxis is administered for 6 months.

High dose cyclophosphamide therapy

Based on the pharmacokinetics of cyclophosphamide,[224] high-dose cyclophosphamide therapy (HiCY) ablates all circulating lymphocytes and spares hematopoietic stem cells (ie, rebooting the immune system from these antigen-naive pluripotent stem cells).[234,235]

HiCY is effective at controlling various refractory autoimmune diseases, including MS, and the Marburg variant of MS.[224,236] HiCY induces MS remission and clinical stability at follow-up from 15 months to 3.5 years, and leads to improvements in clinical and radiologic markers of disease activity, disability, visual function, bladder function, ambulation, fatigue, and quality of life.[237–241] HiCY is more effective for active, inflammatory MS and less so for the progressive forms.[239] If aggressive, refractory disease reemerges, HiCY can be repeated with equal efficacy. The response rate exceeds 90%, but these patients eventually relapse, with only 20% remaining disease free at 5 years following HiCY therapy.[237,238] These remissions are temporary but offer a valuable window to use a standard, less toxic DMT. Standard DMTs may be started 30 days after HiCY,[241] a time when the rebooted immune system may respond more favorably to these agents.

Adverse effects

In general, cyclophosphamide is fairly safe. Frequent side effects include increased mild infections (eg, respiratory, urinary), nausea, vomiting, and alopecia.[242] Serious complications include herpes zoster, pneumonia, hepatotoxicity, gonadal failure, and hemorrhagic cystitis. A curious infusion-related side effect is a nasopharyngeal dysesthesia, termed wasabi nose.[243,244]

Gonadal failure, in both men and women, may result from cyclophosphamide therapy. Infrequently, irreversible infertility occurs. As such, patients should be counseled about sperm or ovarian cryopreservation before therapy. Clinicians should also consider obtaining seminal fluid analysis before and at the end of therapy in men who still desire to have children.

The most worrisome adverse effect of cyclophosphamide therapy is hemorrhagic cystitis, which may lead to cystectomy and/or bladder cancer[244] Our center has always used mesna in order to reduce this risk. The risk of malignancy, particularly bladder cancer, is higher in patients receiving daily oral therapy (in a dose-dependent and/or duration-dependent manner).[245,246] At present, the risk of malignancy in patients with MS treated with IV cyclophosphamide remains unclear; some investigators report an increased bladder cancer risk, particularly in patients who are chronically catheterized,[247] and others have observed no increased risk.[248] It is prudent to be aware of the risk of malignancy (particularly when the cumulative lifetime dose exceeds 80–100 g), and have patients undergo annual mammograms, dermatologic examinations, and urologic evaluations (especially in patients who are chronically catheterized).

Potential laboratory abnormalities include lymphopenia, hypogammaglobulinemia, increased liver transaminase levels, and eosinophilia.[242] Pancytopenia and absolute neutropenia (up to about 8–10 days) always follows HiCY.[236–241] Hematopoietic recovery takes about 2 weeks.[236] Transient alopecia and nausea are almost universal. Infectious complications are fairly common; some serious infections have been reported, including reactivation of cytomegalovirus hepatitis, pneumonia, and *Clostridium difficile* colitis. Febrile neutropenia, which is a complication of HiCY, may warrant hospital admission. Rarely, transient dilated cardiomyopathy and cardiac arrhythmias occur.[236–241]

SUMMARY

The number of DMTs available for MS has increased greatly over the past decade, mirroring the exponential increase in the understanding of the immunopathobiological underpinnings of this complex disease. Every patient with MS is an individual, and deserves a personalized treatment plan. Although financial desires may compel some parties to artificially designate DMTs into treatment tiers and require patients to fail a first-line therapy before they are allowed to receive a more efficacious DMT, such unintelligent, simple-minded bureaucracies are shortsighted and neglect to consider the complexities that make medicine both an art and a science. Such myopic approaches disregard the consequences of failing therapy: MS relapses that result in disabling neurologic deficits that permanently impair the patients' ability to work or care for themselves. Surely the long-term financial burden of such a relapse (to the patient personally, to society, and to the insurance companies) exceeds the short-term savings accrued from depriving patients of a more efficacious DMT. As practitioners of the art of healing, neurologists are duty bound to assess each individual patient, and tailor and devise a suitable plan that is agreed on by both the patient and the physician, based on their risk categories and comorbid conditions.

VIGNETTE 6: SOCIAL WORK AND CASE MANAGEMENT IN THE MS CLINIC

Clinic pearls

Social workers and other team members should work together to ensure that patients maximize their use of national/community resources and receive appropriate and coordinated health/rehabilitation services.

Advocacy on behalf of patients and their families is important.

Communication is key in maintaining healthy relationships when a parent has MS. There are many reasons to encourage patients to talk with their children about MS. This communication ensures that parents are the source of news, validates an issue that the children have already sensed, gives children a sense of control, and allows concerns to be expressed (building trust).

The clinical team may need to assist patients in asking for accommodations and connecting them with state vocational services.

Case vignette

A 40-year-old woman with relapsing-remitting MS calls the social worker for assistance with multiple issues. She is about to start on Tysabri but is worried about her coinsurance amount. She is married with a small child. She is working as a bank account manager. She is having difficulty getting around the bank and traveling because of fatigue and heat sensitivity. She expresses concerns about her cognitive skills not being what they used to be. She has not asked for accommodation or had any testing. The patient and her spouse try to protect their 9-year-old child by not telling him about MS. She admits to feeling down and overwhelmed but denies suicidal ideation.

Clinic approach

The social worker does a psychosocial assessment to determine this patient's needs and corresponding available resources. MS can be particularly difficult because it is most commonly diagnosed in the prime of life when people are establishing their careers and building their families. Most pharmaceutical companies provide patient assistance to patients for their disease-modifying medication, including Tysabri. Patients should be referred to the corresponding company to get help covering their medications.

This patient is seen in clinic and advised to start psychotherapy and an antidepressant. Many companies provide counseling sessions at no cost through employee assistance programs. Neurocognitive testing is recommended once the patient's mood is better because this could affect the results. This patient was advised to acquire cooling equipment and discuss some antifatigue options with her provider. Given that the patient has exceeded the 1-year threshold for employment she is able to apply for family medical leave . This program allows employees with serious conditions up to 12 weeks of leave per year that can be taken in blocks or on an intermittent basis. In this current situation intermittent leave is requested to protect her position at the bank and allow for appointments. Social workers can work collaboratively with counselors at state vocational rehabilitation programs to discuss accommodation ideas. It was decided in this case that a closer parking spot and less traveling would be beneficial. The Job Accommodation Network is an excellent resource for patients and health care providers in discussing workplace accommodations and how to ask for them.

Patients who have MS and their families should be encouraged to continue to talk openly with their clinical teams and to bring their young children or concerns to their next appointments to ask questions. Patients should also be encouraged to think about long-term and short-term plans that should be place in for what-if situations. Children should be assured that MS is not contagious and there is nothing they did to cause the illness. This patient was encouraged to bring her child to her next appointment. She will also be scheduled for follow-up to check on work issues and mood. She will be referred for neurocognitive testing in the future. Neuropsychologists can give patients strategies to compensate for any deficits. Additional accommodations may also be recommended.

The National MS Society, Multiple Sclerosis Foundation, and the Multiple Sclerosis Association of America are all excellent organizations for patients and their families. These national organizations provide education to patients and families, peer support, self-help groups, and support for professionals, and they have various programs that assist patients.

REFERENCES

1. Interferon beta-1b is effective in relapsing-remitting multiple sclerosis. I. Clinical results of a multicenter, randomized, double-blind, placebo-controlled trial. The IFNB Multiple Sclerosis Study Group. Neurology 1993;43:655–61.
2. Paty DW, Li DK. Interferon beta-1b is effective in relapsing-remitting multiple sclerosis. II. MRI analysis results of a multicenter, randomized, double-blind, placebo-controlled trial. UBC MS/MRI Study Group and the IFNB Multiple Sclerosis Study Group. Neurology 1993;43:662–7.
3. Jacobs LD, Cookfair DL, Rudick RA, et al. Intramuscular interferon beta-1a for disease progression in relapsing multiple sclerosis. The Multiple Sclerosis Collaborative Research Group (MSCRG). Ann Neurol 1996;39:285–94.
4. PRISMS (Prevention of Relapses and Disability by Interferon beta-1a Subcutaneously in Multiple Sclerosis) Study Group. Randomised double-blind placebo-controlled study of interferon beta-1a in relapsing/remitting multiple sclerosis. PRISMS (Prevention of Relapses and Disability by Interferon beta-1a Subcutaneously in Multiple Sclerosis) Study Group. Lancet 1998;352:1498–504.
5. Kappos L. European Study Group on interferon beta-1b in secondary progressive MS. Placebo-controlled multicentre randomised trial of interferon beta-1b in treatment of secondary progressive multiple sclerosis. Lancet 1998;352:1491–7.
6. Simon JH, Jacobs LD, Campion M, et al, for the Multiple Sclerosis Collaborative Research Group. Magnetic Resonance studies of intramuscular interferon β-1a for the relapsing multiple sclerosis. Ann Neurol 1998;43:79–87.
7. Li DK, Paty DW. Magnetic resonance imaging results of the PRISMS trial: a randomized, double-blind, placebo-controlled study of interferon-β1a in relapsing-remitting multiple sclerosis. Ann Neurol 1999;46:197–206.
8. SPECTRIMS Study Group. Randomized controlled trial of interferon-beta-1a in secondary progressive MS: clinical results. Neurology 2001;56:1496–504.

9. Cohen JA, Cutter GR, Fischer JS, et al. Benefit of interferon beta-1a on MSFC progression in secondary progressive MS. Neurology 2002;59:679–87.

10. Leuschen MP, Filipi M, Healey K. A randomized open label study of pain medications (naproxen, acetaminophen and ibuprofen) for controlling side effects during initiation of IFN beta-1a therapy and during its ongoing use for relapsing-remitting multiple sclerosis. Mult Scler 2004;10:636–42.

11. Panitch H, Miller A, Paty D, et al. Interferon beta-1b in secondary progressive MS: results from a 3 year controlled study. Neurology 2004;63:1788–95.

12. Trojano M, Liguori M, Paolicelli D, et al. Interferon beta in relapsing-remitting multiple sclerosis: an independent postmarketing study in southern Italy. Mult Scler 2003;9:451–7.

13. Milanese C, La Mantia L, Palumbo R, et al. A post-marketing study on interferon beta 1b and 1a treatment in relapsing-remitting multiple sclerosis: different response in drop-outs and treated patients. J Neurol Neurosurg Psychiatry 2003;74:1689–92.

14. Haas J, Firzlaff M. Twenty-four-month comparison of immunomodulatory treatments - a retrospective open label study in 308 RRMS patients treated with beta interferons or glatiramer acetate (Copaxone). Eur J Neurol 2005;12:425–31.

15. Rio J, Tintore M, Nos C, et al. Interferon beta in relapsing-remitting multiple sclerosis. An eight year experience in a specialist multiple sclerosis centre. J Neurol 2005;252:795–800.

16. Limmroth V, Malessa R, Zettl UK, et al. Quality assessment in multiple sclerosis therapy (QUASIMS): a comparison of interferon beta therapies for relapsing-remitting multiple sclerosis. J Neurol 2007;254:67–77.

17. Kappos L, Clanet M, Sandberg-Wollheim M, et al. Neutralizing antibodies and efficacy of interferon beta-1a: a 4-year controlled study. Neurology 2005;65:40–7.

18. Durelli L, Verdun E, Barbero P, et al. Every-other-day interferon beta-1b versus once-weekly interferon beta-1a for multiple sclerosis: results of a 2-year prospective randomised multicentre study (INCOMIN). Lancet 2002;359:1453–60.

19. Panitch H, Goodin DS, Francis G, et al. Randomized, comparative study of interferon beta-1a treatment regimens in MS: the EVIDENCE Trial. Neurology 2002;59:1496–506.

20. Pachner A, Dail D, Pak E, et al. The importance of measuring IFNbeta bioactivity: monitoring in MS patients and the effect of anti-IFNbeta antibodies. J Neuroimmunol 2005;166:180–8.

21. Sorensen P, Deisenhammer F, Duda P, et al. Guidelines on use of anti-IFN-beta antibody measurements in multiple sclerosis: report of an EFNS Task Force on IFN-beta antibodies in multiple sclerosis. Eur J Neurol 2005;12:817–27.

22. Calabresi PA, Kieseier BC, Arnold DL, et al. Pegylated interferon β-1a for relapsing-remitting multiple sclerosis (ADVANCE): a randomised, phase 3, double-blind study. Lancet Neurol 2014;13(7):657 65.

23. Rubio Fernandez D, Rodriguez Del Canto C, Marcos Galan V, et al. Contribution of endermology to improving indurations and panniculitis/lipoatrophy at glatiramer acetate injection site. Adv Ther 2012;29:267–75.

24. Anderson J, Bell C, Bishop J, et al. Demonstration of equivalence of a generic glatiramer acetate (Glatopa™). J Neurol Sci 2015;359:24–34.

25. Johnson KP, Brooks BR, Cohen JA, et al. Copolymer 1 reduces relapse rate and improves disability in relapsing-remitting multiple sclerosis: results of a phase III

multicenter, double blind placebo-controlled trial. The Copolymer 1 Multiple Sclerosis Study Group. Neurology 1995;45:1268–76.

26. Comi G, Filippi M, Wolinsky JS. European/Canadian multicenter, double-blind, randomized, placebo-controlled study of the effects of glatiramer acetate on magnetic resonance imaging–measured disease activity and burden in patients with relapsing multiple sclerosis. European/Canadian Glatiramer Acetate Study Group. Ann Neurol 2001;49:290–7.

27. Mikol DD, Barkhof F, Chang P, et al. Comparison of subcutaneous interferon beta-1a with glatiramer acetate in patients with relapsing multiple sclerosis (the REbif vs Glatiramer Acetate in Relapsing MS Disease [REGARD] study): a multicentre, randomised, parallel, open-label trial. Lancet Neurol 2008;7: 903–14.

28. O'Connor P, Filippi M, Arnason B, et al. 250 microg or 500 microg interferon beta-1b versus glatiramer acetate in relapsing-remitting multiple sclerosis: a prospective, randomized, multicentre study. Lancet Neurol 2009;8:889–97.

29. Boster A. Efficacy, safety, and cost-effectiveness of glatiramer acetate in the treatment of relapsing-remitting multiple sclerosis. Ther Adv Neurol Disord 2011;4:319–32.

30. Drago F, Brusati C, Mancardi G, et al. Localized lipoatrophy after glatiramer acetate injection in patients with relapsing-remitting multiple sclerosis. Arch Dermatol 1999;135:1277–8.

31. Mancardi GL, Murialdo A, Drago F, et al. Localized lipoatrophy after prolonged treatment with copolymer 1. J Neurol 2000;247:220–1.

32. Hwang L, Orengo I. Lipoatrophy associated with glatiramer acetate injections for the treatment of multiple sclerosis. Cutis 2001;68:287–8.

33. Edgar CM, Brunet DG, Fenton P, et al. Lipoatrophy in patients with multiple sclerosis on glatiramer acetate. Can J Neurol Sci 2004;31:58–63.

34. Chun J, Hartung HP. Mechanism of action of oral fingolimod (FTY720) in multiple sclerosis. Clin Neuropharmacol 2010;33:91–101.

35. Cohen JA, Chun J. Mechanisms of fingolimod's efficacy and adverse effects in multiple sclerosis. Ann Neurol 2011;69:759–77.

36. Mehling M, Johnson TA, Antel J, et al. Clinical immunology of the sphingosine 1-phosphate receptor modulator fingolimod (FTY720) in multiple sclerosis. Neurology 2011;76:S20–7.

37. Kappos L, Radue EW, O'Connor P, et al, FREEDOMS Study Group. A placebo-controlled trial of oral fingolimod in relapsing multiple sclerosis. N Engl J Med 2010;362:387–401.

38. Cohen JA, Barkhof F, Comi G, et al, TRANSFORMS Study Group. Oral fingolimod or intramuscular interferon for relapsing multiple sclerosis. N Engl J Med 2010;362:402–15.

39. Kappos L, Antel J, Comi G, et al, FTY720 D2201 Study Group. Oral fingolimod (FTY720) for relapsing multiple sclerosis. N Engl J Med 2006;355:1124–40.

40. Willis MA, Cohen JA. Fingolimod therapy for multiple sclerosis. Semin Neurol 2013;33:37–44.

41. Collins W, Cohen J, O'Connor P, et al. Long-term safety of oral fingolimod d (FTY720) in relapsing multiple sclerosis: integrated analyses of phase 1 and phase 3 studies (P843). Mult Scler 2010;16(Suppl 10):S295.

42. Schmouder R, Serra D, Wang Y, et al. FTY720: placebo-controlled study of the effect on cardiac rate and rhythm in healthy subjects. J Clin Pharmacol 2006;46: 895–904.

43. DiMarco JP, O'Connor P, Cohen JA, et al. First-dose effect of fingolimod: pooled safety data from two phase 3 studies (TRANSFORMS and FREEDOMS). Mult Scler 2010;16(Suppl 10):S290.

44. Faber H, Fischer HJ, Weber F. Prolonged and symptomatic bradycardia following a single dose of fingolimod. Mult Scler 2013;19:126–8.

45. Espinosa PS, Berger JR. Delayed fingolimod-associated asystole. Mult Scler 2011;17:1387–9.

46. Lindsey JW, Haden-Pinneri K, Memon NB, et al. Sudden unexpected death on fingolimod. Mult Scler 2012;18:1507–8.

47. Jain N, Bhatti MT. Fingolimod-associated macular edema: incidence, detection, and management. Neurology 2012;78:672–80.

48. Francis G, Kappos L, O'Connor P, et al. Temporal profile of lymphocyte counts and relationship with infections with fingolimod therapy. Mult Scler 2014;20: 471–80.

49. Gross CM, Baumgartner A, Rauer S, et al. Multiple sclerosis rebound following herpes zoster infection and suspension of fingolimod. Neurology 2012;79: 2006–7.

50. Pfender N, Jelcic I, Linnebank M, et al. Reactivation of herpesvirus under fingolimod: a case of severe herpes simplex encephalitis. Neurology 2015;84: 2377–8.

51. Ratchford JN, Costello K, Reich DS, et al. Varicella-zoster virus encephalitis and vasculopathy in a patient treated with fingolimod. Neurology 2012;79:2002–4.

52. Lovrik KB, Bogen B, Corthay A. Fingolimod blocks immunosurveillance of myeloma and B-cell lymphoma resulting in cancer development in mice. Blood 2012;119:2176–7.

53. Alshaker H, Sauer L, Monteil D, et al. Therapeutic potential of targeting SK1 in human cancers. Adv Cancer Res 2013;117:143–200.

54. Visser F, Wattjes MP, Pouwels PJW, et al. Tumefactive multiple sclerosis lesions under fingolimod treatment. Neurology 2012;79:2000–2.

55. Castrop F, Kowarik MS, Albrecht H, et al. Severe multiple sclerosis relapse under fingolimod therapy: incident or coincidence? Neurology 2012;78:928–30.

56. Leypoldt F, Munchau A, Moeller F, et al. Hemorrhaging focal encephalitis under fingolimod (FTY720) treatment: a case report. Neurology 2009;72:1022–4.

57. Havla JB, Pellkofer HL, Meinl I, et al. Rebound of disease activity after withdrawal of fingolimod (FTY720) treatment. Arch Neurol 2012;69:262–4.

58. Hakiki B, Portaccio E, Giannini M, et al. Withdrawal of fingolimod treatment for relapsing-remitting multiple sclerosis: report of six cases. Mult Scler 2012;18: 1636–9.

59. Ghezzi A, Rocca MA, Baroncini D, et al. Disease reactivation after fingolimod discontinuation in two multiple sclerosis patients. J Neurol 2013;260:327–9.

60. Piscolla E, Hakiki B, Pasto L, et al. Rebound after fingolimod suspension in a pediatric-onset multiple sclerosis patient. J Neurol 2013;260:1675–7.

61. Claussen MC, Korn T. Immune mechanisms of new therapeutic strategies in MS: teriflunomide. Clin Immunol 2012;142:49–56.

62. Gold R, Wolinsky JS. Pathophysiology of multiple sclerosis and the place of teriflunomide. Acta Neurol Scand 2011;124:75–84.

63. Kappos L, Comi G, Confavreux C, et al. The efficacy and safety of teriflunomide in patients with relapsing MS: results from TOWER, a phase III, placebo-controlled study. Paper presented at the 28th Congress of the European Committee for Treatment and Research in Multiple Sclerosis (ECTRIMS). Lyon (France), October 10–13, 2012.

64. Vermersch P, Czlonkowska A, Grimaldi LME, et al. A multicenter, randomized, parallel-group, rater-blinded study comparing the effectiveness and safety of teriflunomide and subcutaneous interferon beta-1a in patients with relapsing multiple sclerosis. Paper presented at the 28th Congress of the European Committee for Treatment and Research in Multiple Sclerosis (ECTRIMS). Lyon (France), October 10–13, 2012.

65. Confavreux C, Li DK, Freedman MS, et al. Long-term follow-up of a phase 2 study of oral teriflunomide in relapsing multiple sclerosis: safety and efficacy results up to 8.5 years. Mult Scler 2012;18:1278–89.

66. Rahmlow M, Shuster EA, Dominik J, et al. Leflunomide-associated progressive multifocal leukoencephalopathy. Arch Neurol 2008;65:1538–9.

67. O'Connor PW, Li D, Freedman MS, et al. A phase II study of the safety and efficacy of teriflunomide in multiple sclerosis with relapses. Neurology 2006;66: 894–900.

68. Phillips JT, Fox RJ. BG-12 in multiple sclerosis. Semin Neurol 2013;33:56–65.

69. Gold D, Kappos L, Arnold DL, et al. Placebo-controlled phase 3 study of oral BG-12 for relapsing multiple sclerosis. N Engl J Med 2012;367:1098–107.

70. Fox RJ, Miller DH, Phillips JT, et al. Placebo-controlled phase 3 study of oral BG-12 or glatiramer in multiple sclerosis. N Engl J Med 2012;367:1087–97.

71. Hanson J, Gille A, Offermanns S. Role of HCA_2 (GPR109A) in nicotinic acid and fumaric acid ester-induced effects on the skin. Pharmacol Ther 2012;136:1–7.

72. Ermis U, Weis J, Schulz JB. PML in a patient treated with fumaric acid. N Engl J Med 2013;368:1657–8.

73. van Oosten BW, Killestein J, Barkhof F, et al. PML in a patient treated with dimethyl fumarate from a compounding pharmacy. N Engl J Med 2013;368: 1658–9.

74. Pavlovic D, Patera AC, Nyberg F, et al. Progressive multifocal leukoencephalopathy: current treatment options and future perspectives. Ther Adv Neurol Disord 2015;8:255–73.

75. Stuve O, Bennett JL. Pharmacological properties, toxicology and scientific rationale for the use of natalizumab (Tysabri) in inflammatory diseases. CNS Drug Rev 2007;13:79–95.

76. Hynes RO. Integrins: bidirectional, allosteric signaling machines. Cell 2002;110: 673–87.

77. Polman C, O'Connor P, Havrdova E, et al. A randomized, placebo-controlled trial of natalizumab for relapsing multiple sclerosis. N Engl J Med 2006;354:899–910.

78. Hutchinson M, Kappos L, Calabresi PA, et al. The efficacy of natalizumab in patients with relapsing multiple sclerosis: subgroup analyses of AFFIRM and SENTINEL. J Neurol 2009;256:405–15.

79. Rudick RA, Stuart WH, Calabresi PA, et al, SENTINEL Investigators. Natalizumab plus interferon beta-1a for relapsing multiple sclerosis. N Engl J Med 2006;354:911–23.

80. Kappos L, O'Connor PW, Polman CH, et al. Clinical effects of natalizumab on multiple sclerosis appear early in treatment course. J Neurol 2013;260:1388–95.

81. Cree BA, Stuart WH, Tornatore CS, et al. Efficacy of natalizumab therapy in patients of African descent with relapsing multiple sclerosis: analysis of AFFIRM and SENTINEL data. Arch Neurol 2005;62:1681–3.

82. Ghezzi A, Pozzilli C, Grimaldi LM, et al. Safety and efficacy of natalizumab in children with multiple sclerosis. Neurology 2010;75:912–7.

83. Rinaldi F, Calabrese M, Seppi D, et al. Natalizumab strongly suppresses cortical pathology in relapsing-remitting multiple sclerosis. Mult Scler 2012;18:1760–7.

84. Gunnarsson M, Malmestrom C, Axelsson M, et al. Axonal damage in relapsing multiple sclerosis is markedly reduced by natalizumab. Ann Neurol 2011;69: 83–9.
85. Campbell JD, McQueen B, Miravalle A, et al. Comparative effectiveness of early natalizumab treatment in JC virus-negative relapsing-remitting multiple sclerosis. Am J Manag Care 2013;19:278–85.
86. Calabresi PA, Giovannoni G, Confavreux C, et al. The incidence and significance of anti-natalizumab antibodies: results from AFFIRM and SENTINEL. Neurology 2007;69:1391–403.
87. Oliver-Martos B, Orpex-Zafra T, Urbaneja P, et al. Early development of anti-natalizumab antibodies in MS patients. J Neurol 2013;260:2343–7.
88. Sorensen PS, Koch-Henriksen N, Jensen X. Neutralizing antibodies against interferon-beta do not predispose antibodies against natalizumab. Neurology 2011;76:759–60.
89. Zohren F, Toutzaris D, Klärner V, et al. The monoclonal anti-VLA-4 antibody natalizumab mobilizes CD34+ hematopoietic progenitor cells in humans. Blood 2008;111:3893–5.
90. Bonig H, Wundes A, Chang KH, et al. Increased numbers of circulating hematopoietic stem/progenitor cells are chronically maintained in patients treated with the CD49d blocking antibody natalizumab. Blood 2008;111:3439–41.
91. Abbas M, Lalive PH, Chofflon M, et al. Hypereosinophilia in patients with multiple sclerosis treated with natalizumab. Neurology 2011;77:1561–4.
92. Fine AJ, Sorbello A, Kortepeter C, et al. Central nervous system herpes simplex and varicella zoster virus infections in natalizumab-treated patients. Clin Infect Dis 2013;57:849–52.
93. Fragoso YD, Brooks JB, Gomes S, et al. Report of three cases of herpes zoster during treatment with natalizumab. CNS Neurosci Ther 2013;19:280–1.
94. Kwiatkowski A, Gallois J, Bilbault N, et al. Herpes encephalitis during natalizumab treatment in multiple sclerosis. Mult Scler 2012;18:909–11.
95. Bloomgren G, Richman S, Hotermans C, et al. Risk of natalizumab-associated progressive multifocal leukoencephalopathy. N Engl J Med 2012;366:1870–80.
96. Major E. Progressive multifocal leukoencephalopathy in patients on immunomodulatory therapies. Annu Rev Med 2010;61:35–47.
97. Bellizzi A, Nardis C, Anzivino E, et al. Human polyomavirus JC reactivation and pathogenetic mechanisms of progressive multifocal leukoencephalopathy and cancer in the era of monoclonal antibody therapies. J Neurovirol 2012;18:1–11.
98. Tan CS, Koralnik IJ. Progressive multifocal leukoencephalopathy and other disorders caused by JC virus: clinical features and pathogenesis. Lancet Neurol 2010;9:425–37.
99. Jensen PN, Major EO. A classification scheme for human polyomavirus JCV variants based on the nucleotide sequence of the noncoding regulatory region. J Neurovirol 2001;7:280–7.
100. Marshall LJ, Major EO. Molecular regulation of JC virus tropism: insights into potential therapeutic targets for progressive multifocal leukoencephalopathy. J Neuroimmune Pharmacol 2010;5:404–17.
101. Bellizzi A, Anzivino E, Rodio DM, et al. New insights on human polyomavirus JC and pathogenesis of progressive multifocal leukoencephalopathy. Clin Dev Immunol 2013;2013:839719.
102. Baldwin KJ, Hogg JP. Progressive multifocal leukoencephalopathy in patients with multiple sclerosis. Curr Opin Neurol 2013;26:318–23.

103. Yousry IA, Pelletier D, Cadavid D, et al. Magnetic resonance imaging pattern in natalizumab-associated progressive multifocal leukoencephalopathy. Ann Neurol 2012;72:779–87.

104. Gorelik L, Lerner M, Bixler S, et al. Anti-JC virus antibodies: implications for PML risk stratification. Ann Neurol 2010;68:295–303.

105. Gagne Brosseau MS, Stobbe G, Wundes A. Natalizumab-related PML 2 weeks after negative anti-JCV antibody assay. Neurology 2016;86:484–6.

106. Olsson T, Achiron A, Alredsson L, et al. Anti-JC virus antibody prevalence in multinational multiple sclerosis cohort. Mult Scler 2013;19:1533–8.

107. Bozic C, Richman D, Plavina T, et al. Anti-John Cunningham virus antibody prevalence in multiple sclerosis patients: baseline results of STRATIFY-1. Ann Neurol 2011;70:742–50.

108. Neumann F, Zohren F, Haas R. The role of natalizumab in hematopoietic stem cell mobilization. Expert Opin Biol Ther 2009;9:1099–106.

109. Major EO, Frohman E, Douek D. JC viremia in natalizumab-treated patients with multiple sclerosis. N Engl J Med 2013;368:2240–1.

110. Berger JR, Houff SA, Gurwell J, et al. JC virus antibody status underestimates infection rates. Ann Neurol 2013;74:84–90.

111. Perkins MR, Ryschkewitsch C, Liebner JC, et al. Changes in JC virus-specific T cell responses during natalizumab treatment in natalizumab-associated progressive multifocal leukoencephalopathy. PLoS Pathog 2012;8(11):e1003014.

112. Berger JR, Centonze D, Comi G, et al. Considerations on discontinuing natalizumab for the treatment of multiple sclerosis. Ann Neurol 2010;68:409–13.

113. O'Connor PW, Goodman A, Kappos L, et al. Disease activity return during natalizumab treatment interruption in patients with multiple sclerosis. Neurology 2011;76:1858–65.

114. Stuve O, Cravens PD, Frohman EM, et al. Immunologic, clinical, and radiologic status 14 months after cessation of natalizumab therapy. Neurology 2009;72:396–401.

115. Killestein J, Vennegoor A, Strijbis EM, et al. Natalizumab drug holiday in multiple sclerosis: poorly tolerated. Ann Neurol 2010;68:392–5.

116. Miravalle A, Jensen R, Kinkel RP. Immune reconstitution inflammatory syndrome in patients with multiple sclerosis following cessation of natalizumab therapy. Arch Neurol 2011;68:186–91.

117. Kleinschmidt-Demasters BK, Miravalle A, Schowinsky J, et al. Update on PML and PML-IRIS occurring in multiple sclerosis patients treated with natalizumab. J Neuropathol Exp Neurol 2012;71:604–17.

118. Miller DH, Khan OA, Sheremata WA, et al. A controlled trial of natalizumab for relapsing multiple sclerosis. N Engl J Med 2003;348:15–23.

119. Sangalli F, Moiola L, Radaelli M, et al. Starting immunomodulation shortly after natalizumab discontinuation: initial impressions. Mult Scler 2010;16:S142.

120. Kebrat A, Le Page E, Leray E, et al. Assessment of disease activity within 6 months after natalizumab discontinuation: and observational study of 28 consecutive relapsing-remitting multiple sclerosis patients. Mult Scler 2010;16:S128.

121. Jander S, Turowski B, Kieseier BC, et al. Emerging tumefactive multiple sclerosis after switching therapy from natalizumab to fingolimod. Mult Scler 2012;18:1650–2.

122. Daelman L, Maitrot A, Maarouf A, et al. Severe multiple sclerosis reactivation under fingolimod 3 months after natalizumab withdrawal. Mult Scler 2012;18:1647–9.

123. Jokubaitis VG, Li V, Kalincik T, et al. Fingolimod after natalizumab and the risk of short-term relapse. Neurology 2014;82:1204–11.

124. Rinaldi F, Seppi D, Calabrese M, et al. Switching therapy from natalizumab to fingolimod in relapsing-remitting multiple sclerosis: clinical and magnetic resonance imaging findings. Mult Scler 2012;18:1640–3.

125. de Seze J, Ongagna J-C, Collongues N, et al. Reduction of the washout time between natalizumab and fingolimod. Mult Scler 2013;19:1248.

126. Khatri BO, Man S, Giovannoni G, et al. Effect of plasma exchange in accelerating natalizumab clearance and restoring leukocyte function. Neurology 2009;72:402–9.

127. Zhovtis-Ryerson L, Frohman TC, Foley J, et al. Extended interval dosing of natalizumab in multiple sclerosis. J Neurol Neurosurg Psychiatry 2016. [Epub ahead of print].

128. Coles AJ. Alemtuzumab treatment of multiple sclerosis. Semin Neurol 2013;33: 66–73.

129. Coles AJ, Twyman CL, Arnold DL, et al. Alemtuzumab for patients with relapsing multiple sclerosis after disease-modifying therapy: a randomised controlled phase 3 trial. Lancet 2012;380:1829–39.

130. Cohen JA, Coles AJ, Arnold DL, et al. Alemtuzumab versus interferon beta 1a as first-line treatment for patients with relapsing-remitting multiple sclerosis: a randomised controlled phase 3 trial. Lancet 2012;380:1819–28.

131. The CAMMS223 Trial Investigators. Alemtuzumab vs. interferon beta-1a in early multiple sclerosis. N Engl J Med 2008;359:1786–801.

132. Costelloe L, Jones J, Coles A. Secondary autoimmune diseases following alemtuzumab therapy for multiple sclerosis. Expert Rev Neurother 2012;12:335–41.

133. Cossburn M, Pace AA, Jones J, et al. Autoimmune disease after alemtuzumab treatment for multiple sclerosis in a multicenter cohort. Neurology 2011;77: 573–9.

134. Clatworthy MR, Wallin EF, Jayne DR. Anti-glomerular basement membrane disease after alemtuzumab. N Engl J Med 2008;359:768–9.

135. Williamson EM, Berger JR. Central nervous system infections with immunomodulatory therapies. Continnuum (Minneap Minn) 2015;21:1577–98.

136. Coles AJ, Fox E, Vladic A, et al. Alemtuzumab more effective than interferon β-1a at 5-year follow-up of CAMMS223 clinical trial. Neurology 2012;78: 1069–78.

137. Touhy O, Costelloe L, Hill-Cawthorne G, et al. Alemtuzumab treatment of multiple sclerosis: long-term safety and efficacy. J Neurol Neurosurg Psychiatry 2015;86:208–15.

138. Reff ME, Carner K, Chambers KS, et al. Depletion of B cells in vivo by a chimeric mouse human monoclonal antibody to CD20. Blood 1994;83:435–45.

139. Cross AH, Klein RS, Piccio L. Rituximab combination therapy in relapsing multiple sclerosis. Ther Adv Neurol Disord 2012;5:311–9.

140. Bar-Or A, Calabresi P, Arnold D, et al. Rituximab in relapsing-remitting multiple sclerosis: a 72-week, open-label, phase I trial. Ann Neurol 2008;63:395–400.

141. Hauser S, Waubant E, Arnold D, et al. B-cell depletion with rituximab in relapsing-remitting multiple sclerosis. N Engl J Med 2008;358:676–88.

142. Naismith TA, Piccio L, Lyons J, et al. Rituximab add-on therapy for breakthrough relapsing multiple sclerosis: a 52-week phase II trial. Neurology 2010;74: 1860–7.

143. Hawker K, O'Connor P, Freedman M, et al. Rituximab in patients with primary progressive multiple sclerosis: results of a randomized double-blind placebo-controlled multicenter trial. Ann Neurol 2009;66:460–71.

144. Carson KR, Evens AM, Richey EA, et al. Progressive multifocal leukoencephalopathy after rituximab therapy in HIV-negative patients: a report of 57 cases from the Research on Adverse Drug Events and Reports project. Blood 2009; 113:4834–40.

145. Carson KR, Bennett CL. Rituximab and progressive multi-focal leukoencephalopathy: the jury is deliberating. Leuk Lymphoma 2009;50:323–4.

146. Casetta I, Iuliano G, Filippini G. Azathioprine for multiple sclerosis. Cochrane Database Syst Rev 2007;(4):CD003982.

147. Etemadifar M, Janghorbani M, Shaygannejad V. Comparison of interferon beta products and azathioprine in the treatment of relapsing-remitting multiple sclerosis. J Neurol 2007;254:1723–8.

148. Yates CR, Krynetski EY, Loennechen T, et al. Molecular diagnosis of thiopurine S-methyltransferase deficiency: genetic basis for azathioprine and mercaptopurine intolerance. Ann Intern Med 1997;126:608–14.

149. Frohman EM, Havrdova E, Levinson B, et al. Azathioprine myelosuppression in multiple sclerosis: characterizing thiopurine methyltransferase polymorphisms. Mult Scler 2006;12:108–11.

150. Confavreux C, Saddier P, Grimaud J, et al. Risk of cancer from azathioprine therapy in multiple sclerosis: a case–control study. Neurology 1996;46:1607–12.

151. Lhermitte F, Marteau R, Roullet E. Not so benign long-term immunosuppression in multiple sclerosis. Lancet 1984;1:276–7.

152. Cohen JA, Imrey PB, Calabresi PA, et al. Results of the Avonex Combination Trial (ACT) in relapsing–remitting MS. Neurology 2009;72:535–41.

153. Gray OM, McDonnell GV, Forbes RB. A systematic review of oral methotrexate for multiple sclerosis. Mult Scler 2006;12:507–10.

154. Allison AC, Kowalski WJ, Muller CD, et al. Mechanisms of action of mycophenolate mofetil. Ann N Y Acad Sci 1993;696:63–87.

155. Blaheta RA, Leckel K, Wittig B, et al. Mycophenolate mofetil impairs transendothelial migration of allogeneic CD4 and CD8 T-cells. Transplant Proc 1999;31: 1250–2.

156. Becker BN. Mycophenolate mofetil. Transplant Proc 1999;31:2777–8.

157. Barten MJ, van Gelder T, Gummert JF, et al. Novel assays of multiple lymphocyte functions in whole blood measure: new mechanisms of action of mycophenolate mofetil in vivo. Transpl Immunol 2002;10:1–14.

158. Stosic-Grujicic S, Maksimovic-Ivanic D, Miljkovic D, et al. Inhibition of autoimmune diabetes by mycophenolate mofetil is associated with down-regulation of TH1 cytokine-induced apoptosis in the target tissue. Transplant Proc 2002; 34:2955–7.

159. Ahrens N, Salama A, Haas J. Mycophenolate-mofetil in the treatment of refractory multiple sclerosis. J Neurol 2001;248:713–4.

160. Vermersch P, Waucquier N, Michelin E, et al. Combination of IFN beta-1a (Avonex) and mycophenolate mofetil (Cellcept) in multiple sclerosis. Eur J Neurol 2007;14:85–9.

161. Remington GM, Treadaway K, Frohman T, et al. A one-year prospective, randomized, placebo-controlled, quadruple-blinded, phase II safety pilot trial of combination therapy with interferon beta-1a and mycophenolate mofetil in early relapsing-remitting multiple sclerosis. Ther Adv Neurol Disord 2010;3:3–13.

162. Frohman EM, Brannon K, Racke MK, et al. Mycophenolate mofetil in multiple sclerosis. Clin Neuropharmacol 2004;27:80–3.

163. Etemadifar M, Kazemi M, Chitsaz A, et al. Mycophenolate mofetil in combination with interferon beta-1a in the treatment of relapsing-remitting multiple sclerosis: a preliminary study. J Res Med Sci 2011;16:1–5.

164. Frohman EM, Cutter G, Remington G, et al. A randomized, blinded, parallel-group, pilot trial of mycophenolate mofetil (CellCept) compared with interferon beta-1a (Avonex) in patients with relapsing-remitting multiple sclerosis. Ther Adv Neurol Disord 2010;3:15–28.

165. Kieseier BC, Jeffrey DR. Chemotherapeutics in the treatment of multiple sclerosis. Ther Adv Neurol Disord 2010;3:277–91.

166. Millefiorini E, Gasperini C, Pozzilli C, et al. Randomized placebo-controlled trial of mitoxantrone in relapsing-remitting multiple sclerosis: 24-month clinical and MRI outcome. J Neurol 1997;244:153–9.

167. van de Wyngaert FA, Beguin C, D'Hooghe MB, et al. A double-blind clinical trial of mitoxantrone versus methylprednisolone in relapsing, secondary progressive multiple sclerosis. Acta Neurol Belg 2001;101:210–6.

168. Hartung HP, Gonsette R, König N, et al. Mitoxantrone in Multiple Sclerosis Study Group (MIMS). Mitoxantrone in progressive multiple sclerosis: a placebo-controlled, double-blind, randomised, multicentre trial. Lancet 2002;360: 2018–25.

169. Krapf H, Morrissey SP, Zenker O, et al. for the MIMS Study Group. Effect of mitoxantrone on MRI in progressive MS: results of the MIMS trial. Neurology 2005; 65:690–5.

170. Morrissey SP, Le Page E, Edan G. Mitoxantrone in the treatment of multiple sclerosis. Int MS J 2005;12:74–87.

171. Houtchens MK, Kolb CM. Multiple sclerosis and pregnancy: therapeutic considerations. J Neurol 2013;260(5):1202–14.

172. Edan G, Brochet B, Clanet M. Safety profile of mitoxantrone in a cohort of 802 multiple sclerosis patients: a 4 years follow-up study. Neurology 2004;62:A493.

173. Cohen BA, Mikol DD. Mitoxantrone treatment of multiple sclerosis: safety considerations. Neurology 2004;63:S28–32.

174. La Mantia L, Milanese C, Mascoli N, et al. Cyclophosphamide for multiple sclerosis. Cochrane Database Syst Rev 2002;(4):CD002819.

175. Watson AR, Rance CP, Bain J. Long term effects of cyclophosphamide on testicular function. Br Med J 1985;291:1457–60.

176. Lu E, Wang BW, Guimond C, et al. Disease-modifying drugs for multiple sclerosis in pregnancy: a systematic review. Neurology 2012;79:1130–5.

177. Fragoso YD, Finkelsztejn A, Kaimen-Maciel DR, et al. Long-term use of glatiramer acetate by 11 pregnant women with multiple sclerosis: a retrospective, multicentre case series. CNS Drugs 2010;24:969–76.

178. Amato MP, Portaccio E, Ghezzi A, et al. Pregnancy and fetal outcomes after interferon-beta exposure in multiple sclerosis. Neurology 2010;75:1794–802.

179. Hellwig K, Haghikia A, Gold R. Pregnancy and natalizumab: results of an observational study in 35 accidental pregnancies during natalizumab treatment. Mult Scler 2011;17:958–63.

180. Fazekas F, Lublin FD, Li D, et al. Intravenous immunoglobulin in relapsing-remitting multiple sclerosis: a dose-finding trial. Neurology 2008;4:265–71.

181. Dudesek A, Zettl U. Intravenous immunoglobulins as therapeutic options in the treatment of multiple sclerosis. J Neurol 2006;253:50–8.

182. Achiron A, Rotstein Z, Noy S, et al. Intravenous immunoglobulin treatment in the prevention of childbirth associated acute exacerbations in multiple sclerosis - a pilot study. J Neurol 1996;243:25–8.

100. Orvieto H, Achiron R, Rotstein Z, et al. Pregnancy and multiple sclerosis. a 2-year experience. Eur J Obstet Gynecol Reprod Biol 1999;82:191–4.

184. Filippini G, Brusaferri F, Sibley WA, et al. Corticosteroids or ACTH for acute exacerbations in multiple sclerosis. Cochrane Database Syst Rev 2000;(4):CD001331.

185. Miller H, Newell DJ, Ridley A. Treatment of acute exacerbations with corticotrophin (A.C.T.H.). Lancet 1961;2:1120–2.

186. Rose AS, Kuzma JW, Kurtzke JF, et al. Cooperative study in the evaluation of therapy in multiple sclerosis. ACTH vs. placebo. Final report. Neurology 1970; 20:1–59.

187. Milligan NM, Newcombe R, Compston DAS. A double-blind controlled trial of high dose methylprednisolone in patients with multiple sclerosis: 1. Clinical effects. J Neurol Neurosurg Psychiatry 1987;50:511–6.

188. Filipovic SR, Drulovic J, Stojsavljevic N, et al. The effects of high-dose intravenous methylprednisolone on event-related potentials in patients with multiple sclerosis. J Neurol Sci 1997;152:147–53.

189. Sellebjerg F, Frederiksen JL, Nielsen PM, et al. Double-blind, randomized, placebo-controlled study of oral, high-dose methylprednisolone in attacks of MS. Neurology 1998;51:529–34.

190. Martinez-Caceres EM, Barrau MA, Brieva L, et al. Treatment with methylprednisolone in relapses of multiple sclerosis patients: immunological evidence of immediate and short-term but not long-lasting effects. Clin Exp Immunol 2002; 127:165–71.

191. Beck RW, Cleary PA, Anderson MM Jr, et al. A randomized, controlled trial of corticosteroids in the treatment of acute optic neuritis. The Optic Neuritis Study Group. N Engl J Med 1992;326:581–8.

192. Ramo-Tello C, Grau-Lopez L, Giner P, et al. A multicentre, randomized clinical and MRI study of highdose oral versus intravenous methylprednisolone in MS. Mult Scler 2011;17:S91–2.

193. Martinelli V, Pulizzi A, Annovazzi P, et al. A single blind, randomised MRI study comparing high-dose oral and intravenous methylprednisolone in treating MS relapses. Neurology 2009;73:1842–8.

194. Morrow SA, Stoian CA, Dmitrovic J, et al. The bioavailability of iv methylprednisolone and oral prednisone in multiple sclerosis. Neurology 2004;63:1079 80.

195. Alam SM, Kyriakides T, Lawden M, et al. Methylprednisolone in multiple sclerosis: a comparison of oral with IV therapy at equivalent high dose. J Neurol Neurosurg Psychiatry 1993;56:1219–20.

196. O'Brien JA, Ward AJ, Patrick AR, et al. Cost of managing an episode of relapse in multiple sclerosis in the United States. BMC Health Serv Res 2003;3:17.

197. Bergh FT, Kumpfel T, Schumann E, et al. Monthly intravenous methylprednisolone in relapsing-remitting multiple sclerosis – reduction of enhancing lesions, T2 lesion volume and plasma prolactin concentrations. BMC Neurol 2006;6:19.

198. Goodkin DE, Kinkel RP, Weinstock-Guttman B, et al. A phase II study of I.V. methylprednisolone in secondary-progressive multiple sclerosis. Neurology 1998;51:239–45.

199. de Seze J, Chapelotte M, Delalande S, et al. Intravenous corticosteroids in the postpartum period for reduction of acute exacerbations in multiple sclerosis. Mult Scler 2004;10:596–7.

200. Zivadinov R, Rudick RA, De Masi R, et al. Effects of IV methylprednisolone on brain atrophy in relapsing-remitting MS. Neurology 2001;57:1239–47.

201. Sorensen PS, Mellgren SI, Svenningsson A, et al. NORdic trial of oral methyl-prednisolone as add-on therapy to interferon beta-1a for treatment of relapsing-remitting multiple sclerosis. Lancet Neurol 2009;8:519–29.
202. Pozzilli C, Antonini G, Bagnato F, et al. Monthly corticosteroids decrease neutralizing antibodies to IFNbeta1-b: a randomized trial in multiple sclerosis. J Neurol 2002;249:50–6.
203. Ce P, Gedizlioglu M, Gelal F, et al. Avascular necrosis of the bones: an overlooked complication of pulse steroid treatment of multiple sclerosis. Eur J Neurol 2006;13:857–61.
204. Schroder A, Linker RA, Gold R. Plasmapheresis for neurological disorders. Expert Rev Neurother 2009;9:1331–9.
205. Weiner HL, Dau PC, Khatri BO, et al. Double-blind study of true vs. sham plasma exchange in patients treated with immunosuppression of acute attacks of multiple sclerosis. Neurology 1989;39:1143–9.
206. Weinshenker BG, O'Brien PC, Petterson TM, et al. A randomized trial of plasma exchange in acute central nervous system inflammatory demyelinating disease. Ann Neurol 1999;46:878–86.
207. Khatri BO, McQuillen MP, Harrington GJ, et al. Chronic progressive multiple sclerosis: double-blind controlled study of plasmapheresis in patients taking immunosuppressive drugs. Neurology 1985;35:312–9.
208. Gordon PA, Carroll DJ, Etches WS, et al. A double-blind controlled pilot study of plasma exchange versus sham apheresis in chronic progressive multiple sclerosis. Can J Neurol Sci 1985;12:39–44.
209. The Canadian cooperative trial of cyclophosphamide and plasma exchange in progressive multiple sclerosis. The Canadian Cooperative Multiple Sclerosis Study Group. Lancet 1991;337:441–6.
210. Sorensen PS, Wanscher B, Szpirt W, et al. Plasma exchange combined with azathioprine in multiple sclerosis using serial gadolinium-enhanced MRI to monitor disease activity: a randomized single-masked cross-over pilot study. Neurology 1996;46:1620–5.
211. Lee G, Arepally GM. Anticoagulation techniques in apheresis: from heparin to citrate and beyond. J Clin Apher 2012;27:117–25.
212. Sorensen PS, Haas J, Sellebjerg F, et al. IV immunoglobulins as add-on treatment to methylprednisolone for acute relapses in MS. Neurology 2004;63: 2028–33.
213. Visser LH, Bookman R, Tijseen CC, et al. A randomized, double-blind, place-controlled pilot study of IV immune globulins in combination with IV methylprednisolone in the treatment of relapses in patients with MS. Mult Scler 2004;10: 89–91.
214. Elovaara I, Kuusisto H, Wu X, et al. Intravenous immunoglobulins are a therapeutic option in the treatment of multiple sclerosis relapse. Clin Neuropharmacol 2011;34:84–9.
215. Luchinetti C, Bruck W, Parisi J, et al. Heterogeneity of multiple sclerosis lesions: implications for the pathogenesis of demyelination. Ann Neurol 2000;47:707–17.
216. Noseworthy JH, O'Brien PC, Petterson TM, et al. A randomized trial of intravenous immunoglobulin in inflammatory demyelinating optic neuritis. Neurology 2001;56:1514–22.
217. Achiron A, Gabbay U, Gilad R, et al. Intravenous immunoglobulin treatment in multiple sclerosis. Effect on relapses. Neurology 1998;50:398–402.
218. Fazekas F, Deisenhammer F, Strasser-Fuchs S, et al. Randomised placebo controlled trial of monthly intravenous immunoglobulin therapy in

relapsing-remitting multiple sclerosis. Austrian Immunoglobulin in Multiple Sclerosis Study Group. Lancet 1997;349:589–93.

219. Lewanska M, Siger-Zajdel M, Selmaj K. No difference in efficacy of two different doses of intravenous immunoglobulins in MS: clinical and MRI assessment. Eur J Neurol 2002;9:565–72.

220. Sorensen PS, Wanscher B, Jensen CV, et al. Intravenous immunoglobulin G reduces MRI activity in relapsing multiple sclerosis. Neurology 1998;50:1273–81.

221. Achiron A, Kisner I, Dolev M, et al. Effect of intravenous immunoglobulin treatment on pregnancy and postpartum-related relapses in multiple sclerosis. J Neurol 2004;251:1133–7.

222. Confavreux C. Intravenous immunoglobulins, pregnancy and multiple sclerosis. J Neurol 2004;251:1138–9.

223. Haas J, Hommes O. A dose comparison study of IVIG in postpartum relapsing-remitting multiple sclerosis. Mult Scler 2007;13:900–8.

224. Smith DR, Balashov KE, Hafler DA, et al. Immune deviation following pulse cyclophosphamide/methylprednisolone treatment of multiple sclerosis: increased interleukin-4 production and associated eosinophilia. Ann Neurol 1997;42:313–8.

225. Hauser S, Dawson D, Lehrich J, et al. Intensive immunosuppression in progressive multiple sclerosis: a randomized, three-arm study of high-dose intravenous cyclophosphamide, plasma exchange, and ACTH. N Engl J Med 1983;308:173–80.

226. Carter JL, Hafler DA, Dawson DM, et al. Immunosuppression with high-dose IV cyclophosphamide and ACTH in progressive multiple sclerosis: cumulative 6-year experience in 164 patients. Neurology 1988;38:9–14.

227. Perini P, Calabrese M, Tiberio M, et al. Mitoxantrone versus cyclophosphamide in secondary-progressive multiple sclerosis: a comparative study. J Neurol 2006;253:1034–40.

228. Noseworthy JH, Ebers GC, Gent M, et al. The Canadian cooperative trial of cyclophosphamide and plasma exchange in progressive multiple sclerosis. Lancet 1991;337:441–6.

229. Likosky WH, Fireman B, Elmore R, et al. Intense immunosuppression in chronic progressive multiple sclerosis: the Kaiser study. J Neurol Neurosurg Psychiatry 1991;54:1055–60.

230. Smith DR, Weinstock-Guttman B, Cohen JA, et al. A randomized, blinded trial of combination therapy with cyclophosphamide in patients with active MS on interferon-beta. Mult Scler 2005;11:573–82.

231. Patti F, Cataldi ML, Nicolletti F, et al. Combination of cyclophosphamide and interferon-beta halts progression in patients with rapidly transitional multiple sclerosis. J Neurol Neurosurg Psychiatry 2001;71:404–7.

232. Patti F, Reggio E, Palermo F, et al. Stabilization of rapidly worsening multiple sclerosis for 36 months in patients treated with interferon beta plus cyclophosphamide followed by interferon beta. J Neurol 2004;251:1502–6.

233. Reggio E, Nicoletti A, Fiorilla T, et al. The combination of cyclophosphamide plus interferon beta as rescue therapy could be used to treat relapsing-remitting multiple sclerosis patients: twenty-four months follow-up. J Neurol 2005;252:1255–61.

234. Patti F, Lo Fermo S. Lights and shadows of cyclophosphamide in the treatment of multiple sclerosis. Autoimmune Dis 2011;2011:961702.

235. Drachman DB, Jones RJ, Brodsky RA. Treatment of refractory myasthenia: "Rebooting" with high dose cyclophosphamide. Ann Neurol 2003;53:7–9.

236. Nozaki K, Abou-Fayssal N. High dose cyclophosphamide treatment in Marburg variant multiple sclerosis. A case report. J Neurol Sci 2010;296:121–3.
237. Dezern AE, Petri M, Drachman DB, et al. High-dose cyclophosphamide without stem cell rescue in 207 patients with aplastic anemia and other autoimmune disease. Medicine (Baltimore) 2011;90:89–98.
238. Gladstone DE, Zamkoff KW, Krupp L, et al. High-dose cyclophosphamide for moderate to severe refractory multiple sclerosis. Arch Neurol 2006;63:1388–93.
239. Krishnan C, Kaplin AI, Brodsky RA, et al. Reduction of disease activity and disability with high-dose cyclophosphamide in patients with aggressive multiple sclerosis. Arch Neurol 2008;65:1044–51.
240. Schwartzman RJ, Simpkins N, Alexander GM, et al. High dose cyclophosphamide in the treatment of multiple sclerosis. CNS Neurosci Ther 2009;15:118–27.
241. Gladstone DE, Peyster R, Baron E, et al. High-dose cyclophosphamide for moderate to severe refractory multiple sclerosis: 2-year follow-up (Investigational New Drug No. 65863). Am J Ther 2011;18:23–30.
242. Portaccio E, Zipoli V, Siracusa G, et al. Safety and tolerability of cyclophosphamide 'pulses' in multiple sclerosis: a prospective study in a clinical cohort. Mult Scler 2003;9:446–50.
243. Janow GL, Illowite NT, Wahezi DM. Wasabi nose: an underreported complication of cyclophosphamide infusions. Clin Rheumatol 2011;30:1003–5.
244. Stillwell TJ, Benson RC Jr. Cyclophosphamide-induced hemorrhagic cystitis. A review of 100 patients. Cancer 1988;61:451–7.
245. Radis CD, Kahl LE, Baker GL, et al. Effects of cyclophosphamide on the development of malignancy and on long-term survival of patients with rheumatoid arthritis. A 20-year followup study. Arthritis Rheum 1995;38:1120–7.
246. Monach PA, Arnold LM, Merkel PA. Incidence and prevention of bladder toxicity from cyclophosphamide in the treatment of rheumatic diseases: a data-driven review. Arthritis Rheum 2010;62:9–21.
247. De Ridder D, van Poppel H, Demonty L, et al. Bladder cancer in patients with multiple sclerosis treated with cyclophosphamide. J Urol 1998;159:1881–4.
248. Le Bouc R, Zephir H, Majed B, et al. No increase in cancer incidence detected after cyclophosphamide in a French cohort of patients with progressive multiple sclerosis. Mult Scler 2012;18:55–63.

Syncope: Case Studies

Inna Kleyman, MD, Louis H. Weimer, MD*

KEYWORDS

- Syncope • Vasovagal • Orthostatic hypotension • Cardiogenic syncope
- Autonomic dysfunction • Dysautonomia

KEY POINTS

- Syncope is a sudden transient loss of consciousness and is a common medical problem often evaluated by medical practitioners.
- Vasovagal syncope is a form of neurally mediated reflex syncope and is diagnosed by history of a specific trigger and a positive response on tilt-table testing.
- Carotid sinus hypersensitivity has cardioinhibitor and vasodepressor subtypes, and the former is often treated with cardiac pacing.
- Autonomic neuropathies can be caused by a variety of conditions, including diabetes, hereditary, toxic/metabolic, infectious, autoimmune, and paraneoplastic disorders.
- Neurodegenerative disorders, such as Parkinson disease, multisystem atrophy, and pure autonomic failure, are an important cause of orthostatic hypotension, which in severe cases can lead to syncope.

INTRODUCTION

Syncope, or the sudden loss of consciousness, is a common presenting symptom for evaluation by general practitioners, cardiologists, and neurologists. Syncope is not a unique diagnosis but rather a common manifestation of several disorders of diverse mechanisms. Ultimately, loss of consciousness results from insufficient cerebral perfusion pressure. It is differentiated from other causes of altered consciousness, such as seizures, metabolic disturbances, and psychiatric events. Syncope typically occurs when patients are upright and can be preceded by presyncope, a constellation of warning symptoms. These warning symptoms include a general sense of feeling unwell, the sensation of dizziness or light-headedness, nausea, and weakness. Patients may feel detached from their surroundings and immediately before losing consciousness can experience a graying of vision or muffling of sounds. To others, they may appear as pale, diaphoretic, or tachypneic. Loss of consciousness is typically

The authors have nothing to disclose.
Department of Neurology, Columbia University College of Physicians and Surgeons, Neurological Institute of New York, 710 West 168th Street, New York, NY 10032, USA
* Corresponding author.
E-mail address: Lhw1@cumc.columbia.edu

accompanied by generalized loss of tone and collapse to the ground. The episodes are brief, lasting seconds to a few minutes. With severe cerebral hypoperfusion, brief convulsions in the limbs may be observed. In general, the blood pressure (BP) and heart rate quickly recover when the patient is in the supine position, and consciousness and awareness rapidly return. Patients will generally recall the events leading up to the episode, but may have a short period of fatigue or disorientation.

Syncope is a common medical problem and has a lifetime prevalence of about 42% with an annual incidence of 6%.[1] Its frequency varies based on age group, but ranges from 15% to 39%.[2,3] It is an important cause of falls and trauma, especially in the elderly population.

In this article, the evaluation and management of the most common causes of syncope are discussed, including neurally mediated syncope, cardiogenic syncope, orthostatic hypotension (OH), and autonomic dysfunction with orthostatic intolerance.

REFLEX SYNCOPE

Reflex syncope is the most common type of syncope. There is often a clear precipitant, and major subtypes include neurally mediated, vasovagal, situational, carotid sinus hypersensitivity, and atypical forms. Of these subtypes, vasovagal syncope (VVS) is the most prevalent. The diagnosis is based on a history of associated triggers and typical symptoms; residual findings after the event are typically absent. However, the diagnosis is supported by the exclusion of other causes of syncope and by a characteristic response to upright tilt-table testing, discussed in more detail later.

Case 1

A 19-year-old previously healthy woman was referred to you for evaluation after her second episode of loss of consciousness. The first event occurred 6 months prior when she went to brush her teeth shortly after waking in the morning and lost consciousness in the bathroom. She hit her head on the bathtub during the fall but quickly recovered to baseline. She recalled feeling "woozy" and sweaty immediately before passing out. The second episode occurred last week when she was standing on a very slow line in the cafeteria. She began to feel light-headed, and her friends noticed that she appeared pale. She fell to the ground and was unconscious for less than 1 minute and woke up to a group of people crouching around her. This time she was taken to the Emergency Department where basic laboratory tests and electrocardiogram (ECG) were normal. She had a supine BP of 106/70 mm Hg, heart rate of 69, and a standing BP of 99/68 mm Hg, heart rate of 79. Her neurologic examination was normal. She received intravenous fluids and was discharged with outpatient follow-up. You referred her for tilt-table testing, which showed abrupt bradycardia following a significant hypotensive response after 18 minutes at 70° upright position (Fig. 1A). She was started on sodium chloride tablets and counseled on lifestyle modifications with no recurring episodes over the next year.

VASOVAGAL SYNCOPE

Case 1 illustrates VVS, which is a form of neurally mediated syncope and is the most common cause of transient loss of consciousness.[1] Typical VVS is transient loss of consciousness triggered by emotional distress (fear, pain, disgust) or orthostatic stress (prolonged standing). There are prodromal symptoms due to activation of the autonomic nervous system, and these can include nausea, vomiting, diaphoresis, pallor, feeling cold or warm, palpitations, salivation, and rarely, urinary incontinence. Transient hypoperfusion to the brain and retina can also cause dizziness and visual graying. These symptoms can also sometimes be present in the recovery phase.[4] Recovery is usually rapid without confusion or focal neurologic deficits. VVS typically occurs in younger people and is more frequent in women but can occur at any age.[5,6]

The basic mechanism is a sudden withdrawal of sympathetic tone leading to paradoxic vasodilation and hypotension. In some cases, a vagal surge produces bradycardia; if cerebral perfusion drops sufficiently, loss of consciousness occurs.[7,8] In central episodes of the "emotional" quality, afferent triggers probably originate within the cerebral cortex and activate pathways relaying information from the cortex to hypothalamic centers and to medullary cardiovascular nuclei, controlling parasympathetic and sympathetic outflow. In the brainstem, the nucleus of the solitary tract and ventrolateral medulla regulate efferent autonomic tone.[9] However, the precise pathways and mechanisms that underlie these physiologic changes remain incomplete. Noradrenergic and cholinergic sympathetic overactivity (tachycardia, palpitations, sweating) may be followed by vagal enhancement (nausea, pallor, fatigue, and bradycardia).

Several neurohumoral factors, including epinephrine, endorphins, and adenosine, have been studied in relation to the vasovagal pathway. Adenosine is a naturally occurring purine nucleoside that is a byproduct of adenosine triphosphate (ATP) breakdown in humans. It has cardiac effects similar to acetylcholine and counteracts the effects of the sympathetic neurotransmitters epinephrine and norepinephrine.[10,11] Studies have examined the use of an ATP test as a potential diagnostic tool in patients with unexplained syncope. A positive test is defined as a cardiac pause or asystole following the infusion of ATP and is proposed to identify underlying cardioinhibitory neurally mediated syncope or latent conducting system disease.[12,13] Data suggest that a positive ATP test may help identify a proportion of people with unexplained syncope that may benefit from pacing therapy, and further studies, including a double-blind randomized controlled study, are currently underway.[14,15]

The clinical manifestations of VVS in older patients can mimic cardiogenic syncope, and distinguishing the 2 is essential. For example, in the elderly, prodromal symptoms tend to be less prevalent and shorter in duration. Older patients are also more likely to experience atypical VVS, which refers to individuals who lack an evident trigger before losing consciousness, but are subsequently found to have a positive tilt test.[5,16] Several mechanisms have been proposed for the different presentation of VVS in the elderly and include a decline in parasympathetic activity with age, reduced β-adrenergic response, and small change in circulating adrenaline in the upright position.[17,18]

Another clinical entity, psychogenic pseudosyncope (PPS), can present as a complex phenotype that mimics VVS. These episodes are similar to vasovagal events but have atypical features, such as high attack frequency, typically without injury, delayed recovery of consciousness, absence of prodrome, atypical triggers, eye closure, and apparent prolonged loss of consciousness.[19] Although BP, heart rate, or both are low during VVS, these parameters tend to be high during PPS. PPS can be seen preceding or following VVS during tilt-table testing in a pattern referred to as VVS/PPS.[20]

Importantly, VVS can also present as an otherwise unexplained fall. Not all patients recall the loss of consciousness and may mistake a spell for a simple mechanical fall. If a cardiac cause is not apparent in the initial evaluation, tilt testing and carotid sinus massage can be useful. Two studies examined the role of tilt-table testing and carotid sinus massage in the evaluation of patients presenting with unexplained falls or unexplained syncope (presence of prodromal symptoms). They found that the combination of both tests produced a positive response in about 60% of patients. Although orthostatic hypotension (OH) is likely the most common cause of unexplained falls, these data suggest some patients with unexplained falls may have atypical VVS or carotid sinus syncope with retrograde amnesia.[21–23]

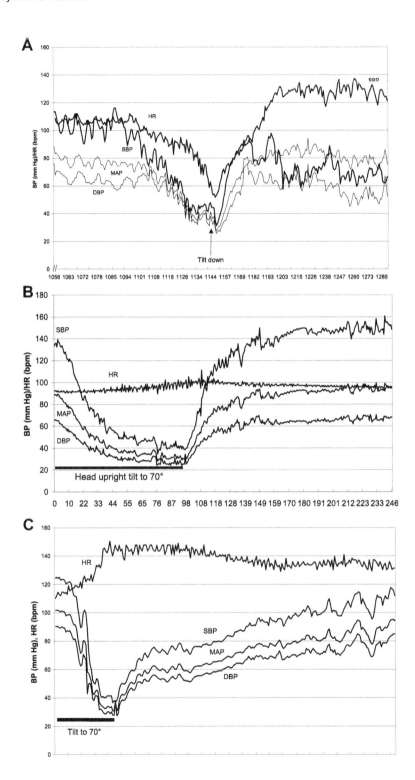

VVS is rare in the supine position because of preservation of cerebral perfusion when recumbent. When syncope occurs in the supine position, a cardiac cause should be investigated first and other causes considered only if a cardiac cause is excluded. One type of syncope that can occur in the supine position is "sleep syncope," which is transient loss of consciousness that occurs after waking up in the middle of the night. It has been reported predominantly in middle-aged women and tends to begin with autonomic symptoms (sweating, nausea, palpitations, and feeling warm). More than half of these patients reported VVS during daytime hours, and tilt testing was positive in 64%.[24–26] A form of autosomal-dominant VVS has also recently been described.[27]

If a clear trigger is established by history and if there is no overt heart disease or other competing diagnosis, further workup may not be indicated. However, if a precipitating factor is uncertain, tilt-table testing can aid in making the diagnosis.

TILT-TABLE TESTING

Tilt-table testing is a standard and widely available method of evaluation of unexplained syncope. Standing causes the gravitational shift of blood into the venous capacitance system of the legs and pelvis, which in turn reduces venous return. Prolonged standing causes fluid movement into interstitial spaces and lack of muscular pumping to aid with venous return. In healthy people, compensatory mechanisms cause an increase in vascular resistance and heart rate to help maintain adequate cerebral perfusion. Tilt testing can provide a similar but more controlled orthostatic stress to evaluate for susceptibility to vasovagal reactions.

Attempts to standardize guidelines have suggested the following protocol: patients should fast for 2 hours before the test and should rest in a supine position for 20 to 30 minutes before tilting; continuous beat-to-beat arterial BP should be monitored; a tilt table with a foot support should be used; the upright phase should take place at 60° to 70° for a maximum of 20 minutes, and if is nondiagnostic at that point, a pharmacologic agent such as nitroglycerin or isoproterenol may be administered; some laboratories extend passive tilt to 30 to 40 minutes. The end point is defined as the induction of syncope or imminent syncope or completion of the planned duration of tilting (including drug provocation). The test is considered positive if it induces syncope due to systemic hypotension, ideally with the reproduction of the patient's spontaneous symptoms.[28,29] Prompt return of the patient to the supine position should follow the syncopal episode.

A positive test may be associated with different BP and heart rate patterns. A common pattern shows an initial phase of rapid reflex adaptation to being upright with a relative stabilization of BP and heart rate, suggesting normal baroreceptor function. A classic pattern in a positive test shows a stable state until abrupt onset of the

Fig. 1. Head-upright tilt-table studies with beat-to-beat heart rate and BP monitoring. (*A*) Reflex syncope with bradycardia and hypotension occurring spontaneously at minute 18 of 70° passive tilt (case 1). (*B*) Severe OH with minimal heart rate response. Syncope occurred suddenly without warning symptoms or signs (case 4). (*C*) Acute autonomic neuropathy with rapid imminent syncope within seconds of upright tilt. Marked sinus tachycardic response in this form with cardiovagal preservation (case 5). DBP, diastolic blood pressure; HR, heart rate; MAP, mean arterial pressure; SBP, systolic blood pressure. (*From* Weimer LH, Williams O. Syncope and orthostatic intolerance. Med Clin North Am 2003;87(4):835–65; with permission.)

vasovagal reaction, which is typically observed in young and healthy patients with VVS. Another commonly seen pattern is characterized by the lack of a steady-state adaptation to the upright position, and instead, a variable period of relative stability followed by a progressive drop in BP and limited heart rate response. This "vasodepressor" pattern may be due to compromised ability to adapt to postural stress and is seen more commonly in older patients.[28] Beat-to-beat BP recording can aid in detecting cardioinhibitory patterns, namely an asystolic period that triggers the BP decline and may be amenable to pacing and is discussed in more detail later.

Case 2

A 60-year-old man with hypertension and insulin-dependent diabetes was referred to cardiology clinic for evaluation of recurrent syncopal episodes. The first episode occurred several years ago and has recurred about 3 times per year. A typical episode begins with sudden light-headedness and diaphoresis while sitting down followed by loss of consciousness upon walking. The syncopal episode lasts seconds with no observed seizure activity and no subsequent confusion. A few episodes have occurred while driving, and the most recent resulting in a car accident during which he sustained no major injuries. Examination revealed an obese man with a supine BP of 150/90 mm Hg, heart rate of 74, and a 2-minute standing BP of 139/79 mm Hg, heart rate of 75. Cardiac examination revealed an I/VI systolic ejection murmur, and ECG showed normal sinus rhythm with left ventricular hypertrophy. Neurologic examination was normal. Prior workup had included a normal computed tomographic head scan and prolonged Holter monitoring with frequent premature ventricular depolarizations. Echocardiography showed no significant valvular dysfunction and slightly reduced ejection fraction. Carotid sinus massage was performed under continuous electrocardiographic monitoring, and light pressure on either carotid sinus resulted in mild sinus bradycardia (pulse decreasing from 74 to 60 beats per minute). Firmer pressure over the right and left carotid sinuses caused sinus asystole with a ventricular escape rate of 25 after a 2500-ms pause. The patient reported feeling light-headed during the bradycardia.[30]

CAROTID SINUS HYPERSENSITIVITY

Case 2 demonstrates an example of carotid sinus hypersensitivity (or carotid sinus syndrome), which is defined as a decrease in heart rate and/or BP in response to carotid sinus massage. It can be triggered by local pressure over the carotid region from head turning, shaving, or wearing a tight collar, although other more subtle head positions such as looking down while descending stairs can be provocative. The loss of consciousness is typically sudden and recovery is spontaneous, but significant injuries from falls can occur. It is an important consideration in patients with unexplained syncope, especially those aged older than 60 years.[31]

The carotid sinus is a baroreceptor that responds to stretching of the arterial wall, which leads to increased vagal tone and decreased sympathetic activity.[32] Several pathophysiologic mechanisms have been proposed, including atherosclerotic vascular changes and noncompliance with age, peripheral denervation of the sternocleidomastoid muscle (causing preferential afferent signals from the carotid sinus and not the muscle with head turning), and sympathetic upregulation due to generalized autonomic disorder.[33–35]

Carotid sinus hypersensitivity is diagnosed when carotid sinus massage causes a greater than 3-second asystole (in the cardioinhibitory subtype) or greater than 50 mm Hg drop in BP (in the vasodepressor subtype).[1] The current guidelines recommend performing carotid massage for 5 to 10 seconds at the anterior margin of the sternocleidomastoid muscle at the level of the cricoid cartilage with continuous electrocardiography and BP monitoring. If a positive result is not obtained, the procedure is repeated on the other side and should be performed in both the supine and the upright positions.[29] Carotid massage should be used with caution or avoided entirely in patients with prior stroke or myocardial infarction, previous ventricular tachyarrhythmia, cerebrovascular disease, or carotid bruits.[36]

Permanent pacing is common clinical practice in the treatment of the cardioinhibitory subtype of carotid sinus hypersensitivity. Multiple randomized trials have evaluated the benefit of pacing in this condition, but have yielded varying results. Dual-chamber pacing has been proposed to be optimal to single-chamber atrial and ventricular devices.[37–41] The prognosis following pacemaker placement is generally favorable, but up to 20% of patients have recurrent symptoms after 5 years.[42] One possible explanation for this is that a proportion of patients with the cardioinhibitory pattern develop the vasodepressor subtype after treatment.[43] Carotid sinus denervation, via irradiation or during carotid endarterectomy, has also been evaluated as a potential treatment option but has not been established, with large clinical trials lacking.[44] No established therapy exists for the vasodepressor subtype of carotid sinus hypersensitivity, but small trials have suggested benefit with the use of midodrine and fludrocortisone.[45,46] In general, a patient with the cardioinhibitory subtype has a high likelihood of recurrent syncope (35%–55%) without pacemaker implantation, and a pacemaker can reduce these chances, although minor symptoms including presyncope can persist.[47]

SITUATIONAL SYNCOPE

Situational syncope refers to forms of neurally mediated syncope associated with a particular context (micturition, defecation, coughing, laughing, swallowing, instrumentation, sneezing). Many of these circumstances are associated with the Valsalva maneuver, causing increased transthoracic pressure with decreased venous return. The proposed mechanism in micturition or defecation syncope invokes the sudden decompression of the bladder, causing stimulation of genitourinary or gastrointestinal receptors. These afferent stimuli are transmitted to the nucleus tractus solitarius in the medulla, which is associated with the dorsal and ambiguus nuclei of the vagus nerve, resulting in enhanced efferent parasympathetic tone.[48,49] Defecation syncope is more common in older women, and micturition syncope is more common in middle-aged men.[50] Swallow (deglutition) syncope is thought to occur via an aberrant vagal reflex when vagal afferents in the esophagus are stimulation by dilation during swallowing, leading to cerebral hypoperfusion via cardiac arrhythmia or vasodepression.[51]

One prospective study investigated the response to head-up tilt testing in patients with situational syncope and found similar rates of positive tilt-test results between patients with situational syncope and those with VVS.[52]

Case 3

A 42-year-old woman presents for evaluation of "seizurelike episodes" witnessed by her family over the past 2 years. She does not recall any aura or warning symptoms, and she abruptly loses consciousness, typically while standing. Observers have noted that her eyes roll back and her whole body stiffens and limbs jerk a few times for a few seconds. She recovers quickly to baseline and has no associated tongue biting, but on at least 2 occasions she had urinary incontinence. She sustained several injuries, including a recent head laceration requiring stitches. She has a history of febrile seizures as a child and an uncle with epilepsy. On examination, she is found to have a supine BP of 118/76 mm Hg, heart rate of 74, 3-minute upright BP of 100/69 mm Hg, heart rate of 81. Her neurologic examination is normal. Prior evaluation has included an ECG with normal sinus rhythm and 2-day continuous electroencephalogram (EEG) monitoring with normal sleep and waking states. No typical events were captured on EEG. MRI brain scan was unremarkable. She was started on Levetiracetam (Keppra) by her primary care physician with no improvement in the frequency of the episodes. You arrange for prolonged ambulatory EEG monitoring that captures a typical episode showing no epileptiform discharges but the presence of sinus pauses up to 8 seconds on the ECG lead with significant EEG slowing. Subsequent head-up tilt testing revealed a cardioinhibitory pattern, and she was referred for pacemaker placement.

CONVULSIVE SYNCOPE

Case 3 describes convulsive syncope, which can be easily confused with seizures because both conditions can manifest with whole body stiffening, myoclonic or clonic movements, and loss of consciousness. Convulsive syncope is typically caused by prolonged cerebral hypoperfusion. The syncopal episode itself is generally brief and with rapid recovery. There may be no preceding prodrome, but some people report nausea, light-headedness, or diaphoresis before losing tone. Jerking movements are typically multifocal and nonsustained or rhythmic, unlike a seizure. The phenomenon is more common if the patient is artificially held upright by a well-meaning bystander and not allowed to recline. Urinary incontinence may be present. A video review of the clinical features of syncope induced in healthy volunteers showed that automatisms, head turning, and upward rolling of the eyes, similar to that seen in seizures, can also occur.[53] Convulsive syncope is estimated to account for around 12% of patients presenting with syncope.[54]

Continuous EEG monitoring during cerebral hypoperfusion shows characteristic patterns depending on the duration of low blood flow, with prolonged events causing near flattening of waveforms.[55] EEG findings are similar regardless of the underlying cause. An EEG obtained within 24 hours of a convulsive episode can aid in differentiating syncope from seizure because up to 50% of patients with a generalized tonic clonic seizure show an abnormality. An EEG within 48 hours shows abnormalities in only 21% to 34% of patients presenting with a seizure. Younger patients are more likely than older patients to have electroencephalographic abnormalities.[56] Video monitoring in a safe monitoring environment that captures a typical episode is perhaps the most useful tool in differentiating between a seizure, convulsive syncope, and nonepileptic seizures.

If seizure is excluded, a cardiac cause for convulsive syncope should always be considered.[57] Identifying an underlying arrhythmia early in the clinical course is vital to choosing the appropriate treatment. Neurally mediated syncope can also cause seizurelike activities, and one study found that 8% of patients with neurally mediated syncope developed seizurelike activities during head-up tilt testing.[58] Complicated cases may require a broad diagnostic approach that includes a combination of cardiac evaluation, EEG, and tilt testing; simultaneous studies are performed at some sites. Very rarely, a condition known as asystolic (bradycardic) seizures can occur. Most seizures are associated with tachycardia, typically starting before other clinical or even EEG signs. In these rare patients, the seizure affects a critical central pathway that triggers severe bradycardia or a significant sinus pause and leads to syncope. These patients need treatment of both conditions and often both a pacemaker and anticonvulsants.[59–62]

ORTHOSTATIC HYPOTENSION

OH is a drop in BP in upright positions. It is a common problem, especially in the elderly, and can be due to a variety of underlying conditions (intravascular volume depletion, antihypertensive therapy, severe anemia, and physical deconditioning). Neurogenic orthostatic hypotension (NOH) is less common and is caused by a failure to increase sympathetic vasomotor nerve outflow and an inability to raise peripheral vascular resistance when standing.[63] NOH is a feature of several disorders affecting autonomic neurons, including neurodegenerative diseases, peripheral neuropathies, and genetic conditions, which are discussed later in this article.

The physiologic response to standing in normal individuals is triggered by distal blood pooling, leading to a transient decrease in cardiac output and BP, which decreases baroreceptor activity, producing increased sympathetic outflow, peripheral resistance, and venous return. Norepinephrine is the principal mediator of this response.[64]

Orthostatic intolerance is characterized by symptoms of cerebral hypoperfusion, including light-headedness, blurred vision, weakness, reduced concentration, and loss of consciousness in the setting of positional changes despite preserved systemic BP. In elderly patients, presyncopal symptoms may be atypical and can manifest as vague cognitive impairment, vertigo, or "coat-hanger" pattern neck and shoulder pain.[65] Occasionally, there can be focal neurologic symptoms, which may be due to asymmetric hypoperfusion of the 2 hemispheres as demonstrated in prior studies.[66,67]

Detection of NOH may require repeated measurements on different days, and measurements taken in the morning tend to be more sensitive.[68] There is variability in the selection of a time interval to measure BP after standing, but the range is typically between 1 and 3 minutes; patients with early autonomic insufficiency may have a delayed return to baseline pressure after standing. The most widely accepted definition is based on the consensus of the American Academy of Neurology and the American Autonomic Society published in 1996, which defines OH as the reduction of systolic BP by at least 20 mm Hg or diastolic BP by at least 10 mm Hg within 3 minutes of standing or upright tilt-table testing to at least 60°.[69] The problem with this definition is that many individuals have symptoms of orthostatic that begin after 3 to 10 minutes from the positional change,[70] suggesting that a significant proportion of patients with OH are missed on routine bedside assessments of orthostasis.

The concept of delayed orthostatic hypotension (DOH) has been an area of interest in recent studies. One report documented a similar frequency of OH and DOH in patients referred for autonomic testing.[71] DOH has been associated with both parasympathetic and sympathetic adrenergic dysfunction, but of a lesser severity than standard definitions of OH. Thus, it is not yet clear whether DOH is a milder form of orthostatic intolerance or whether it may be an early presentation of OH. A recent longitudinal study found that over a period of 10 years, 54% of individuals with DOH went on to develop OH and that a substantial number developed neurodegenerative diseases, most commonly α-synucleinopathies.[72] The study also found an increase in mortality in those who progressed to develop OH, particularly in patients who had diabetes.

Case 4

A 70-year-old woman with non-insulin-dependent type 2 diabetes diagnosed 13 years ago was referred to you for evaluation of syncopal episodes. These events began a year ago and are typically preceded by a feeling of general weakness and graying of her vision. She loses consciousness for several seconds and regains awareness quickly, but has sustained multiple injuries during the falls. These events have become more frequent and recently started occurring after eating large meals. Even without syncope, meals now tend to cause nausea, bloating, and severe fatigue. On review of systems, she also endorses rare urinary incontinence, diarrhea, and dry mouth. She also has dry eyes but thinks this began after laser surgery used to treat diabetes-related retinopathy. She has no other known complications of her diabetes except tingling in her feet, which her primary doctor attributed to neuropathy. On examination, her supine BP was 174/89 mm Hg, heart rate was 74, and after 3 minutes of standing, BP was 112/64 mm Hg, heart rate was 84. Her general examination revealed distal trophic changes of the skin with hair loss in the ankles, and neurologic examination showed reduced sensation to temperature, pinprick, and vibration in the feet to mid shins bilaterally. She had normal strength and absent ankle reflexes. Initial workup included an ECG with nonspecific changes and an echocardiogram with mild left ventricular hypertrophy. Autonomic testing revealed reduced heart rate variability with deep breathing and OH with minimal heart rate compensation on 70° upright tilt (see **Fig. 1**B). She also had abnormal heart rate and BP responses to the Valsalva maneuver. She was initially treated with conservative management, including nighttime bed tilt, compression stockings, and fluid intake, but continued to have syncopal episodes. Fludrocortisone was started and titrated to 0.3 mg/d with a reduction in frequency of her episodes. Midodrine was subsequently added but caused an elevation in her supine BP and was discontinued. Pyridostigmine was added as an adjunct agent with near resolution of the syncopal events.

CHRONIC AUTONOMIC NEUROPATHY

Case 4 illustrates an example of a type of chronic autonomic neuropathy related to diabetes. Diabetic and prediabetic autonomic neuropathy is the most common cause of autonomic neuropathy in the United States and can affect multiple systems, including cardiovascular, gastrointestinal, genitourinary, neuroendocrine, papillary, and sudomotor, causing diverse manifestations.[73] OH in diabetes is thought to be a consequence of efferent sympathetic vasomotor denervation that results in reduced vasoconstriction of the peripheral vascular beds, in turn causing excessive pooling in the splanchnic, pelvic, and other dependent areas with standing.[74] Reduced cardiac acceleration and cardiac output, especially in association with exercise, may also contribute.[75]

Prediabetes is emerging as an important cause of autonomic neuropathy. This condition preferentially damages small-diameter nerve fibers, causing both distal painful neuropathy and impaired autonomic function. The most common autonomic symptoms endorsed by patients with impaired glucose tolerance are dry mouth or eyes, cold feet, light-headedness, erectile dysfunction (in men), and urine incontinence (predominantly in women). There is suggestion that report of these symptoms may even precede objective abnormalities on autonomic testing.[76] Several studies have reported autonomic dysfunction in individuals with impaired glucose tolerance, including reduced cardiac parasympathetic function (measured by heart rate variability with deep respiration and the Valsalva ratio), abnormal sudomotor function (measured by the quantitative sudomotor axon reflex test and the skin sympathetic reflex), abnormal circadian BP regulation, and enhanced sympathetic activity.[77–84] Autonomic symptoms can also paradoxically get worse with correction of hyperglycemia after starting insulin or oral medications, a phenomenon known as treatment-induced neuropathy.[85] Treatment-induced neuropathy and autonomic dysfunction tend to improve after months of continued glucose control.

Other important conditions that can cause chronic autonomic neuropathy include amyloidosis, hereditary, infectious, and toxic neuropathies. Primary and familial (mainly transthyretin [TTR] mutation) amyloidosis are the 2 most prevalent forms. Primary amyloidosis is caused by the abnormal production and deposition of a monoclonal κ or λ light chain. Familial amyloidoses are autosomal-dominant disorders caused by mutations in several identified genes, with TTR mutations most likely to cause autonomic dysfunction. The presence of autonomic neuropathy in primary amyloidosis has recently been suggested to be an independent negative prognostic factor for survival, stressing the importance of early diagnosis and potential treatment with autologous stem cell transplantation (ASCT).[86] Patients who are not eligible for ASCT are treated with chemotherapeutic alkylating agents, corticosteroids, and other immunomodulatory drugs. Treatment of familial amyloidosis is typically with liver transplantation, but newer therapeutic agents to improve the genetic output are undergoing clinical trials.[87,88]

Toxic autonomic neuropathy can be caused by marine toxins (box jellyfish, ciguatoxins), and arsenic, mercury, thallium, acrylamide, and chemotherapy agents (vincristine). Infectious causes include human immunodeficiency virus, botulism, Chagas disease, diphtheria, and leprosy. Hereditary conditions other than amyloidosis that can cause autonomic neuropathy include Fabry disease, Allgrove syndrome, Tangier disease, multiple endocrine neoplasia type 2b, mitochondrial neurogastrointestinal encephalomyopathy, and the hereditary sensory autonomic neuropathies, including type III, familial dysautonomia.[89] Dopamine β-hydroxylase deficiency is a genetic disorder causing an absence of norepinephrine and epinephrine, resulting in severe OH, noradrenergic failure, and impaired exercise tolerance.[90]

Case 5

A 34-year-old woman is referred to you for evaluation of syncope beginning 1 month ago. She loses consciousness when standing or sitting up quickly, and episodes typically last a couple of seconds. They began suddenly last month and now occur multiple times per day, limiting her ability to go to work. She has no prior history of presyncope or syncope. She also reports loss of appetite, constipation, nausea, and dry mouth over the same time period. Nausea and vomiting are severe and problematic. Her examination reveals supine BP of 118/70 mm Hg, heart rate of 80, 2-minute standing BP of 89/59 mm Hg, heart rate of 82, with reported near-syncope. Her neurologic examination is normal with the exception of dilated and poorly reactive pupils. ECG was unremarkable. Autonomic function testing showed generalized autonomic failure (see Fig. 1C), and based on this result, you order a paraneoplastic panel that eventually reports a significantly elevated titer of ganglionic nicotinic acetylcholine receptor (AChR) antibodies. She was initially treated with 8 courses of intravenous immunoglobulin (IVIg) twice a week without significant improvement. She was started on plasma exchange and subsequently mycophenolate mofetil before showing improvement after several months. After 1 year, her antibody titer was undetectable, and she had significant clinical improvement but had residual gastrointestinal symptoms.

ACUTE AND SUBACUTE AUTONOMIC NEUROPATHY

This case demonstrates autoimmune autonomic ganglionopathy, also known as acute pandysautonomia or autoimmune autonomic neuropathy. This condition is characterized by the selective of involvement of autonomic nerve fibers or ganglia causing severe acute or subacute autonomic failure over a period of days or weeks.[91] Sympathetic failure manifests as severe OH and anhidrosis, whereas parasympathetic failure causes urinary retention, gastrointestinal dysmotility (early satiety, constipation, diarrhea, postprandial pain), dry mouth, sexual dysfunction, an impaired pupillary response to light and accommodation, and a fixed heart rate.[92,93] Autoantibodies specific for nicotinic AChRs in the autonomic ganglia may serve as markers of various forms of immune-mediated autonomic neuropathy.[94] Nicotinic AChRs normally mediate synaptic transmission through autonomic ganglia in both the sympathetic and the parasympathetic systems.[95] High levels of ganglionic-receptor binding antibodies correlate with the severity of autonomic dysfunction, and the titers decrease or become undetectable with improvement in autonomic function.[94] Some cases with negative antibodies can also respond to immunomodulatory therapy, suggesting that there are other unidentified antibodies targeting autonomic pathways (eg, N-type calcium channel antibodies).[96,97]

Autoimmune autonomic ganglionopathy, with or without the presence of antibodies, has also been described following infections (including upper respiratory tract and gastrointestinal), vaccination, surgical procedures, and treatment with interferons.[98–101] The clinical course can be monophasic, relapsing-remitting, or chronic and refractory to treatment. Some patients anecdotally respond to monotherapy with IVIg or plasma exchange, while those more severely affected may need prolonged therapy with immunosuppressant agents, such as mycophenolate mofetil or rituximab, to maintain clinical improvement. One case of very chronic autonomic failure associated with high ganglionic antibodies titers highly responsive to plasmapheresis is reported.[102] Many anecdotal reports of benefit from IVIg are known; a multicenter randomized trial with IVIg was initiated, but few patients were identified and enrolled.

Acute inflammatory demyelinating polyneuropathy (AIDP), or Guillain-Barre syndrome, is the most common immune-mediated neuropathy throughout the world and causes autonomic dysfunction in about two-thirds of affected patients.[103,104] Some patients even develop OH before motor or sensory manifestations.[105] The most worrisome dysautonomia results from sympathetic overactivity, causing tachycardia, sustained hypertension, cardiac arrhythmia, and labile BP, although AIDP can overactivate or depress both the sympathetic and the parasympathetic systems.

Paraneoplastic syndromes are a rare but important consideration in acute and subacute autonomic neuropathy that in severe cases can lead to OH and syncope. The most commonly associated malignancies are small-cell and non–small-cell lung, gastrointestinal, ovarian, and breast carcinomas, Hodgkin and non-Hodgkin lymphoma, and thymoma.[106] Paraneoplastic autonomic neuropathy can either precede or follow the diagnosis of malignancy. Several antibodies are identified in paraneoplastic autonomic neuropathies, including antineuronal nuclear antibody, type 1 (or anti-Hu), AChR α-3, collapsin response mediator protein-5, voltage-gated potassium channel, P/Q calcium channel, and Purkinje cell antibody-2.[107] Treatment of these disorders involves management of the underlying malignancy as well as immunomodulating therapy targeted at the paraneoplastic syndrome.

Case 6

A 61-year-old man with a history of hypertension was referred to you for the evaluation of falls beginning 2 years ago. Initially, the falls were attributed to tripping and gait instability, but more recently his family has noticed that he loses consciousness during these events. Occasionally, there is urinary incontinence during the episodes, but he has also had worsening urinary incontinence in general over the past year. He has had erectile dysfunction for the past 3 years. He has no rest tremor. On examination, he had supine BP of 155/90 mm Hg, heart rate of 74, and standing BP of 92/68 mm Hg, heart rate of 80.

His neurologic examination revealed mild bradykinesia and left wrist rigidity, no rest or action tremor but subtle dysmetria on the left, and a positive pull test. His initial workup already included an ECG with evidence of left ventricular hypertrophy, MRI brain with periventricular white matter disease and mild generalized atrophy, and normal blood work. His antihypertensives were discontinued by his primary care physician with some improvement in the syncopal episodes. He improved even further on fludrocortisone and midodrine therapy, but this effect plateaued after 2 months. He developed more parkinsonian features and eventually lost the ability to ambulate.

PARKINSONISM AND AUTONOMIC FAILURE

Case 6 illustrates that neurodegenerative disorders, especially α-synuclein-related conditions, can present with autonomic insufficiency. The neurodegenerative disorders that cause NOH can be grouped into those that affect central autonomic pathways sparing the peripheral postganglionic fibers (ie, multiple system atrophy [MSA]) and those with an intact central network but with loss of autonomic fibers (ie, Parkinson disease [PD] and pure autonomic failure). Pure autonomic failure, PD, and MSA are classified into a category called synucleinopathies because they share a similar pathophysiology of α-synuclein deposition.[108] The location of abnormal deposition within the autonomic nervous system manifests in varied clinical ways. MSA, as illustrated in the case above, can have either parkinsonian or cerebellar predominant features and is associated with the most severe autonomic dysfunction; nearly all patients develop at least one autonomic manifestation. This finding has been attributed to multiple factors, including loss of spinal preganglionic sympathetic neurons, disruption of brainstem regulatory networks, cell loss in the hypothalamus, and involvement of the ventrolateral medulla.[109,110] MSA typically has a poor response to levodopa therapy.[111]

Pure autonomic failure is an example of primary peripheral autonomic dysfunction and is characterized by slowly progressive isolated autonomic failure without concomitant neurologic features. It is associated with Lewy body inclusions in peripheral sympathetic and parasympathetic fibers, preganglionic and postganglionic autonomic neurons, and brainstem nuclei.[112] PD also primarily involves the peripheral form of autonomic failure. OH is reported less frequently and in less severe forms of PD, but autonomic failure may be severe in a subset of patients and is designated PD with autonomic failure. Exacerbation of OH with levodopa therapy has long been recognized, although this effect is probably modest in most cases, and the relationship is not as clear in recent studies.[113]

TREATMENT OF ORTHOSTATIC HYPOTENSION

The management of OH depends on the frequency and severity of events. Patients with milder cases should be educated regarding avoidance of triggers, including hot showers and quick positional changes. They should be encouraged to increase salt and water intake. Physical maneuvers, such as leg crossing, standing on toes, and buttock clenching, can effectively increase venous return.[114] Compression stockings and abdominal binders can also be beneficial, but most find them cumbersome, which limits utility. Raising the head of the bed by 4 inches can cause a slight gravitational stress while sleeping, which lowers BP and reduces nighttime sodium and water excretion. This measure improves nocturia and increases intravascular volume upon waking.[115] Eating small frequent meals can reduce postprandial hypotension. Patients should be encouraged to exercise, especially in the recumbent position, such as using a stationary bicycle, rowing machine, or swimming. Tilt training has been shown to be effective.[116]

More severe cases may require pharmacologic management with agents that can expand intravascular volume or increase peripheral vascular resistance. Fludrocortisone is a synthetic mineralocorticoid that increases sodium and water reabsorption in the kidneys and expands intravascular volume. Although It is not US Food and Drug Administration (FDA) -approved, it is one of the first-line agents used for treatment of NOH. Side effects include hypokalemia, ankle edema, and supine hypertension. Midodrine, a selective α1-adrenoreceptor agonist, is another first-line agent that has been studied in several randomized trials and is FDA approved for the treatment of NOH.[117–119] A systematic review of the data concluded that midodrine might have a positive impact on clinical outcomes in both OH and reflex syncope, but the overall quality of the data is low/moderate.[120] The side effects of midodrine are urinary urgency or retention, pilomotor reactions, and supine hypertension. The second medication to be approved by the FDA is droxidopa, a synthetic amino acid that is converted into norepinephrine by the enzyme aromatic amino acid decarboxylase (or dopa-decarboxylase), the same enzyme that converts L-dopa to dopamine. Droxidopa increases BP and prevents cerebral perfusion pressure from dropping enough to cause symptoms of cerebral hypoperfusion. Multicenter clinical trials showed that droxidopa significantly improved symptoms of dizziness, vision disturbance, weakness, and fatigue due to NOH.

Other medications are less established. Atomoxetine blocks the reuptake of norepinephrine and can increase BP in some patients.[121] Pyridostigmine is a cholinesterase inhibitor that potentiates cholinergic neurotransmission in sympathetic ganglia. One randomized controlled study showed that it significantly improves standing BP (especially diastolic pressure) in patients with OH without worsening supine hypertension,[122] making it a favorable agent to use in elderly or hypertensive patients in whom fludrocortisone or midodrine may be intolerable.

Case 7

A 29-year-old woman presents for evaluation of episodes of palpitations, "brain fog," and generalized weakness. Most episodes begin shortly after standing and are improved after sitting or lying down. Sometimes she feels panicked and shaky. Symptoms are worse in hot temperatures, including in saunas and after taking a shower. She had one episode of loss of consciousness while taking a hot shower last week. Her sister noticed that she appears confused and pale at times, which improves when sitting down. Over the past year, she also complains of generalized fatigue and worsening anxiety. She was recently prescribed an anxiolytic medication to take during these episodes out of concern for panic attacks, but the medication tends to make her symptoms worse. On your examination, supine BP was 114/68 mm Hg, heart rate was 76, 3-minute standing BP was 106/60 mm Hg, heart rate was 126. With standing, she developed typical symptoms of palpitations, nausea, and compulsion to lie down. On general examination, she was noted to have mild dependent swelling and cyanosis in the feet, and her neurologic examination was normal. Her laboratory testing showed normal serum aldosterone, cortisol, and metanephrine levels. Autonomic testing showed signs of impaired vasoconstriction with robust heart rate responses to Valsalva and deep breathing maneuvers.

IDIOPATHIC ORTHOSTATIC INTOLERANCE

This last case describes a patient with postural orthostatic tachycardia syndrome (POTS), a form of chronic orthostatic intolerance in which an excessive increase in heart rate is seen during upright posture, without a significant drop in BP. Posturally induced symptoms include light-headedness or dizziness, impaired cognition, blurred vision, palpitations, fatigue, tremulousness, and shortness of breath. POTS is not a unique diagnostic entity, rather the phenotype of several heterogeneous pathophysiological processes. The current criteria define POTS as a heart rate increase of greater than 30 beats per minute within 5 minutes of standing (or head-up tilt testing) without hypotension (a drop >20 mm Hg in systolic or >10 mm Hg in diastolic BP).[123] There must also be a concomitant history of chronic (>6 months) orthostatic symptoms without other cause. VVS and POTS overlap clinically and a head-up tilt test can be helpful in differentiating between the entities. Patients with VVS maintain their BP for several minutes following head-up tilt and then experience a rapid drop in BP as cardiac output and stroke volume decrease. The resulting cerebral hypoperfusion can cause sudden loss of consciousness.[124] Patients with POTS maintain their BP when tilted up, but orthostatic tachycardia is enhanced as sympathetic tone increases in response to reduced circulating blood volume. As the heart rate increases, patients may begin to report presyncopal symptoms, but actual loss of consciousness is rare.[124,125]

REFERENCES

1. Task Force for the Diagnosis and Management of Syncope, European Society of Cardiology (ESC), Moya A, et al. Guidelines for the diagnosis and management of syncope (version 2009). Eur Heart J 2009;30(21):2631–71.
2. Lewis DA, Dhala A. Syncope in the pediatric patient: the cardiologist's perspective. Pediatr Clin North Am 1999;46(2):205–19.
3. Serletis A, Rose S, Sheldon AG, et al. Vasovagal syncope in medical students and their first-degree relatives. Eur Heart J 2006;27(16):1965–70.
4. Alboni P, Brignole M, Menozzi C, et al. Clinical spectrum of neurally mediated reflex syncopes. Europace 2004;6(1):55–62.
5. Del Rosso A, Alboni P, Brignole M, et al. Relation of clinical presentation of syncope to the age of patients. Am J Cardiol 2005;96(10):1431–5.
6. Sheldon RS, Sheldon AG, Connolly SJ, et al. Age of first faint in patients with vasovagal syncope. J Cardiovasc Electrophysiol 2006;17(1):49–54.
7. Mosqueda-Garcia R, Furlan R, Tank J, et al. The elusive pathophysiology of neurally mediated syncope. Circulation 2000;102(23):2898–906.
8. Jardine DL. Vasovagal syncope: new physiologic insights. Cardiol Clin 2013; 31(1):75–87.
9. Alboni P, Furlan R. Vasovagal syncope. Spring International Publishing; 2015. p. 53–95.
10. Saadjian AY, Lévy S, Franceschi F, et al. Role of endogenous adenosine as a modulator of syncope induced during tilt testing. Circulation 2002;106(5): 569–74.
11. Koeppen M, Eckle T, Eltzschig HK. Selective deletion of the A1 adenosine receptor abolishes heart-rate slowing effects of intravascular adenosine in vivo. PLoS One 2009;4:e6784.
12. Matthews IG, Sutton R, Blanc JJ, et al. The adenosine triphosphate test in the diagnosis of unexplained syncope: a test looking for a home. Europace 2014; 16(12):1703–5.
13. Parry SW, Chadwick T, Gray JC, et al. The intravenous adenosine test: a new test for the identification of bradycardia pacing indications? A pilot study in subjects with bradycardia pacing indications, vasovagal syncope and controls. QJM 2009;102(7):461–8.

14. Brignole M, Menozzi C, Moya A, et al. Pacemaker therapy in patients with neurally mediated syncope and documented asystole third international study on syncope of uncertain etiology (ISSUE-3): a randomized trial. Circulation 2012;125(21):2566–71.

15. Parry SW. Adenosine testing to DEtermine the need for Pacing Therapy with the additional use of an Implantable Loop Recorder (ADEPT-ILR study)—the efficacy of permanent pacing in patients presenting to emergency medical services with syncope and a positive intravenous adenosine: a randomised, double-blind, placebo-controlled, cross-over trial. ISRCT62199741.

16. van Dijk JG, Thijs RD, van Zwet E, et al. The semiology of tilt-induced reflex syncope in relation to electroencephalographic changes. Brain 2014;137(2): 576–85.

17. Pfeifer MA, Weinberg CR, Cook D, et al. Differential changes of autonomic nervous system function with age in man. Am J Med 1983;75(2):249–58.

18. Rowe JW, Troen BR. Sympathetic nervous system and aging in man. Endocr Rev 1980;1(2):167–79.

19. Blad H, Lamberts RJ, Gert van Dijk J, et al. Tilt-induced vasovagal syncope and psychogenic pseudosyncope overlapping clinical entities. Neurology 2015; 85(23):2006–10.

20. Tannemaat MR, van Niekerk J, Reijntjes RH, et al. The semiology of tilt-induced psychogenic pseudosyncope. Neurology 2013;81(8):752–8.

21. Paling D, Vilches-Moraga A, Akram Q, et al. Carotid sinus syndrome is common in very elderly patients undergoing tilt table testing and carotid sinus massage because of syncope or unexplained falls. Aging Clin Exp Res 2011;23(4):304–8.

22. Rafanelli M, Ruffolo E, Chisciotti VM, et al. Clinical aspects and diagnostic relevance of neuroautonomic evaluation in patients with unexplained falls. Aging Clin Exp Res 2014;26(1):33–7.

23. Alboni P. The different clinical presentations of vasovagal syncope. Heart 2015; 101(9):674–8.

24. Krediet CTP, Jardine DL, Cortelli P, et al. Vasovagal syncope interrupting sleep? Heart 2004;90(5):e25.

25. Jardine DL, Krediet CT, Cortelli P, et al. Fainting in your sleep? Clin Auton Res 2006;16(1):76–8.

26. Busweiler L, Jardine DL, Frampton CM, et al. Sleep syncope: important clinical associations with phobia and vagotonia. Sleep Med 2010;11(9):929–33.

27. Klein KM, Bromhead CJ, Smith KR, et al. Autosomal dominant vasovagal syncope clinical features and linkage to chromosome 15q26. Neurology 2013; 80(16):1485–93.

28. Benditt DG, Richard S. Tilt-table testing in the evaluation of syncope. J Cardiovasc Electrophysiol 2005;16(3):356–8.

29. Brignole M, Alboni P, Benditt DG, et al. Guidelines on management (diagnosis and treatment) of syncope–update 2004. Eur Heart J 2004;25(22):2054–72.

30. Coplan NL, Paul S. Carotid sinus hypersensitivity: case report and review of the literature. Am J Med 1984;77(3):561–5.

31. Humm AM, Mathias CJ. Unexplained syncope—is screening for carotid sinus hypersensitivity indicated in all patients aged> 40 years? J Neurol Neurosurg Psychiatry 2006;77(11):1267–70.

32. Luck JC, Hoover RJ, Biederman RW, et al. Observations on carotid sinus hypersensitivity from direct intraneural recordings of sympathetic nerve traffic. Am J Cardiol 1996;77(15):1362–5.

33. von zur Muhlen F, Quan W, D'Agate DJ, et al. A study of carotid sinus massage and head-up tilt table testing in patients with syncope and near-syncope. J Invasive Cardiol 2002;14(8):477–82.

34. Blanc JJ, L'Heveder G, Mansourati J, et al. Assessment of a newly recognized association carotid sinus hypersensitivity and denervation of sternocleidomastoid muscles. Circulation 1997;95(11):2548–51.

35. Tan MP, Kenny RA, Chadwick TJ, et al. Carotid sinus hypersensitivity: disease state or clinical sign of ageing? Insights from a controlled study of autonomic function in symptomatic and asymptomatic subjects. Europace 2010;12(11): 1630–6.

36. Lacerda G, Pedrosa RC, Lacerda RC, et al. Complications related to carotid sinus massage in 502 ambulatory patients. Arq Bras Cardiol 2009;92:78–87.

37. Claesson JE, Kristensson BE, Edvardsson N, et al. Less syncope and milder symptoms in patients treated with pacing for induced cardioinhibitory carotid sinus syndrome: a randomized study. Europace 2007;9(10):932–6.

38. Parry SW, Steen N, Bexton RS, et al. Pacing in elderly recurrent fallers with carotid sinus hypersensitivity: a randomised, double-blind, placebo controlled crossover trial. Heart 2009;95(5):405–9.

39. Ryan DJ, Nick S, Colette SM, et al. Carotid sinus syndrome, should we pace? A multicentre, randomised control trial (Safepace 2). Heart 2010;96(5):347–51.

40. Sutton R. Pacing in patients with carotid sinus and vasovagal syndromes. Pacing Clin Electrophysiol 1989;12(7):1260–3.

41. McIntosh SJ, Lawson J, Bexton RS, et al. A study comparing VVI and DDI pacing in elderly patients with carotid sinus syndrome. Heart 1997;77(6):553–7.

42. Gaggioli G, Brignole M, Menozzi C, et al. A positive response to head-up tilt testing predicts syncopal recurrence in carotid sinus syndrome patients with permanent pacemakers. Am J Cardiol 1995;76(10):720–2.

43. Lagi A, Sergio C, Simone C. Recurrent syncope in patients with carotid sinus hypersensitivity. ISRN Cardiol 2012;2012:216206.

44. Fachinetti P, Bellocchi S, Dorizzi A, et al. Carotid sinus syndrome: a review of the literature and our experience using carotid sinus denervation. J Neurosurg Sci 1998;42(4):189.

45. Moore A, Watts M, Sheehy T, et al. Treatment of vasodepressor carotid sinus syndrome with midodrine: a randomized, controlled pilot study. J Am Geriatr Soc 2005;53(1):114–8.

46. Da Costa D, McIntosh S, Kenny RA. Benefits of fludrocortisone in the treatment of symptomatic vasodepressor carotid sinus syndrome. Br Heart J 1993;69(4): 308–10.

47. Amin V, Behzad BP. Carotid sinus syndrome. Cardiol Rev 2015;23(3):130–4.

48. Benditt DG. Neurally mediated syncopal syndromes: pathophysiological concepts and clinical evaluation. Pacing Clin Electrophysiol 1997;20(2):572–84.

49. Kapoor WN, Jacqueline P, Michael K. Defecation syncope: a symptom with multiple etiologies. Arch Intern Med 1986;146(12):2377–9.

50. Bae MH, Kang JK, Kim NY, et al. Clinical characteristics of defecation and micturition syncope compared with common vasovagal syncope. Pacing Clin Electrophysiol 2012;35(3):341–7.

51. Gawrieh S. Swallow syncope. Principles of deglutition. New York: Springer; 2013. p. 445–8.

52. Livanis EG, Leftheriotis D, Theodorakis GN, et al. Situational syncope. Pacing Clin Electrophysiol 2004;27(7):918–23.

53. Lempert T, Bauer M, Schmidt D. Syncope: a videometric analysis of 56 episodes of transient cerebral hypoxia. Ann Neurol 1994;36(2):233–7.
54. McKeon A, Carl V, Norman D. Seizure versus syncope. Lancet Neurol 2006;5(2): 171–80.
55. Gastaut H, Fischer-Williams M. Electro-encephalographic study of syncope: its differentiation from epilepsy. Lancet 1957;270(7004):1018–25.
56. King MA, Newton MR, Jackson GD, et al. Epileptology of the first-seizure presentation: a clinical, electroencephalographic, and magnetic resonance imaging study of 300 consecutive patients. Lancet 1998;352(9133):1007–11.
57. Patel SJ, Jackson G, Marshall A. Convulsive syncope in young adults: think of a cardiac cause. Int J Clin Pract 2001;55(9):639–40.
58. Song PS, Kim JS, Park J, et al. Seizure-like activities during head-up tilt test-induced syncope. Yonsei Med J 2010;51(1):77–81.
59. Reeves AL, Nollet KE, Klass DW, et al. The ictal bradycardia syndrome. Epilepsia 1996;37(10):983–7.
60. Tinuper P, Bisulli F, Cerullo A, et al. Ictal bradycardia in partial epileptic seizures. Brain 2001;124(12):2361–71.
61. Devinsky O, Steven P, Gopal T. Bradycardia and asystole induced by partial seizures: a case report and literature review. Neurology 1997;48(6):1712–4.
62. Locatelli ER, Varghese JP, Shuaib A, et al. Cardiac asystole and bradycardia as a manifestation of left temporal lobe complex partial seizure. Ann Intern Med 1999;130(7):581–3.
63. Goldstein DS, Yehonatan S. Neurogenic orthostatic hypotension a pathophysiological approach. Circulation 2009;119(1):139–46.
64. Benarroch EE. The arterial baroreflex functional organization and involvement in neurologic disease. Neurology 2008;71(21):1733–8.
65. Robertson D, Kincaid DW, Haile V, et al. The head and neck discomfort of autonomic failure: an unrecognized aetiology of headache. Clin Auton Res 1994; 4(3):99–103.
66. Lankford J, Numan M, Hashmi SS, et al. Cerebral blood flow during HUTT in young patients with orthostatic intolerance. Clin Auton Res 2015;25(5):277–84.
67. Wyller VB, Due R, Saul JP, et al. Usefulness of an abnormal cardiovascular response during low-grade head-up tilt-test for discriminating adolescents with chronic fatigue from healthy controls. Am J Cardiol 2007;99(7):997–1001.
68. Weiss A, Grossman E, Beloosesky Y, et al. Orthostatic hypotension in acute geriatric ward: is it a consistent finding? Arch Intern Med 2002;162(20):2369–74.
69. Kaufmann H. Consensus statement on the definition of orthostatic hypotension, pure autonomic failure and multiple system atrophy. Clin Auton Res 1996;6(2): 125–6.
70. Campos ACR, de Almeida NA, Ramos AL, et al. Orthostatic hypotension at different times after standing erect in elderly adults. J Am Geriatr Soc 2015; 63(3):589–90.
71. Gibbons CH, Freeman R. Delayed orthostatic hypotension: a frequent cause of orthostatic intolerance. Neurology 2006;67(1):28–32.
72. Gibbons CH, Freeman R. Clinical implications of delayed orthostatic hypotension: a 10-year follow-up study. Neurology 2015;85(16):1362–7.
73. Freeman R. The peripheral nervous system and diabetes. In: Weir G, Kahn R, King GL, editors. Joslin's Diabetes Mellitus. Philadelphia: Lippincott; 2002.
74. Low PA, Walsh JC, Huang CY, et al. The sympathetic nervous system in diabetic neuropathy. Brain 1975;98(3):341–56.

75. Albers AR, Marc ZK, Gary JB. Stress testing in patients with diabetes mellitus diagnostic and prognostic value. Circulation 2006;113(4):583–92.

76. Zilliox L, Peltier AC, Wren PA, et al. Assessing autonomic dysfunction in early diabetic neuropathy the survey of autonomic symptoms. Neurology 2011; 76(12):1099–105.

77. Isak B, Oflazoglu B, Tanridag T, et al. Evaluation of peripheral and autonomic neuropathy among patients with newly diagnosed impaired glucose tolerance. Diabetes Metab Res Rev 2008;24(7):563–9.

78. Putz Z, Tabák AG, Tóth N, et al. Noninvasive evaluation of neural impairment in subjects with impaired glucose tolerance. Diabetes Care 2009;32(1):181–3.

79. Laitinen T, Lindström J, Eriksson J, et al. Cardiovascular autonomic dysfunction is associated with central obesity in persons with impaired glucose tolerance. Diabet Med 2011;28(6):699–704.

80. Smith AG, Russell J, Feldman EL, et al. Lifestyle intervention for pre-diabetic neuropathy. Diabetes care 2006;29(6):1294–9.

81. Grandinetti A, Chow DC, Sletten DM, et al. Impaired glucose tolerance is associated with postganglionic sudomotor impairment. Clin Auton Res 2007;17(4): 231–3.

82. Putz Z, Németh N, Istenes I, et al. Autonomic dysfunction and circadian blood pressure variations in people with impaired glucose tolerance. Diabetic Med 2013;30(3):358–62.

83. Straznicky NE, Grima MT, Sari CI, et al. Neuroadrenergic dysfunction along the diabetes continuum a comparative study in obese metabolic syndrome subjects. Diabetes 2012;61(10):2506–16.

84. Flaa A, Aksnes TA, Kjeldsen SE, et al. Increased sympathetic reactivity may predict insulin resistance: an 18-year follow-up study. Metabolism 2008;57(10): 1422–7.

85. Gibbons CH, Freeman R. Treatment-induced diabetic neuropathy: a reversible painful autonomic neuropathy. Ann Neurol 2010;67(4):534–41.

86. Dingli D, Tan TS, Kumar SK, et al. Stem cell transplantation in patients with autonomic neuropathy due to primary (AL) amyloidosis. Neurology 2010;74(11): 913–8.

87. Gertz MA. Immunoglobulin light chain amyloidosis: 2013 update on diagnosis, prognosis, and treatment. Am J Hematol 2013;88(5):416–25.

88. Ando Y, Coelho T, Bork JL, et al. Guideline of transthyretin-related hereditary amyloidosis for clinicians. Orphanet J Rare Dis 2013;8:31.

89. Iodice V, Paola S. Autonomic neuropathies. Continuum (Minneap Minn) 2014; 20(5 Peripheral Nervous System Disorders):1373–97.

90. Senard JM, Philippe R. Dopamine beta-hydroxylase deficiency. Orphanet J Rare Dis 2006;1(7):1–4.

91. Klein CM, Vernino S, Lennon VA, et al. The spectrum of autoimmune autonomic neuropathies. Ann Neurol 2003;53(6):752–8.

92. Sandroni P, Phillip AL. Other autonomic neuropathies associated with ganglionic antibody. Auton Neurosci 2009;146(1):13–7.

93. Fischer PR, Sandroni P, Pittock SJ, et al. Isolated sympathetic failure with autoimmune autonomic ganglionopathy. Pediatr Neurol 2010;43(4):287–90.

94. Vernino S, Low PA, Fealey RD, et al. Autoantibodies to ganglionic acetylcholine receptors in autoimmune autonomic neuropathies. N Engl J Med 2000;343(12): 847–55.

95. Huot G, Burgunder JM, Lauterburg TF, et al. Expression of neuronal nicotinic acetylcholine receptor subunit genes in the rat autonomic nervous system. Eur J Neurosci 1994;6(3):478–85.

96. Iodice V, Kimpinski K, Vernino S, et al. Efficacy of immunotherapy in seropositive and seronegative putative autoimmune autonomic ganglionopathy. Neurology 2009;72(23):2002–8.

97. Kimpinski K, Iodice V, Vernino S, et al. Association of N-type calcium channel autoimmunity in patients with autoimmune autonomic ganglionopathy. Auton Neurosci 2009;150(1):136–9.

98. Sandroni P, Vernino S, Klein CM, et al. Idiopathic autonomic neuropathy: comparison of cases seropositive and seronegative for ganglionic acetylcholine receptor antibody. Arch Neurol 2004;61(1):44–8.

99. Koike H, Hashimoto R, Tomita M, et al. The spectrum of clinicopathological features in pure autonomic neuropathy. J Neurol 2012;259(10):2067–75.

100. Vernino S, Sandroni P, Singer W, et al. Invited article: autonomic ganglia target and novel therapeutic tool. Neurology 2008;70(20):1926–32.

101. Yokote H, Saitou Y, Kanda T, et al. Pure pandysautonomia associated with interferon-alpha therapy. J Neurol 2007;254(7):961–2.

102. Schroeder C, Vernino S, Birkenfeld AL, et al. Plasma exchange for primary autoimmune autonomic failure. N Engl J Med 2005;353(15):1585–90.

103. Hughes RAC, David RC. Guillain-Barre syndrome. Lancet 2005;366(9497): 1653–66.

104. Burns TM. Guillain-Barré syndrome. Semin Neurol 2008;28:152–67.

105. Zhang Q, Gu Z, Jiang J, et al. Orthostatic hypotension as a presenting symptom of the Guillain–Barré syndrome. Clin Auton Res 2010;20(3):209–10.

106. Sharp L, Steven V. Paraneoplastic neuromuscular disorders. Muscle Nerve 2012;46(6):839–40.

107. Vernino S. Antibody testing as a diagnostic tool in autonomic disorders. Clin Auton Res 2009;19(1):13–9.

108. McDonell KE, Cyndya AS, Daniel OC. Clinical relevance of orthostatic hypotension in neurodegenerative disease. Curr Neurol Neurosci Rep 2015;15(12): 1–12.

109. Benarroch EE. New findings on the neuropathology of multiple system atrophy. Auton Neurosci 2002;96(1):59–62.

110. Cersosimo MG, Eduardo EB. Autonomic involvement in Parkinson's disease: pathology, pathophysiology, clinical features and possible peripheral biomarkers. J Neurol Sci 2012;313(1):57–63.

111. Magalhaes M, Wenning GK, Daniel SE, et al. Autonomic dysfunction in pathologically confirmed multiple system atrophy and idiopathic Parkinson's disease–a retrospective comparison. Acta Neurol Scand 1995;91(2):98–102.

112. Hague K, Lento P, Morgello S, et al. The distribution of Lewy bodies in pure autonomic failure: autopsy findings and review of the literature. Acta Neuropathol 1997;94(2):192–6.

113. Goldstein DS, Eldadah BA, Holmes C, et al. Neurocirculatory abnormalities in Parkinson disease with orthostatic hypotension independence from levodopa treatment. Hypertension 2005;46(6):1333–9.

114. Krediet CT, van Lieshout JJ, Bogert LW, et al. Leg crossing improves orthostatic tolerance in healthy subjects: a placebo-controlled crossover study. Am J Physiol Heart Circ Physiol 2006;291(4):H1768–72.

115. MacLean AR, Edgar VA. Orthostatic hypotension and orthostatic tachycardia: treatment with the head-up bed. J Am Med Assoc 1940;115(25):2162–7.

116. Reybrouck T, Heidbüchel H, Van de Werf F, et al. Tilt training: a treatment for malignant and recurrent neurocardiogenic syncope. Pacing Clin Electrophysiol 2000;23(4):493 8.

117. Qingyou Z, Du J, Tang C. The efficacy of midodrine hydrochloride in the treatment of children with vasovagal syncope. J Pediatr 2006;149(6):777–80.

118. Liu XY, Wang C, Wu LJ, et al. Efficacy of midodrine hydrochloride in the treatment of children with vasovagal syncope. Zhonghua yi xue za zhi 2009; 89(28):1951–4 [in Chinese].

119. Romme JJ, van Dijk N, Go-Schön IK, et al. Effectiveness of midodrine treatment in patients with recurrent vasovagal syncope not responding to non-pharmacological treatment (STAND-trial). Europace 2011;13(11):1639–47.

120. Izcovich A, González Malla C, Manzotti M, et al. Midodrine for orthostatic hypotension and recurrent reflex syncope: a systematic review. Neurology 2014; 83(13):1170–7.

121. Ramirez CE, Okamoto LE, Arnold AC, et al. Efficacy of atomoxetine versus midodrine for the treatment of orthostatic hypotension in autonomic failure. Hypertension 2014;64(6):1235–40.

122. Singer W, Sandroni P, Opfer-Gehrking TL, et al. Pyridostigmine treatment trial in neurogenic orthostatic hypotension. Arch Neurol 2006;63(4):513–8.

123. Freeman R, Wieling W, Axelrod FB, et al. Consensus statement on the definition of orthostatic hypotension, neurally mediated syncope and the postural tachycardia syndrome. Auton Neurosci 2011;161(1):46–8.

124. Raj SR, Samuel TC. Medical therapy and physical maneuvers in the treatment of the vasovagal syncope and orthostatic hypotension. Prog Cardiovasc Dis 2013; 55(4):425–33.

125. Garland EM, Jorge EC, Satish RR. Postural tachycardia syndrome: beyond orthostatic intolerance. Curr Neurol Neurosci Rep 2015;15(9):1–11.

Distal Myopathies

Case Studies

Aziz Shaibani, MD

KEYWORDS

- Distal • Myopathy • Weakness • Myofibrillar

KEY POINTS

- Distal weakness is an important presentation to the neurology clinics and the differential diagnosis is wide.
- Diagnostic process requires differentiation of myopathic causes of distal weakness from nonmyopathic causes such as neuropathies, myasthenia gravis, and motor neuron diseases.
- The most common causes of myopathic muscle weakness are inclusion body myositis, myotonic dystrophy, and facioscapulohumeral muscular dystrophy.
- Myofibrillar myopathy and distal muscular dystrophy are rare causes of distal myopathy and their differentiation depends on the clinical, pathologic, and genetic profiles.

 Video content accompanies this article at http://www.neurologic.theclinics. com.

CASE 1: DYSPHAGIA AND HANDS WEAKNESS (SEE FIG. 1 FOR VIDEO 1)

A 67-year-old woman presented with a 5-year history of gait imbalance and dysphagia. Examination is shown. Creatine kinase (CK) level was 800 U/L and electromyogram (EMG) revealed mixed short and long duration potentials in the proximal and distal arm and leg muscles bilaterally. Discontinuation of atorvastatin and treatment with oral steroids reduced the CK level to 300 U/L and led to improvement of the stamina for a couple of months. No objective changes in the muscle strength were noted.

Regarding the case

1. CK reduction with steroids argues against inclusion body myositis (IBM)
2. The pathologic condition is due to statins
3. Statins may have worsened weakness produced by IBM
4. She is a good candidate for intravenous gamma globulin (IVIG)
5. The pattern of weakness is not typical for IBM

Disclosure Statement: No disclosures.

Department of Medicine, Nerve and Muscle Center of Texas, Baylor College of Medicine, 6624 Fannin # 1670, Houston, TX 77030, USA

E-mail address: shaibani@bcm.edu

http://dx.doi.org/10.1016/j.ncl.2016.04.014
0733-8619/16/$ – see front matter © 2016 Elsevier Inc. All rights reserved.
neurologic.theclinics.com

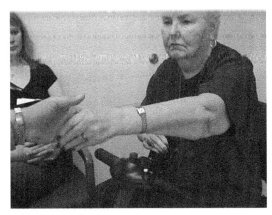

Fig. 1. Dysphagia and hands weakness.

IBM

- The pattern of weakness in this case is very typical for IBM, which should be highly suspected just after shaking hand with the patient (fish mouth handshake appearance due to weakness of finger flexors).

- The practice of adjusting the dose of prednisone based on the CK level is not recommended because steroids stabilize the cell membrane and reduce the CK level regardless of the cause.
  - Strength measurement and functional scales are the most valid outcome measures in monitoring progression and recovery of myopathies.

- Statins can cause different kinds of myopathies, including toxic myopathy and autoimmune necrotizing myopathy, with positive antibodies against 3-hydroxy-3-methylglutaryl coenzyme A (HMG-CoA) reductase.
  - Also, statins may unmask an underlying metabolic or mitochondrial myopathy because 30% of statin-induced myopathies showed evidence of an underlying metabolic defect such as carnitine palmitoyl transferase (CPT)-2, myoadenylate deaminase (MAD), or phosphorylase deficiencies.
  - Some of these myopathies may improve after discontinuation of the statins but it may take several months for maximum recovery. Others need to be treated with steroids and or other immunosuppressive agents.
  - An IBM phenotype is not reported in association with statins therapy. Myopathies may be worsened by statins.
- Neither IVIG nor prednisone, azathioprine, or any other immunomodulatory agent was proven to be effective in treating IBM.
  - Some authorities advocate a 3 months of steroids therapy for patients who show a CK level of more than 20 times normal and intense endomysial inflammation in muscle biopsy. In the author's experience, if improvement happens it is transient and steroids do not change the natural history of the disease.

Reference

Machado PM, Dimachkie MM, Barohn RJ. Inclusion body myositis: a new insight and potential therapy. Curr Opin Neurol 2014;27:591–8.

CASE 2: CHRONIC DYSPHAGIA AND HANDS STIFFNESS (SEE FIG. 2 FOR VIDEO 2)

A 65-year-old woman presented with 10-year history of frequent falls and slowly progressive dysphagia and facial weakness. She had several syncopal episodes few years earlier and a pacemaker was inserted. She had no significant family history. CK level was 95 U/L. Her examination is shown.

Which of the following features was not in favor of IBM but in favor of myotonic dystrophy (DM)?

1. Female patient
2. White race
3. Quadriceps weakness
4. Facial weakness
5. Syncope

DM

- The picture was very suggestive of IBM, including chronic course, weakness of the finger flexors and quadriceps muscles, facial weakness, dysphagia, and mild CK elevation. Syncope could be incidental or due to heart block that is associated with DM, one of the mimicking conditions.
- EMG revealed diffuse waxing and waning 150 Hz discharges and myopathic units. Reexamination revealed mild percussion myotonia. Muscle biopsy was cancelled and instead mutation analysis for DM type 1 (DM1) was requested and it revealed a CTG repeat expansion to 1200 repeats in the DMPK gene, confirming the diagnosis of DM1.

- Examination for percussion and grip myotonia is often deleted from evaluation, although it can provide very relevant and sometimes unexpected information.

- IBM is the most common myopathy after age 50 years and myotonic dystrophy (DM) is the most common muscular dystrophy in adults. Although DM is an autosomal dominant disease, symptoms in the parents can be very subtle (unreported) compare with offspring due to the genetic phenomenon of anticipation.

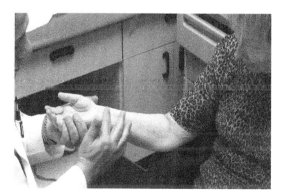

Fig. 2. Chronic dysphagia and hands stiffness.

- Cardiac conduction abnormalities are very common in DM and they contribute to mortality. Most patients will need a pacemaker by age 50 years and, therefore, serial monitoring with electrocardiogram (ECG) for detection of conduction detects is important.
- Sometimes, syncope due to heart block is the presenting feature of DM.

Reference

Machuca-Tzili L, Brook D, Hilton-Jones D. Clinical and molecular aspects of the myotonic dystrophies: a review. Muscle Nerve 2005;32(1):1–18.

CASE 3: FACIAL WEAKNESS, DYSPHAGIA, AND DISTAL WEAKNESS (SEE FIG. 3 FOR VIDEO 3)

A 70-year-old woman presented with 5-year history of right hand grip weakness that spread to the left hand after 2 years. She then developed dysphagia and weight loss. The leg muscles strength was normal. CK level was 450 U/L. EMG showed many short and long duration units in the biceps and wrist flexors.

The combination of chronic facial weakness, dysphagia, and distal arms weakness is typically seen in

1. IBM
2. Facioscapulohumeral muscular dystrophy (FSHD)
3. DM
4. Polymyositis (PM)
5. Amyotrophic lateral sclerosis (ALS)

IBM phenotypes

- Chronic dysphagia and facial weakness are seen in DM, IBM, PM, FSHD, and some congenital myopathies and myasthenia gravis (MG).
- If weakness of finger flexors is added, IBM and DM are the qualified disorders.
- IBM has many phenotypes; quadriceps sparing occurs in 5% to 10% of cases.
- Mild CK elevation is common in all the mentioned possibilities.
- A careful examination for percussion and grip myotonia and for waxing and waning EMG discharges is important. If found, a blood test for DMPK mutation would be more appropriate than a muscle biopsy. Otherwise, a muscle biopsy

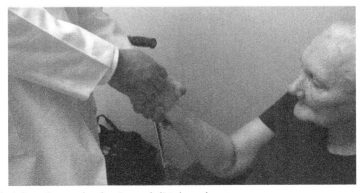

Fig. 3. Facial weakness, dysphagia, and distal weakness.

would be indicated to look for red-rimmed vacuoles (RRVs) and cytoplasmic inclusion bodies that are the pathologic hallmark of IBM.

- MG may cause distal weakness but it almost always affects wrist extensors and not finger flexors.
- FSHD is more likely to cause distal legs weakness (feet extensors) than hands weakness. Dysphagia is not common.
- Sometimes, although the clinical picture is suggestive of IBM, the muscle biopsy shows endomysial inflammation without RRV or inclusions (PM picture). Some experts tend to treat these cases as PM, particularly if the CK is significantly elevated. Almost always, these cases behave like IBM and the lack of degenerative features in the biopsy is common in the initial inflammatory phase of the disease.

- IBM can be confused with ALS due to progressive hands weakness and bulbar dysfunction. Long finger flexors and not intrinsic hand muscles are the target in IBM. Dysarthria almost always precedes dysphagia in ALS.

Reference

Dabby R, Lange DJ, Trojaborg W, et al. Inclusion body myositis mimicking motor neuron disease. Arch Neurol 2001;58(8):1253–6.

CASE 4: SCAPULAR WINGING AND FOOT DROP (SEE FIG. 4 FOR VIDEO 4)

A 61-year-old woman presented with the shown findings that evolved over years. CK level was 650 U/L.

The most appropriate next testing includes

1. Muscle biopsy
2. FSHD mutation analysis
3. Lumbar spine MRI
4. Emerin gene mutation analysis
5. Nerve conduction study (NCS)

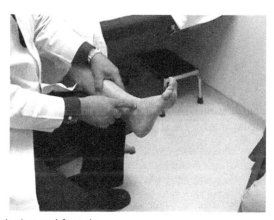

Fig. 4. Scapular winging and foot drop.

The following features are typically seen in FSHD:

1. Asymmetric onset
2. Distal weakness
3. Scapular winging
4. Facial weakness
5. Inflammatory muscle pathologic condition.

Myopathic foot drop

- Painless asymmetrical foot drop, scapular winging, and myopathic EMG suggest FSHD. Neurogenic and myopathic scapuloperoneal syndromes are also possible. This patient had contraction of D4Z4 allele, confirming the diagnosis of FSHD.
- Unilateral or bilateral foot drop may be caused by muscle disease.
- Factors that would suggest a myopathic foot drop include
  - Preserved bulk or even compensatory hypertrophy of the extensor digitorum brevis due to the lack of involvement of the intrinsic foot muscles (unlike neurogenic causes when these muscles are affected early)
  - Lack of sensory symptoms or signs
  - Preservation of sural responses
  - Lack of denervation of the tibialis anterior (spontaneous activity may be seen as a part of irritative myopathy)
  - The presence of other features of muscle disease, such as proximal weakness and scapular winging.
- FSHD is a common inherited muscle disease in which tibialis anterior muscles are affected early, leading to unilateral or bilateral foot drop, usually in association with scapular winging and facial weakness. Twenty percent of cases do not show facial weakness.
- Foot drop can be the presenting symptom of FSHD, which may lead to diagnostic confusion with peroneal neuropathy, L5 radiculopathy, and sometimes ALS.
- Affected family members may not be aware of their weakness and their examination is usually helpful.

- Asymmetry can be striking in FSHD, leading to unilateral foot drop or facial weakness.

- Inflammation in the muscle biopsy is characteristic leading to misdiagnosis of PM. Muscle biopsy is not required for the diagnosis, which can be made from a blood sample.
- Twenty percent of patients end up on a wheelchair.

CASE 5: SEVERE PROXIMAL AND DISTAL WEAKNESS (SEE FIG. 5 FOR VIDEO 5)

A 70-year-old woman presented with a 10-year history of dysphagia and arms weakness. The power of her quadriceps muscles was 3/5 and she had bilateral foot drop and severe weakness of the fingers flexors. CK level was 400 U/L. EMG revealed long and short duration motor unit potentials (MUPs) in the arms with no spontaneous activity. Sensory responses and motor conduction studies were normal. Muscle biopsy is shown.

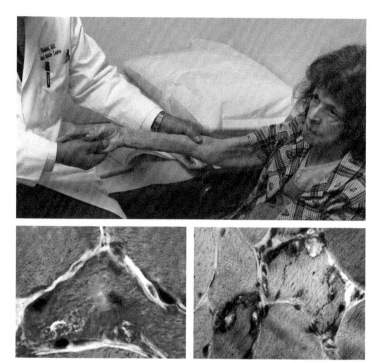

Fig. 5. Severe proximal and distal weakness.

The most likely diagnoses include

1. PM
2. IBM
3. Vasculitis
4. Muscular dystrophy
5. Necrotizing myopathy

End-stage IBM

- The clinical picture is classic of sIBM and muscle pathologic condition confirmed the diagnosis by showing RRVs and cytoplasmic eosinophilic inclusion bodies.
- IBM remains a dismal disease.
- The response to treatment is poor. Progressive weakness is the rule. The older the age of onset, the more rapid the loss of strength and function. Within 10 years of the diagnosis, most people become wheelchair-bound. Patients lose 5% of strength per year.

Complications of IDM and causes of death

1. Loss of ambulation due to severe weakness of the legs
2. Aspiration pneumonia due to severe dysphagia
3. Exposure keratitis from facial weakness
4. Malnutrition due to dysphagia and depression
5. Immobility complications, such as DVT and skin ulceration
   - Life expectancy is normal
     - No increase in the risk of systemic diseases or malignancy.

CASE 6: CHRONIC FACIAL AND HAND GRIP WEAKNESS (SEE FIG. 6 FOR VIDEO 6)

A 50-year-old man presented with chronic progressive weakness of bilateral hand grips and facial muscles.

Weak finger flexors and facial muscles are typically observed in

1. IBM
2. PM
3. DM
4. Facial onset sensorimotor neuropathy
5. FSHD

Facial and finger flexors weakness

- Patients with chronic progressive weakness of the hand grips without sensory symptoms usually belong to one of the following categories:
  - Distal myopathy: purely distal or part of a more generalized myopathy
  - Spinal muscular atrophy (SMA): distal type or part of a more generalized type
  - Lower cervical radiculopathy: pain and numbness may be minimal
  - Lower cord or trunk brachial plexopathy: pain and numbness may be minimal
  - Motor neuropathy, such as multifocal motor neuropathy with conduction blocks.
- Unlike SMA, in myopathic weakness there is usually no atrophy of the intrinsic hands muscles but weakness of the finger flexors and atrophy of the volar forearm muscles.
- Facial weakness limits the diagnosis to the first 2 categories.
- Mild CK elevation is common in both but more than 10 times normal would favor a myopathic condition.
- A good EMG can sort out the myopathic from the neurogenic type (diffuse high firing frequency is commonly seen in SMA and low amplitude short duration united with early recruitment are features of myopathy), although in chronic cases mixed MUPs are difficult to sort out. A muscle biopsy in these cases is useful.
- Among the chronic myopathic causes, the ones that cause facial weakness, finger flexor weakness, and dysphagia are IBM and DM. It is crucial to look for clinical percussion myotonia and the typical facies of the DM and the appropriate family history.

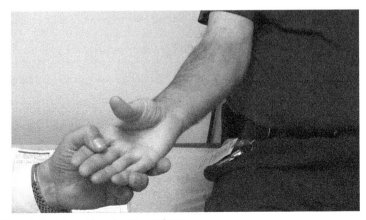

Fig. 6. Chronic facial and hand grip weakness.

- However, due to the phenomenon of anticipation, other family members may only be minimally affected and do not seek medical advice.
- Patients with IBM may get temporalis atrophy, leading to a thin face and may even show paraspinal myotonic discharges or, more often, pseudomyotonic discharges.
- In these cases, a muscle biopsy is crucial. RRVs and intracytoplasmic eosinophilic inclusion bodies of IBM could be easily differentiated from type 1 atrophy and sarcoplasmic masses of DM.

CASE 7: A POLICEMAN WHO COULD NOT PULL THE TRIGGER (SEE FIG. 7 FOR VIDEO 7)

A 50-year-old police officer noticed 3 years earlier difficulty pulling the trigger. Three years before that he gradually developed difficulty dancing and running. His mother was diagnosed with FSHD due to facial and legs weakness. Two aunts and 2 cousins were diagnosed with limb-girdle muscular dystrophy (LGMD). One of them had congestive heart failure. CPK level was 124 U/L and EMG revealed mixed short and long duration potentials in distal and proximal muscles of all extremities and many fibrillations and positive sharp waves. Left biceps biopsy revealed chronic myopathic and neurogenic changes with no inflammation. Rare RRVs were noted.

The following immunohistochemical reaction would be most appropriate:

1. CD8
2. Dysferlin
3. Desmin
4. Calpain
5. Dystroglycan

Hereditary IBM (hIBM) type 1 (myofibrillar myopathy [MFM]1)

- The pattern of weakness (quadriceps, fingers flexors and feet extensors weakness), the chronicity, and RRVs suggested IBM. The age of the patient and the family history (more likely dominant inheritance) suggested hIBM. Spontaneous discharges and history of heart failure suggested hIBM1 (MFM1).

- Rimmed vacuoles are not specific and can be seen in
  - IBM: sporadic and hereditary types
  - Oculopharyngeal muscular dystrophy
  - Distal muscular dystrophies
  - Myofibrillar myopathies.

- IBMs
  - IBM: sporadic
  - Hereditary
    - IBM1 (MFM): mostly autosomal dominant
    - IBM2 (GNE mutation): autosomal recessive, high CK, quadriceps sparing, anterior compartment of the legs
    - IBM3: joint contractures and ophthalmoplegia (myosin heavy chain IIa)
    - IBM plus Paget and dementia (VCP mutations).

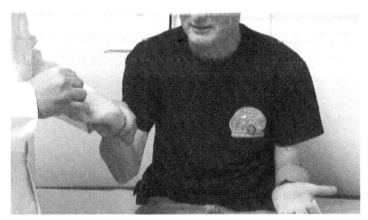

Fig. 7. A policeman who could not pull the trigger.

- hIBM1
  - Autosomal dominant inclusion body myopathy had previously been referred to as IBM1 to distinguish it from autosomal recessive IBM, which is caused by mutation in the GNE gene on chromosome 9p13.3. Since then, autosomal dominant inclusion body myopathy has been found to be a genetically heterogeneous condition and is referred to as MFM.
  - Desmin mutations, chromosome 2q35, dominant or recessive
  - Onset: 25 to 40 years
  - Quadriceps weakness and foot dorsiflexion weakness and sometimes finger flexor weakness
  - Slow progression
  - Congestive cardiac failure in 25% of cases and neuropathy in 20% of cases
  - Normal or mildly elevated CK
  - Light microscopic findings: RRV and myopathic changes, amorphous granular material; electron microscopic findings: Z-disc disintegration.

References

Selcen D, Ohno K, Engel AG. Myofibrillar myopathy: clinical, morphological, and genetic studies in 63 patients. Brain 2004;127(Pt 2):439–51.

Needham M, Mastaglia FL, Garlepp MJ. Genetics of inclusion body myositis. Muscle Nerve 2007;35(5):549–61.

CASE 8: CALVES ATROPHY AND MODERATELY ELEVATED CK LEVEL (SEE FIG. 8 FOR VIDEO 8)

A 30-year-old man who had difficulty walking on his toes since age 15 years. At that time he was found to have a CK level of 2800 U/L and EMG revealed fibrillations in the bilateral calf muscles. He was diagnosed with axonal neuropathy. Gradually, he developed more atrophy of the calves, proximal leg and arm weakness, and weakness of the finger flexors. CK level was 3000 to 4000 U/L and NCS were normal. EMG revealed irritative myopathy involving proximal and distal muscles of the arms and legs. There was no family history of muscle disease. He started using a walker 7 years after the onset of the symptoms. Left biceps biopsy revealed chronic inflammatory myopathic changes.

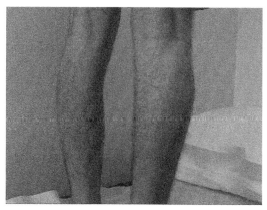

Fig. 8. Calves atrophy and moderately elevated CK level.

The most appropriate immunohistochemical tests on the muscle biopsy are

1. CD4/CD8 antibodies
2. Dysferlin antibodies
3. Dystrophin antibodies
4. Sarcoglycan antibodies

Miyoshi myopathy

- Distal myopathy is a feature of many myopathic disorders, most of them are hereditary.
- Among the sporadic disorders, IBM is the most common myopathy with distal involvement.
- Dystrophic myopathies, such as DM, usually cause distal weakness along with facial and proximal weakness.
- There is a group of hereditary myopathies that are characterized by distal weakness only, at least in the beginning of the disease. These disorders lack molecular understanding and they are classified according to the region affected, mode of inheritance, and age of onset. Many of them are allelic to specific LGMDs. More molecular understanding will likely change the classification in the future.
- Miyoshi myopathy is one of the better-characterized distal muscular dystrophies (distal hereditary myopathies).
  - It starts in early adult life with calves atrophy and weakness and remarkably elevated CK level and myopathic EMG.
  - It is caused by mutation of dysferlin gene and is allelic with LGMD2B.
  - Endomysial inflammation in muscle biopsy may lead to erroneous diagnosis of PM.

- Patients with myopathic calves atrophy and remarkable CK elevation do not need a muscle biopsy unless mutation analysis carried on white cell count fails to reveal absent dysferlin staining.

Reference

Dimachkie M, Barohn R. Distal myopathies. Neurol Clin 2014;32(3):817–42.

CASE 9. BILATERAL FOOT DROP AND QUADRICEPS WEAKNESS (SEE FIG. 9 FOR VIDEO 9)

A 37-year-old man had stopped dancing due to knees unbuckling 10 years earlier. He fell frequently. Gradually he could not arise from a chair without using his hands. His hands grips have gotten weaker. CK level was 4100 U/L. His older brother had similar problems. His parents were healthy.

The most likely causes of quadriceps weakness in this patient are

1. Dysferlinopathy
2. Dystrophinopathy
3. Calpainopathy
4. Myotilinopathy
5. Caveolinopathy

Becker muscular dystrophy (BMD)

- BMD should be considered in the differential diagnoses of several presentations in men, including limb-girdle weakness, isolated quadriceps weakness, asymptomatic hyperCKemia, muscle cramps, rhabdomyolysis, and cardiomyopathy. The diagnosis is not difficult when all these abnormalities exist in the same patients but they may be present individually and, in these cases, the diagnosis is usually delayed.
- The lack of family history is not exclusive because 10% of cases are due to spontaneous mutations.

- Calves hypertrophy is common in BMD and is diagnostically useful. Contrary to common belief, it is caused by real muscle hypertrophy rather than by fatty degeneration.

- The most common presentation is walking difficulty after age 15 years. Fifty percent of patients lose ability to walk by age 40 years.
- CK elevation is usually 20 to 200 times normal. EMG is myopathic in the affected muscles.
- MRI has become a popular tool in the neuromuscular clinic in the last decade. It was used in this case to demonstrate fatty replacement of calf muscles.

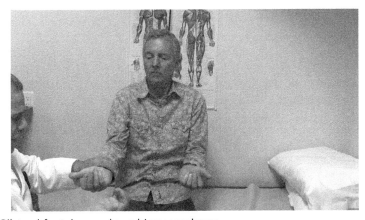

Fig. 9. Bilateral foot drop and quadriceps weakness.

- Muscle biopsy shows dystrophic myopathy. Dystrophin is decreased uniformly or in a patchy pattern, unlike DM in which it is absent. Western blot (WB) analysis typically reveals decreased amount or size of dystrophin.
- There is a 50% chance that the daughters of this man will be carriers. Carriers are usually asymptomatic but they may display mild weakness or muscle pain. The more sensitive way to diagnose carriers is WB analysis and not CK or muscle biopsy.
- Although steroids are commonly used to treat DM patients, they are not recommended in BMD except in very progressive cases.
- There is no promising treatment modality in the horizon. Genetic engineering and stem cell transplantation may provide a glimpse of hope in the future.
- Annual ECG is recommended to detect conduction abnormalities early.

References

Flanigan KM. Duchenne and Becker muscular dystrophies. Neurol Clin 2014;32(3):671–88.

Monforte M. Calf muscle involvement in Becker muscular dystrophy: when size does not matter. J Neurol Sci 2014;347(1–2):301–4.

CASE 10: WRIST AND FINGER FLEXORS WEAKNESS AND MYOPATHIC ELECTROMYOGRAM (SEE FIG. 10 FOR VIDEO 10)

A 65-year-old woman with 15-year history of slowly progressive weakness of the arms and legs as demonstrated in the video. She had no dysphagia and normal quadriceps

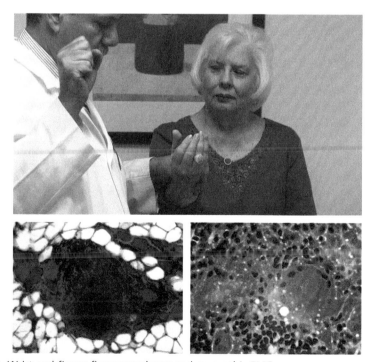

Fig. 10. Wrist and finger flexors weakness and myopathic EMG.

strength. CPK level was normal and EMG revealed mixed small and large MUPs in the bilateral distal arm and leg muscles. Left biceps biopsy is shown.

The most likely diagnoses include

1. IBM
2. PM
3. Granulomatous myositis
4. Vasculitic myositis
5. Parasitic myositis

Granulomatous myopathy

- Muscle biopsy revealed multiple noncaseating granulomata that contained many multinucleated giant cells.

> - Patients with chronic distal hands weakness are usually given different diagnoses, such as carpal tunnel syndrome, cervical radiculopathy, or arthritis, and it may take years before they see a neuromuscular specialist.

- The lack of sensory symptoms and the diffuse nature of the weakness were consistent with
  - Myopathy
  - Motor neuron disease, including Hirayama disease (HD)
  - MG
- Myopathic EMG confirmed the diagnosis of distal myopathy and raised the following possibilities:
  - Distal muscular dystrophies
  - Inclusion body myopathies
  - Myofibrillar myopathies
  - Muscle biopsy reveals unexpected diagnosis. There were several noncaseating granulomas and endomysial inflammation.
- Granulomatous myopathy is a rare form of inflammatory muscle disease:
  - It may present as progressive proximal weakness along with MG and thymoma
  - Or as a chronic distal weakness as a manifestation of sarcoidosis.
  - Frequently, search for sarcoidosis is not productive and the diagnosis of idiopathic granulomatous myopathy is given.
  - CK level is normal to 5X normal level.
  - EMG shows chronic myopathic findings (mixed short and long duration MUPs and early recruitment).
  - Prognosis is not good and, unfortunately, response to immunosuppression or modulation is poor in the distal form.
  - Unlike the proximal variant, the distal idiopathic type does not affect the heart but it may extend to the proximal muscles.

Reference

Jasim S, Shaibani A. Nonsarcoid granulomatous myopathy: two cases and a review of literature. Int J Neurosci C 2013;123(7):516–20.

CASE 11: FAMILIAL HOARSENESS AND FOOT DROP (SEE FIG. 11 FOR VIDEO 11)

A 78-year-old man presented with a 7-year history of slowly progressive hoarseness and painless bilateral foot drop. He had mild proximal leg weakness. There was no

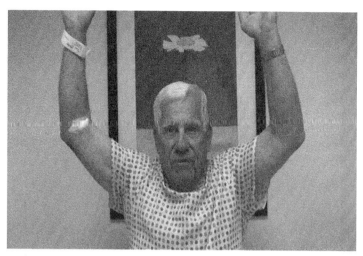

Fig. 11. Familial hoarseness and foot drop.

dysphagia or ptosis. CK level was 400 U/L and EMG showed 30% short duration units in the proximal and distal leg muscles. There were no spontaneous discharges. A twin brother developed similar signs. Muscle biopsy revealed nonspecific myopathic features with several RRVs.

The most likely diagnoses include

1. Oculopharyngeal muscular dystrophy
2. Matrin 3 gene mutation
3. Dysferlinopathy
4. Calpainopathy
5. Caveolinopathy

Diagnosis

Distal myopathy with vocal cord and pharyngeal weakness

- Autosomal dominant disease caused by mutations of matrin 3 gene, which is located on chromosome 5q31 ?
- Reported in North American German and Bulgarian families
- Onset in the third to fifth decade.
- Clinical picture
  - Peroneal weakness and hands weakness
  - Respiratory weakness in 60% of cases
  - Hoarseness in 65% of cases
  - Dysphagia and aspiration common
  - Slowly progressive course
  - Respiratory failure occurs in 60%
- Differential diagnosis
  - SMA
  - Neuronal Charcot-Marie-Tooth disease
  - LGMD2F
  - LGMD1A
- Serum CK is normal to 8 times normal and EMG is myopathic.

- Muscle pathologic conditions include myopathic features and rimmed vacuoles.
- MATR3 variant syndrome: familial ALS.

CASE 12: A FISHERMAN WHO CANNOT PEEL SHRIMP ANYMORE (SEE FIG. 12 FOR VIDEO 12)

A 21-year-old shrimp peeler who developed weakness of his fingers 5 years earlier that progressed to a degree that was not compatible with his job. He had no neck pain, arm numbness, dysphagia, or muscle twitching. Family history was nonrelevant. Examination is shown. CPK was 530 U/L and EMG revealed chronic diffuse denervation of the arms muscles with normal sensory and motor responses. EMG of the legs was normal.

The most likely diagnoses include

1. ALS
2. Hirayama disease (HD)
3. IBM
4. West Nile virus infection
5. Cervical radiculopathy

Case 5: Hirayama disease

- Chronic unilateral or bilateral pure motor weakness of the hand muscles in a young patient is not common. Differential diagnosis includes
  - Cervical cord pathologic conditions, such as syringomyelia (dissociated sensory loss), are typically present.
  - Brachial plexus pathologic condition: sensory findings are usually present.
  - Motor neurons diseases: ALS and SMA.
    - Cervical spines are usually investigated before neuromuscular referrals are made.
    - The lack of pain, radicular or sensory symptoms, normal sensory nerve action potentials, and cervical MRI ruled out most of the mentioned possibilities, except
    - Distal myopathy (usually not unilateral) and SMA.

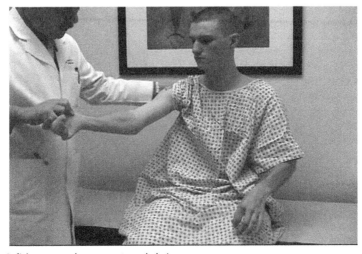

Fig. 12. A fisherman who cannot peel shrimp anymore.

- EMG or NCS demonstration of chronic distal denervation with normal sensory responses and no demyelinating features limited the diagnosis to motor neurone disease.
- Segmental denervation pattern further narrowed the diagnosis to HD.

- HD is a sporadic and focal form of SMA that affects predominantly young men at ages 15 to 25 years.

- Weakness and atrophy usually starts unilaterally in C8-T1 muscles of the hand and forearm, typically in the dominant hand.
  - In a third of cases, the other hand is affected and weakness may spread to the proximal muscles.
  - DTRs are normal or brisk, unlike the most SMA cases were the reflexes are decreased or absent.
  - After progressive course of 6 years or less, the progression plateaus.
  - Extreme exacerbation of weakness in the cold and focal hyperhidrosis are reported.
  - The disease is more common in India.
- Hypothesis: radiological forward displacement of the cervical dural sac and compressive flattening of the cervical cord during flexion suggest that this is a form of cervical myelopathy. The resulting ischemia leads to preferential damage of the motor neurons. Decompressive surgery is unlikely to be effective due to the chronic nature of the neurologic insult.

Reference

Hirayama K, Tokumaru Y. Cervical dural sac and spinal cord in juvenile muscular atrophy of distal upper extremity. Neurology 2000;54:1922–6.

CASE 13: PAINLESS FINGERS DROP (SEE FIG. 13 FOR VIDEO 13)

A 75-year-old man presented with a 2-week history of gradually increasing painless weakness of the left fingers extension followed by weakness of the right fingers extension. He denied weakness of the handgrips or difficulty standing from a chair. He had mild dysphagia but no diplopia. Examination is shown in the video. EMG of the extensor digitorum communis. 20% short duration unites. There was no fibrillation. Past medical history was remarkable for seropositive MG in drug-free remission for 15 years that initially presented with dysarthria, dysphagia, and respiratory failure, and responded to plasmapheresis and oral steroids.

The most likely diagnoses include

1. Welander myopathy
2. C8 radiculopathy
3. Relapse of MG
4. IBM
5. HD

Distal MG

- In MG, proximal, ocular, and bulbar muscles are commonly affected. Distal muscles are typically spared. Less than 10% of cases are associated with distal weakness and 2% of cases present with only distal weakness.

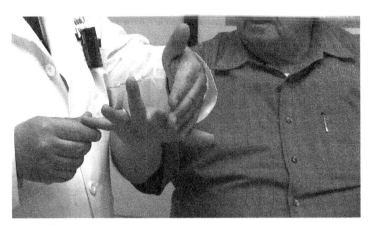

Fig. 13. Painless fingers drop.

- Typical and distal MG are not different in terms of age, gender, and response to treatment.
- Distal weakness in MG usually affects the wrist and fingers extensors and sometimes feet extensors.
- Myopathic units are common and are caused by neuromuscular block of some muscle fibers. CK level is normal. Repetitive stimulation of the ulnar nerve and recording from the abductor digiti quinti usually shows decremental response.

Reference

Werner P, Kiechl S, Löscher W, et al. frequency and clinical course in a large prospective series. Acta Neurol Scand 2003;108(3):209–11.

SUPPLEMENTARY DATA

Supplementary data related to this article can be found at http://dx.doi.org/10.1016/j.ncl.2016.04.014.

Sleep Disorders in Neurologic Practice

A Case-based Approach

Lori Ani Panossian, MD[a], Alon Y. Avidan, MD, MPH[b,*]

KEYWORDS

- Sleep disorders • Narcolepsy • Restless leg syndrome • Sleep apnea
- REM sleep behavior disorder • Insomnia • Circadian rhythm disorders

KEY POINTS

- Patients with neurologic conditions are at increased risk for comorbid sleep disorders, including insomnia, sleep disordered breathing or sleep apnea, circadian rhythm disorder, restless legs syndrome, rapid eye movement–sleep behavior disorder, and narcolepsy.
- Identification and treatment of sleep disorders may improve control of the underlying neurologic condition as well as improve quality of life, and thus comprises a critical component of patient care.
- A reciprocal relationship may exist whereby a sleep disorder can exacerbate a neurologic condition, and the neurologic condition or its treatments can increase risk of a sleep disorder.

CASE A: EPILEPSY AND SLEEP DISORDERED BREATHING

Patients with epilepsy can experience a variety of sleep-related symptoms that may increase the frequency of seizures.

Case Presentation

A 43-year-old woman with a history of epilepsy since childhood presented to neurology clinic for a follow-up visit. She had complex partial seizures with occasional secondary generalization that developed after a bout of meningitis at 8 months of age. She was previously treated with phenobarbital and phenytoin for many years and was later transitioned to carbamazepine monotherapy approximately 10 years ago.

Disclosures: Dr L.A. Panossian has nothing to disclose. Dr A.Y. Avidan is on the speaker's bureaus for Xenoport and Merck and has received honoraria from the American Academy of Neurology, American Academy of Sleep Medicine, American Thoracic Society, and Elsevier

a Sleep Laboratory, East Bay Division, Department of Neurology, Veterans Affairs Northern California Health Care System, 150 Muir Road, Martinez, CA 94553, USA; b Department of Neurology, UCLA Sleep Disorders Center, David Geffen School of Medicine at UCLA, 710 Westwood Boulevard, Room 1-145 RNRC, Los Angeles, CA 90095-1769, USA
* Corresponding author.
E-mail address: avidan@mednet.ucla.edu

Neurol Clin 34 (2016) 565–594
http://dx.doi.org/10.1016/j.ncl.2016.04.003
0733-8619/16/$ – see front matter © 2016 Elsevier Inc. All rights reserved.

neurologic.theclinics.com

Lamotrigine was subsequently added 6 years ago because of poor seizure control. She currently reported approximately 8 to 9 breakthrough seizures per year.

Her chief complaint at the follow-up visit was gradually worsening daytime sleepiness and inadvertent dozing when she was sedentary. On further questioning, she endorsed mild snoring on most nights, restless and poor quality sleep, difficulty falling asleep several times per week, and frequent nighttime awakenings. She had no bed partner but did not think she had any seizures during sleep. Her Epworth Sleepiness Scale (ESS) score was 14 out of 24, indicating excessive sleepiness (normal is <10; **Table 1**). On examination, she had normal waking oxygen saturation, an increased body mass index (BMI) of 31 kg/m^2, neck circumference of 42 cm (16.5 inches), and narrow upper airway anatomy with a modified Mallampati III airway (**Fig. 1**), low-lying soft palate, an elongated uvula, and macroglossia. Her neurologic examination was unremarkable.

Clinical Questions

1. What are some common causes of excessive daytime sleepiness in individuals with epilepsy?
2. What are likely mechanisms by which sleep disturbances may worsen seizures/ increase seizure frequency in patients with epilepsy?
3. In contrast, what mechanisms may confer an increased risk of sleep disordered breathing among patients with epilepsy?

Discussion

Hypersomnolence, a state of recurrent episodes of excessive daytime sleepiness, is frequently encountered among patients with epilepsy and is usually secondary to underlying causes.[1] These causes can include a comorbid sleep disorder such as obstructive sleep apnea (OSA) or insomnia, medication-related adverse effects, psychiatric comorbidities such as depression, or behavioral patterns that may disrupt sleep, such as poor sleep hygiene. Recent data examining sleep in individuals with epilepsy show evidence of fragmented sleep architecture on

Table 1 Epworth Sleepiness Scale	
Situations	**Chance of Dozing**
Sitting and reading	0, 1, 2, 3
Watching television	0, 1, 2, 3
Sitting inactive in a public place (eg, in a theater or a meeting)	0, 1, 2, 3
As a passenger in a car for an hour without a break	0, 1, 2, 3
Lying down to rest in the afternoon when circumstances permit	0, 1, 2, 3
Sitting and talking to someone	0, 1, 2, 3
Sitting quietly after a lunch without alcohol	0, 1, 2, 3
In a car, while stopped for a few minutes in traffic	0, 1, 2, 3

The ESS was developed by researchers in Australia and is widely used by sleep professionals to appraise the degree of excessive sleepiness. Patients are asked "How likely are you to doze off or fall asleep in the following situations, in contrast with feeling just tired?" "This refers to your usual way of life in recent times." Patients are instructed to use the scale to rate the level of their sleepiness in each of the following situations/scenarios: 0, no chance of dozing; 1, slight chance of dozing; 2, moderate chance of dozing; 3, high chance of dozing.
Modified from Johns M. A new method for measuring daytime sleepiness: the Epworth Sleepiness Scale. Sleep 1991;14:540–45.

Class I   Class II

Class III   Class IV

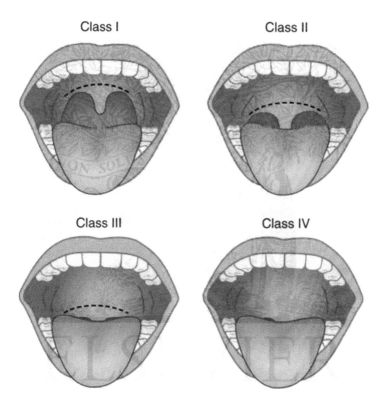

Fig. 1. The Mallampati Airway Classification. During the Mallampati assessment, the patient is instructed to open his or her mouth as wide as possible, while protruding the tongue as far as possible. Patients are instructed to not emit sounds during the assessment. Class I: good visibility of the soft palate and entire uvula; Class II: partial visualization of the soft palate and portion of uvula; Class III: soft palate visible only (may include base of uvula), and; Class IV: soft palate not visible. The system is often used to judge the likelihood of sleep disordered creating, and may be helpful especially in patients who have class III and IV airway.

electroencephalogram (EEG) with increased spontaneous arousals and awaken ings.[2] However, fragmented sleep by electrographic recording does not necessarily correlate with daytime symptoms. Simply having epilepsy is similarly not an independent risk factor for hypersomnia, as shown by comparable scores on objective and subjective measures of sleepiness in untreated patients with epilepsy and healthy controls.[1,3]

In the case described earlier, the patient has features that are suggestive of OSA. The differential diagnosis also includes nocturnal seizures and Insomnia As a premenopausal woman, she does not conform to the demographic profile of a typical patients with OSA given that OSA more commonly occurs in older patient cohorts and in men.[4] Her risk factors for OSA include snoring; obesity; having narrow upper airway anatomy, which predisposes her to upper airway collapse; and having a history of epilepsy.

Epilepsy is independently associated with an increased risk of OSA. Both polysomnography-based and questionnaire-based studies have shown a higher prevalence of OSA among individuals with epilepsy.[5–8] There is evidence that even patients with well-controlled epilepsy have higher OSA rates of between 15% and 30% in polysomnography-based studies, compared with general population estimates of 2% in women and 4% in men.[5,6,9]

Comorbid OSA can have important implications for seizure control as well as quality of life (QOL), cardiovascular risk, and fatigue symptoms. Untreated OSA can worsen seizure control in patients with epilepsy and may provoke spike-wave discharges during sleep.[10,11] Appropriate use of continuous positive airway pressure (CPAP) often improves seizure control and reduces occurrence of interictal discharges, even in medically refractory epilepsy.[5,12]

The mechanism by which epilepsy is associated with OSA has not been clearly elucidated, but studies point to a reciprocal relationship (**Fig. 2**). OSA can worsen seizure control by increasing sympathetic nervous system activity and overall neuronal excitability.[7,13] OSA also causes frequent sleep-wake transitions and sleep fragmentation, which can trigger seizures.[11]

Potential ways that epilepsy can cause sleep apnea include neuronal abnormalities that adversely affect central nervous system (CNS) control of respiration and upper airway tone, weight gain caused by antiepileptic drugs (AEDs) and a less active lifestyle, and AED direct effects on reduction of upper airway muscle tone.[6] There are also some data to suggest that seizures can directly cause apneas, possibly via seizure-induced reduction of upper airway muscle tone and respiratory control. Seizures involving the amygdala are shown to episodically suppress respiration, and therefore could contribute to both sleep apnea and to sudden unexpected death in epilepsy.[14] In support of this hypothesis, a case report showed resolution of sleep apnea after epilepsy surgery in a nonobese 18-year-old man, despite no change in AEDs and a slight postoperative weight gain.[15]

Epilepsy can also lead to daytime hypersomnia for reasons other than sleep disordered breathing. Seizures, sometimes occurring undetected while asleep, may cause postictal somnolence the next day.[16] Moreover, AEDs can disturb sleep architecture and contribute to hypersomnia or insomnia with ensuing daytime sleepiness. AEDs with detrimental sleep effects include phenobarbital, phenytoin, valproic acid, and

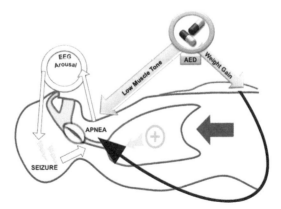

Fig. 2. Epilepsy and obstructive sleep apnea (OSA). Case A: reciprocal relationship between epilepsy and sleep apnea. Antiepileptic drugs (AEDs) can indirectly increase risk of sleep apnea by contributing to weight gain and causing reduced upper airway muscle tone. Furthermore, seizures during sleep can directly induce apneas. Sleep apnea causes frequent electroencephalogram (EEG) microarousals out of sleep, and over the long term can increase overall sympathetic nervous system activity; this can subsequently increase seizure frequency in individuals with epilepsy.

high-dose levetiracetam.[17] However, some AEDs have no effect or can improve sleep architecture, possibly by reducing interictal discharges or subclinical nocturnal seizures.[18,19]

Summary of Case Presentation

In this case, the patient underwent polysomnography testing, which showed moderate to severe OSA with associated episodic moderate oxygen desaturations to a nadir of 81%, from a normal baseline level of 96%. There were no significant interictal discharges or electrographic seizures during sleep during the study. She subsequently initiated treatment with CPAP during sleep. After an initial period of acclimation to CPAP use, at her next follow-up she reported considerable improvement in daytime sleepiness with an improved ESS score of 6 out of 24 and a reduction in nighttime awakenings. She had had no seizures since starting CPAP 3 months prior, and she was optimistic about eventually attempting to wean off 1 of her AEDs.

CASE B: MULTIPLE SCLEROSIS AND INSOMNIA

Sleep disturbance is a frequent complaint among individuals with multiple sclerosis (MS), often leading to worse QOL compared with patients without sleep disturbances.

Case Presentation

A 32-year-old woman with relapsing-remitting MS presented for neurologic follow-up with a chief complaint of severe fatigue during the day and poor sleep at night. She was diagnosed with MS 5 years previously and had been treated since that time with interferon beta-1b. She had had 2 relapses since her initial diagnosis, most recently 18 months ago, with mild residual disability. Recent brain MRI showed several periventricular demyelinating plaques, as well as a small plaque in the spinal cord at C4. Current examination findings included normal vital signs, BMI of 23 kg/m^2, slightly reduced visual acuity of 20/40 on the left, left-sided numbness, mild distal right upper extremity weakness with 4/5 grip strength and mild right lower extremity weakness with 4+/5 strength in the iliopsoas and quadriceps muscles. She also had symptoms of urinary urgency and nocturia with occasional urinary incontinence. She complained of frequent bilateral leg spasms, worse on the right, which were triggered by walking or stretching her limbs. She had trouble falling asleep because of ruminative thoughts and anxiety, and limb discomfort also made it difficult for her to physically relax in bed. She estimated that it took her approximately 2 hours to fall asleep on most nights. She found herself awakening multiple times nightly because of spasms or nocturia, and then had trouble quieting her thoughts in order to go back to sleep. She denied snoring or breathing pauses in sleep. She indicated episodes of irresistible and unintentional sleep attacks during the day. She was distressed by her insomnia, which she thought was contributing to feeling depressed and irritable and causing poor memory and fatigue during the day.

Clinical Questions

1. How common is insomnia in individuals with MS?
2. Does MS cause insomnia?
3. What treatment approaches for insomnia are effective in MS?

Discussion

MS is a chronic condition with associated medical and psychiatric comorbidities that can contribute to a reduced health-related QOL. Prominent among these are sleep disturbances. Chronic insomnia is highly prevalent in MS with reported rates of 22% to 52%.[20,21] Chronic insomnia is defined as at least 3 months of difficulty initiating and/or maintaining sleep, with ensuing impairments in daytime functioning at least 3 times per week.[22] Among patients with MS, insomnia is more prevalent in women, individuals with mood symptoms, and those with multiple medical problems.[20] Insomnia is also associated with poor QOL, highlighting the importance of identifying, evaluating, and treating this common condition.[23]

Insomnia in MS is frequently not intrinsic, but occurs secondary to medical symptoms such as pain, spasticity, and nocturia, and psychiatric disorders such as depression and anxiety.[24] **Fig. 3** Pain and discomfort from spasticity and mobility limitations can contribute to sleep-onset and sleep-maintenance insomnia and daytime fatigue.[25,26] Although not specific for MS, chronic pain conditions can adversely affect sleep EEG architecture by causing alpha intrusions during deep slow wave sleep, more frequent arousals into lighter sleep stages, and reduced sleep efficiency.[27] A reciprocal relationship exists between pain and sleep by which poor or fragmented sleep can also worsen the perception of pain, thereby perpetuating the maladaptive cycle.[28] Nocturia and other symptoms of neurogenic bladder can contribute especially to sleep-maintenance insomnia, with frequent nocturnal awakenings and ensuing difficulty falling back to sleep. Pharmacologic treatment of the underlying bladder dysfunction can help to improve sleep consolidation and reduce daytime fatigue.[29]

Mood disorders also play a prominent role. Patients with MS with depression are much more likely to have insomnia compared with the overall MS population.[30] Effectively treating depression and anxiety with psychotherapy directly correlates with the degree of insomnia improvement, particularly in sleep-onset insomnia.[30] Pharmacologic treatment with antidepressant medication should also be considered as part of a comprehensive approach to managing depression and fatigue symptoms in MS. For example, studies have found that use of duloxetine, a dual serotonin and norepinephrine reuptake inhibitor, was associated with improved mood, lessened fatigue, reduced pain, and improved sleep quality.[31,32]

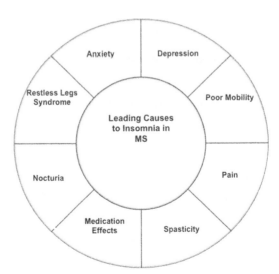

Fig. 3. Multiple sclerosis (MS) and insomnia. Multiple medical and psychiatric comorbidities can interact to contribute to secondary insomnia in individuals with multiple sclerosis.

As in the general population, primary psychophysiologic insomnia can also occur in patients with MS. This phenotype of insomnia is characterized by a learned pattern of maladaptive behaviors and negative associations with regard to sleep, and psychological and physiologic heightened arousal during sleep attempts.[33] An effective nonpharmacologic treatment is a course of cognitive behavior therapy for insomnia (CBTi) that targets both excessive thoughts about sleep inability and negative behaviors that maintain the dysfunctional sleep habits.[34,35]

Medications for sleep can also be used, particularly when treatment of underlying medical and psychological problems have not resulted in a significant improvement in insomnia. However, data regarding their efficacy in MS are sparse and the available studies have yielded mixed results; for example, with eszopiclone causing improved total sleep time but insufficient symptomatic improvement in fatigue.[36] Hypnotic medications for the general population consist of benzodiazepine receptor agonists that act on the gamma-aminobutyric acid A receptor complex, as well as newer generation nonbenzodiazepine receptor agonists with shorter half-lives and fewer side effects, including zolpidem (regular and controlled release), zaleplon, and eszopiclone.[37] Melatonin receptor agonists (ramelteon) may be helpful in patients with sleep-onset insomnia. Doxepin, a histamine H_1 receptor antagonist, has also received US Food and Drug Administration (FDA) approval for the treatment of chronic sleep initiation and maintenance insomnia. The most recently approved hypnotic agent is suvorexant, a hypocretin receptor antagonist, currently available for management of sleep-onset and maintenance insomnia.[38,39]

Other sleep disorders can also co-occur with MS, including (in non–population-based samples) narcolepsy (prevalence of 0%–1.6%), restless legs syndrome (RLS; prevalence of 14%–58%), rapid eye movement (REM) sleep behavior disorder (RBD; prevalence of 2%–3%), and OSA (prevalence of 7%–58%).[40] Although sleep symptoms are present in most patients with MS, often the conditions are not formally diagnosed or sufficiently evaluated by providers.[41,42] Varied rates of awareness and testing by clinical providers may in part explain the wide range of reported prevalences for sleep disorders in MS.

Summary of Case Presentation

In the case discussed earlier, the patient's symptoms of pain, depression, and anxiety were targeted as the first steps in improving sleep. She was started on baclofen for treatment of painful limb spasms and referred to a psychologist for CBTi as well as for fatigue and mood management. At her 6-week follow-up visit, she reported partial improvement in her sleep symptoms. She was able to fall asleep within 30 minutes on most nights, and was less prone to excessively ruminating and worrying about sleep. Spasms were improved with baclofen, which she used primarily in the evenings because it also made her drowsy. She continued to have nocturia 3 to 4 times per night and therefore was given a prescription for oxybutynin, which significantly improved the frequency of nocturia and sleep continuity on subsequent visits.

CASE C: ALZHEIMER DISEASE AND CIRCADIAN RHYTHM DISORDER, ADVANCED SLEEP PHASE TYPE

Sleep disturbances can pose a significant challenge in the management and QOL of patients with dementia. Interventions to improve sleep in this population are important because they can improve nighttime sleep and daytime wakefulness, and reduce caregiver burden.

Case Presentation

An 00-year old man proconts to nourology clinic for initial consultation regarding memory loss. He lives with his daughter, who accompanied him to the appointment. They describe a 5-year history of insidious and slowly progressive memory loss with symptoms of forgetfulness, inability to manage complex tasks such as his finances, confusion when trying to follow directions, and frequent repetitive questioning. He had to stop driving because of several instances of getting lost in familiar areas. A prior neuropsychological testing battery had revealed primarily amnestic mild-to-moderate cognitive impairment with a lesser degree of executive dysfunction, in a pattern most consistent with a neurodegenerative process such as Alzheimer disease (AD). On neurologic examination, his Mini-Mental State Examination score was 23 out of 30 (reflecting mild cognitive impairment) and he had an otherwise unremarkable neurologic examination with no extraocular movement abnormalities, no tremor or motor findings, and intact gait and balance. Brain MRI showed moderate diffuse cerebral atrophy and mild periventricular leukoaraiosis.

His daughter inquired about the possibility of treatment with a cholinesterase inhibitor and whether her father could be prescribed a sleeping medication to help address his early morning awakenings. Further questioning of his sleep pattern indicated that he would doze off intermittently throughout the afternoon and evening in his recliner, but seemed to have significant difficulties maintaining sleeping during the later part of the night and would often be heard pacing around the house after 4 AM. His daughter was very concerned about the risk of falls or accidents as a result of the patient's pre-dawn restlessness.

Clinical Questions

1. What are likely mechanisms for the development of sleep cycle alterations and daytime sleepiness in individuals with AD?
2. What are some potential sequelae and adverse health effects of untreated circadian rhythm disorders among elderly individuals or patients with dementia?

Discussion

Changes in sleep patterns and sleep stage architecture can occur with advancing age. Normal age-related changes after age 60 years can include fragmentation of sleep with frequent brief EEG arousals, decreased sleep efficiency (time spent asleep compared with time spent attempting to sleep), increased time to onset of sleep, and a reduction in the proportion and EEG spectral power of slow wave and REM sleep.[43–45] These disturbances in sleep become even more pronounced among individuals with dementia syndromes such as AD.[46]

Older individuals and particularly those with cognitive impairment are much more likely to experience decreased total sleep time at night, early morning awakenings, and a propensity to nap throughout the day. This alteration in circadian rhythmicity of sleep with a propensity for phase advancement of sleep timing is known as advanced sleep phase syndrome (ASPS).[43,47] Circadian rhythms are generated by biological clocks that use external cues such as light to entrain and coordinate biological processes. Circadian control of sleep-wake cycles is mediated by the suprachiasmatic nucleus (SCN) of the hypothalamus using the pineal gland–produced hormone melatonin.[48] In AD, neurodegeneration of cortical and subcortical areas, including neuronal loss in the SCN, may be responsible for circadian abnormalities such as ASPS as well as the phenomenon of worsened evening confusion and behavioral problems known as sundowning.[43,48]

Patients with AD frequently develop irregular sleep rhythms with difficulty staying asleep for consolidated periods of time, long awakenings at night, and daytime sleepiness requiring frequent naps. These disrupted sleep behaviors can be problematic both for patients and for their caregivers. Patients with AD who are active late at night are at higher risk for falls, accidents, wandering, or confusion. Sleepiness during the day also interferes with caregiving and medication schedules as well as reducing the opportunity for exercise and social interaction. In addition, daytime sleepiness and fragmented or inadequate nighttime sleep can contribute to poor cognitive performance both in patients with AD and in healthy adults because of adverse effects on attention, concentration, and sustained vigilance.[49]

In addition to circadian rhythm disturbance, other sleep disorders can also be associated with AD. There is an increased risk of OSA; CPAP treatment can often improve cognition in individuals with dementia and comorbid OSA.[35] Other comorbid sleep disorders include insomnia, which is usually secondary to factors such as ASPS, pain, nocturia, RLS, or periodic limb movement disorder of sleep (PLMDS).[50] In elderly or institutionalized adults, the increased risk for RLS and PLMD may be associated with reduced iron stores or use of neuroleptic medications, including selective serotonin reuptake inhibitors.[50] RLS and PLMD may contribute to poor sleep, and may be difficult to diagnose in cognitively impaired individuals who cannot provide a reliable history. Poor sleep may also exacerbate the symptoms of many comorbid sleep disorders, including RLS, PLMD, and ASPS[49] (**Fig. 4**).

Several recent studies have found an association between early markers of sleep and circadian disruption and subsequent onset of cognitive impairment, as shown in **Fig. 4**.[51–53] It is possible that sleep architecture changes and circadian abnormalities play a causal role in contributing to the development of dementia in healthy older individuals.[54] Studies in animal models have investigated possible mechanisms for

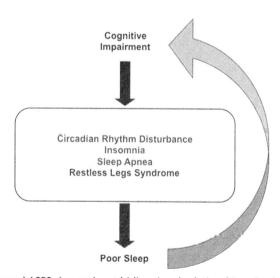

Fig. 4. Alzheimer and ASPS. A prominent bidirectional relationship exists between cognitive impairment and poor sleep. Sleep loss can transiently reduce attention and concentration, and may play a direct role in the development of neurodegenerative disorders such as Alzheimer disease. Individuals with dementia, including Alzheimer disease, are at higher risk for sleep disorders such as circadian rhythm disturbance, insomnia, sleep apnea, and RLS/periodic limb movement disorder, all of which can reduce sleep quality and duration.

this and found evidence that amyloid β accumulation in the brain is under circadian control.[55] Moreover, sleep loss in both animals and humans is associated with increased levels of amyloid-β, which is thought to be the inciting event in the development of AD.[56,57]

Given the prominent bidirectional relationship between sleep regulation and cognitive function, sleep should be an important concern in the management of AD. Circadian rhythm disturbance and ASPS can be treated primarily with behavioral interventions. These interventions include optimizing the patient's environment to ensure adequate natural light exposure and exercise during the day, minimizing prolonged naps and sedentary status during the day, avoiding excessive light exposure and mental or physical stimulation in the evenings, and adjusting the timing of medication administration to facilitate sleep at night when possible.[43] For patients with AD without ASPS, bright light therapy with at least a 30-minute exposure to full-spectrum light using a light box or natural sunlight in the mornings is effective. For patients with ASPS, bright light exposure is helpful during periods of excessive sleepiness in the late afternoon to early evening, because it may help delay the circadian phase in ASPS.[59] Pharmacologic therapies may also have some benefit. Treatment of insomnia with the dietary supplement, melatonin, is frequently used in the evenings for circadian regulation, but some studies have shown no significant benefit in patients with AD.[50,60] Other pharmacologic approaches have been tried with varying degrees of success, including 1 trial of trazodone that showed significant improvement in sleep among patients with AD.[61] Pharmacologic treatments for sleep should be used judiciously in AD with careful consideration of the potential benefit versus the inherit risks and side effect profiles.[50]

Summary of Case Presentation

In the case of the patient with AD, he was diagnosed with ASPS. Behavioral changes focused on activities conducive to improving the circadian desynchronization (ie, a loss of synchrony of the sleep-wake cycle) were initially recommended as a first-line treatment. At the subsequent follow-up visit, his daughter reported mild improvements in nighttime sleep after the patient joined an adult day program to increase his daytime activity and decrease likelihood of napping. He was also taking short walks with his daughter in the late afternoon for increased light exposure. As a safety measure, he was now sleeping downstairs and with a night-light to reduce fall risk in case of nocturnal awakenings. He was advised to take his donepezil dose in the mornings rather than at bedtime to reduce the potential alerting effects of acetylcholinesterase inhibitors.

CASE D: SECONDARY NARCOLEPSY IN A PATIENT WITH NEUROSARCOIDOSIS OF THE HYPOTHALAMUS

Narcolepsy type 1 (NT1; formerly narcolepsy with cataplexy) is a category of CNS hypersomnia reflecting a dysfunction of the hypocretin-producing neurons in the diencephalon. Most patients with NT1 and cataplexy have low or undetectable levels of hypocretin-1 in the cerebrospinal fluid (CSF). Pathologically low hypocretin levels have been reported in patients with underlying diencephalic injuries caused by CNS disorders, including stroke, tumors, neurosarcoidosis, or demyelinating disease.

Case Presentation

A 53-year-old man, who was previously in good health, presented from an outside institution for a higher level of care with alterations in consciousness, with unexplained weight loss, fevers, night sweats, and severe pathologic hypersomnolence.[62] Brain MRI revealed a diencephalic lesion with specific involvement of the hypothalamus demarcated with both T2 and T1 postcontrast hyperintensity (**Fig. 5**) within this region.

Hypothalamic biopsy showed neurosarcoidosis exemplified by noncaseating granulomas and exclusion of other infectious diseases. Physical examination revealed a lethargic, thin man who aroused sporadically to verbal stimuli, and showed a brief attention span of approximately 10 seconds, lapsing back to sleep.[62]

The patient proceeded to undergo a lumbar puncture revealing a CSF hypocretin level of 0 pg/mL. The CSF was otherwise clear and colorless with 2 red blood cells, 3 white blood cells, without evidence for demyelination. Major histocompatibility complex, class II, DQ beta 1 0602 (human leukocyte antigen [HLA]–DQB1*0602) was negative.[62]

Clinical Questions

1. What is the most likely explanation for the patient's severe hypersomnolence?
2. What are the different types of hypersomnias related to a CNS cause?

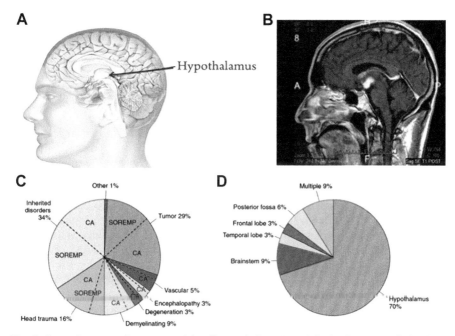

Fig. 5. Secondary narcolepsy caused by diencephalic injury. (*A*) The location of the diencephalon, where the wake-stabilizing hypocretin-producing cells are localized. (*B*) Brain MRI indicated involvement of the hypothalamus, showing postcontrast hyperintensity within the anterior hypothalamus. The patient did not experience any brainstem involvement, nor were any appreciable lesions found in the locus coeruleus or raphe nuclei. (*C, D*) Neurologic diseases and location of brain lesions in 113 cases of secondary narcolepsy. (*C*) Neurologic diseases are shown by category reported as secondary narcolepsy. Reported here are tumors, inherited disorders, and head trauma, which are the 3 most frequent causes. The percentage of cataplexy (CA) or sleep-onset REM periods (SOREMP) is denoted in each category with a dashed line. (*D*) Location of brain lesions in symptomatic patients with narcolepsy associated with brain tumor; the hypothalamus and adjacent structures are the most common location. Included are 113 symptomatic cases of narcolepsy. (*Modified from* Kanbayashi T, Sagawa T, Takemura F, et al. The pathophysiologic basis of secondary narcolepsy and hypersomnia. Curr Neurol Neurosci Rep 2011;11(2):235–41.)

3. What is the differential diagnosis of narcolepsy?
4. What are specific drug treatments for centrally mediated hypersomnia?

Discussion

The International Classification of Sleep Disorders-III (ICSD-III) divides narcolepsy into 2 subtypes: narcolepsy type 1 (NT1; with cataplexy, or associated with low hypocretin levels), and narcolepsy type 2 (NT2; without cataplexy, and with normal hypocretin levels).[63] Secondary narcolepsy caused by a known underlying CNS disorder, as in the case presented earlier, is referred to as NT1 caused by a medical condition (when hypocretin levels are low) or NT2 caused by a medical condition (when hypocretin levels are normal).[63]

Narcolepsy symptoms include severe unremitting hypersomnolence with sleep attacks in 100% of patients, cataplexy (in 60%–70% of patients), sleep paralysis (in 25%–50%), hypnagogic hallucinations (in 20%–40%), disturbed night sleep (in 70%–80%), and automatic behavior (in 20%–40% of patients). Sleep attacks are defined as chronic and irresistible desire to fall asleep at inappropriate opportunities and in inappropriate places (eg, while driving, playing, eating), as illustrated in **Fig. 6**.[64,65] About a third of patients report 3 of the 4 major manifestations of the narcoleptic tetrad (sleep attacks, cataplexy, sleep paralysis, and hypnagogic hallucinations), and about 10% of patients describe all 4 major features occurring together.[66,67]

Cataplexy is pathognomonic for narcolepsy, and is defined as a sudden loss of skeletal muscle tone typically preceded by a prodromal powerful emotional stimulus, such as laughter, excitement, surprise, or anger, leading to a transient loss of skeletal muscle tone.[64,65] Episodes of cataplexy typically last from a few seconds to several minutes; may be partial or complete; and appear to an observer to consist of head nodding, sagging of the jaw, and buckling of the knees. However, consciousness is always preserved, and neurologic examination shows flaccidity of the muscles and markedly reduced or even absent skeletal muscle stretch reflexes. Cataplexy does not always present with the onset of hypersomnolence, but may manifest months to years after the initial onset of sleepiness.[65] Physiologically, during cataplexy, skeletal muscle weakness is generated by decreased excitation of noradrenergic neurons and increased inhibition of motor neurons by gamma-aminobutyric acid–releasing or glycinergic neurons.[68]

Sleep paralysis consists of paralysis of skeletal muscle tone, lasting from a few minutes to as long as 15 to 20 minutes, and occurs either during sleep onset or immediately on awakening. Patients describe frightening spells of complete paralysis, with inability to move or speak with preservation of consciousness. Hallucinations in narcolepsy occur during sleep onset (hypnagogic) or on awakening (hypnopompic) and are reported as vibrant and dramatic visual (and often fear-inducing) hallucinations but could also present as auditory, vestibular, or somesthetic.

Narcolepsy is a manifestation of inability to maintain wakefulness during the day and, paradoxically, inability to maintain sleep during the night: although patients are pathologically sleepy during the day, as many as 70% to 80% report significant disruption of their ability to maintain sleep.[65] Automatic behavior in narcolepsy consists of repeated performance of a single monotonous, repetitive, routine task, such as writing, shopping, or driving, in a dull manner without conscious memory or awareness of the behavior.[65] Automatic behaviors in narcolepsy are thought to emerge from partial sleep episodes, frequent lapses, or microsleeps.

It has been established that HLA-DQB1*0602 is a biomarker for narcolepsy across all ethnic groups. About 12% to 38% of the general population carries this HLA allele, whereas narcolepsy is present in only 0.02% to 0.18% of the population. Hypocretin

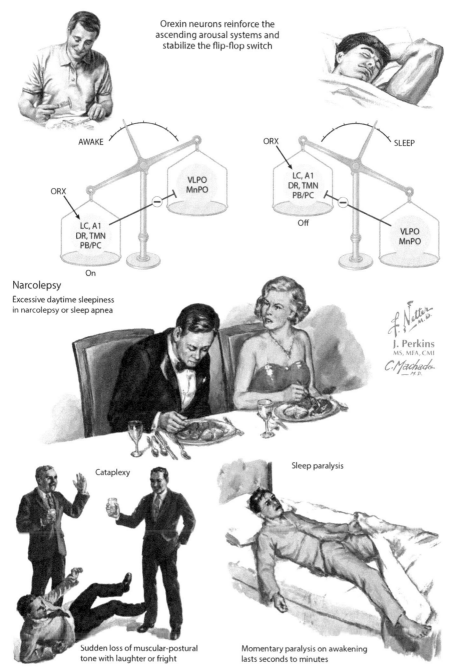

Orexin neurons reinforce the
ascending arousal systems and
stabilize the flip-flop switch

AWAKE

ORX

ORX
LC, A1
DR, TMN
PB/PC

VLPO
MnPO

On

ORX

SLEEP

LC, A1
DR, TMN
PB/PC

Off

VLPO
MnPO

Narcolepsy

Excessive daytime sleepiness
in narcolepsy or sleep apnea

Cataplexy

Sleep paralysis

Sudden loss of muscular-postural
tone with laughter or fright

Momentary paralysis on awakening
lasts seconds to minutes

Fig. 6. Narcolepsy: A Hypothalamic Sleep Disorder. Orexin/Hypocretin (ORX) ventrolateral preoptic nucleus (VLPO), Median preoptic nucleus (MnPO), tuberomammillary nucleus (TMN), the locus coeruleus (LC), parabrachial and precoeruleus (PB/PC) nuclei, Adenosine A1 Receptors (A1), dorsal raphe (DR).

levels are generally normal if the patient is HLA DQB1*0602 negative, unless the patient has a diencephalic lesion that explains the CNS hypersomnia—NT1 caused by a medical condition, as in the patient presented.[63]

The current underlying pathophysiology of narcolepsy-cataplexy syndrome is thought to manifest from an injury or degeneration, possibly through an autoimmune process, of the hypocretin neurons residing in the perifornical and lateral regions of the hypothalamus.[69–71] Narcolepsy-cataplexy syndrome (NT1) thus can be considered a hypocretin deficiency syndrome, which is how the condition is currently referred to in the updated version of the ICSD-III.[63]

The differential diagnosis of hypersomnia is extensive, but includes sleep deprivation and insufficient sleep syndrome (voluntary sleep curtailment); sleep disordered breathing (such as OSA); hypersomnias related to alcohol and medications; circadian rhythm sleep disorders (such as delayed sleep phase syndrome); and medical, neurologic, and psychiatric disorders causing hypersomnolence. Common neurologic diseases presenting with pathologic sleepiness include MS, myotonic dystrophy, and Parkinson disease.

OSA is the most common cause of hypersomnia in patients referred to a sleep laboratory for evaluation. Idiopathic hypersomnia (IH) overlaps with narcolepsy syndrome in that these patients are pathologically sleepy, but, in contrast with narcolepsy, the sleep episodes in IH are prolonged, and the sleep is not refreshing. Cataplexy should be differentiated from atonic seizures (as well as gelastic-atonic seizures characterized by laughing followed by loss of muscle tone), drop attacks, basilar migraines, vertebrobasilar insufficiency, and syncope.

Management of narcolepsy consists of nonpharmacologic and pharmacologic treatment strategies.[64] Behavioral, or nonpharmacologic, treatments include scheduled short daytime power naps typically lasting between 15 and 20 minutes in the early to midafternoon; measures to enhance sleep hygiene, such as maintenance of a regular sleep schedule; and avoidance of sleep deprivation. Strategies to address excessive daytime sleepiness include the use of wake-promoting agents such as modafinil or armodafinil and stimulants such as methylphenidate, dextroamphetamine, or methamphetamine.[64,72,73] Treatment of cataplexy and other REM intrusion events of narcolepsy (such as sleep paralysis and hypnagogic hallucinations) depends on the frequency and severity of these episodes. For cataplexy, treatment with tricyclic antidepressants, serotonin norepinephrine reuptake inhibitors, or selective serotonin reuptake inhibitors (SSRIs) is helpful. However, sodium oxybate (gamma hydroxybutyric acid) is specifically indicated for the treatment of cataplexy as well as daytime sleepiness in the setting of NT1 and NT2.[72,73]

Summary of the Case Presentation

The patient presented with other manifestations of hypothalamic dysfunction, including inability to feed and regulate body temperature, and panhypopituitarism. He was witnessed to experience cataplexy later during the hospital course. The case is an example of symptomatic or secondary narcolepsy, terms used to describe narcolepsy associated with underlying structural, genetic, inflammatory, or vascular abnormality affecting the hypothalamus and leading to severe CNS hypersomnolence with or without cataplexy or abnormal CSF hypocretin levels. Depending on the presence of cataplexy or reduced CSF hypocretin levels, NT1 or NT2 may be diagnosed. As illustrated in **Fig. 5**, leading CNS causes of secondary narcolepsy include diencephalic and midbrain tumors, cerebrovascular disease, traumatic brain injury, MS, vascular malformations, encephalitis, cerebral trauma, and paraneoplastic syndrome with anti-Ma2.[74–79]

CASE E: RESTLESS LEGS SYNDROME MANIFESTING WITH SLEEP-ONSET INSOMNIA, POOR QUALITY OF LIFE, AND EXCESSIVE SLEEPINESS

Also known as Willis-Ekbom disease (WED), RLS is a sleep-related neurologic disorder that affects about 5% to 10% of the adult population. It has specific diagnostic clinical criteria and effective treatment strategies that make screening and management of this condition critical in sleep medicine practice.

Case Presentation

A 71-year-old man presents to the sleep disorders clinic with bothersome complaints of irresistible urge to constantly move his legs and significant sleep-onset insomnia occurring on a nightly basis. He is observed to engage in vigorous stretching and flexing of his legs, and to have difficulties remaining still during long drives and prolonged international flights to visit his daughter and her family, who live overseas. His wife describes that he constantly moves his legs back and forth in the evening and has bothersome and frequent leg jerks throughout the night. He is presenting to clinic because his symptoms are now intolerable. Activities that improve or alleviate the symptoms include stretching the legs, getting out of bed, walking, and massaging his legs. His wife says that the leg jerks also severely disrupt her sleep during the night.

Clinical Questions

1. What are the diagnostic criteria for RLS?
2. What is the most likely cause for the reported leg jerks?
3. What are the specific treatment strategies for RLS?
4. What are the key treatment-related side effects that must be reviewed with every patient with RLS?

Discussion

RLS is also known as WED, which credits the British physician Sir Thomas Willis (1621–1675), who first noted the disorder during his studies of the human nervous system, and the Swedish neurologist Dr Karl-Axel Ekbom (1907–1977), who originally named the condition RLS.[80,81]

Five essential diagnostic criteria used for diagnosing RLS/WED are (1) an urge or a compulsion to move the legs, (2) worsening of this discomfort in the evening, (3) temporary relief of the discomfort by movement, (4) worsening of symptoms during rest, and (5) symptoms that are not solely caused by another medical or behavioral condition.[80,81] The condition manifests as insomnia, and can significantly impair health-related QOL by worsening pain, vitality, and social functioning. The reduced QOL for individuals with RLS/WED is comparable with that of patients with serious chronic medical conditions, such as hypertension and diabetes.[82,83]

RLS is a prevalent sleep disorder, affecting about 10% of the general population[84–86] and often presents, as in the patient described earlier, with difficulties initiating sleep.[87] RLS is further classified into primary, if no identifiable cause can be established, or secondary, when a comorbid neurologic or medical condition is identified.[88,89] Patients with primary RLS/WED have greater than a 50% probability of having a first-degree relative with this condition.[90–92]

Up to 80% of patients with RLS/WED also experience undesirable nocturnal myoclonic movements known as periodic limb movements of sleep (PLMS), as shown in **Fig. 7**, consisting of rhythmic, stereotyped movements of the legs during sleep.[93] PLMS can be asymptomatic, or may induce sleep disruption, insomnia, and excessive daytime sleepiness. The combination of PLMS and symptoms of disrupted sleep is

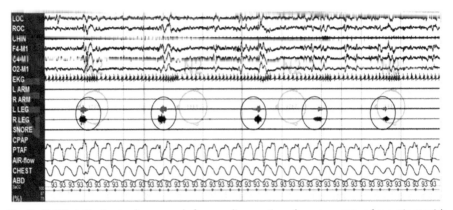

Fig. 7. PLMS. A 2-minute sleep epoch from a diagnostic polysomnogram of a patient with PLMS associated with an irresistible urge to move her legs. Her husband reports that she has frequent nighttime kicking and jerking movements that disrupt his sleep. A succession of 5 periodic limb movements are shown (circled in purple), occurring in the right and left legs (anterior tibialis muscles). According to the American Academy of Sleep Medicine, periodic leg movements are diagnosed when more than 15 leg movements per hour of sleep are captured. Four or more consecutive movements are required and the interval between movements is typically 20 to 40 seconds. The movements should appear at sequence of 4 or more separated by an interval of more than 5 and less than 90 seconds and have an amplitude of greater than or equal to 25% of toe dorsiflexion during the calibration. Reference electrodes (F4, C4, O2) are referenced to mastoid electrode (M1) or average (AVG). ABD, abdominal respiratory effort; CHEST, chest respiratory effort; Chin, Chin electromyogram; EKG, electrocardiogram; L, left; LOC, left electro-oculogram; PTAF, nasal pressure; R, right; R LEG, right anterior tibias surface electromyogram; ROC, right electro-oculogram; SNORE, snore sensor air flow, nasal and oral airflow; Spo$_2$, pulse oximetry.

known as the syndrome of PLMDS. PLMDS represents a separate diagnosis from RLS, although the two frequently co-occur.

The pathophysiology of RLS/WED and PLMDS is based on studies of brain iron and dopamine metabolism, which suggest a CNS cause involving 3 major contributors to the disease: iron, dopamine (DA), and glutamate. However, recent data indicate that brain iron deficiency acting partially through hypoxic pathway activation, induces increased presynaptic and synaptic DA, which produces postsynaptic downregulation that overcorrects for the normal evening and nocturnal decrease in dopamine-promoting RLS/WED.[94]

The differential diagnosis of RLS/WED is critical to establish, because many other conditions, such as nocturnal leg cramps (NLC), positional discomfort, peripheral neuropathy, akathisias, and neurogenic and vascular claudication, can complicate the diagnosis by meeting 4 diagnostic criteria for RLS (1, 2, 3, and 4 mentioned earlier) and hence mimic RLS.[95–97] Definitive RLS/WED diagnosis now requires exclusion of these other conditions (criterion 5 listed earlier).[95] To further elucidate the differential diagnosis of RLS/WED, clinicians may ask patients about the circadian time predilection (which is often more specific to RLS), painful palpable muscle contraction or cramping (more unique to NLC), an inner body as opposed to peripheral restlessness in patients who are on neuroleptics drugs (more specific to akathisias), and amelioration with rest (symptomatic of vascular claudication).[96,98,99]

As mentioned earlier, the specific cause of the patient's leg jerks is most likely relate to PLMS, which are described as a series of stereotyped leg movements consisting of dorsiflexion of the foot and extension of the big toe, occurring at a typical frequency of every 20 to 40 seconds throughout the night, but primarily during non-REM (NREM) sleep. Patients with PLMDS typically report disturbed sleep continuity, insomnia, reduced sleep quality, or hypersomnia secondary to nighttime arousals. Although PLMDS can be suspected based on a clinical history or reports by bed partners of disruptive limb movements, the condition requires formal polysomnographic diagnosis.

Management strategies for RLS/WED include both nonpharmacologic and specific pharmacologic intervention strategies.[100,101] Conservative, behavioral, nonpharmacologic approaches are appropriate first options and include the removal of medications or substances known to induce/worsen RLS/WED. Examples include discontinuation of substances such as tobacco, alcohol, and caffeine and removal of medications such as dopamine antagonists, antiemetics, lithium, and antidepressants (particularly SSRIs, tricyclic antidepressants).[96,100–102] Iron deficiency can exacerbate RLS symptoms and therefore iron should be supplemented if appropriate when serum ferritin levels decrease to less than 50 ng/mL (50 µg/L).[96] It is suggested that any patient with newly diagnosed RLS/WED or patients with RLS with a recent exacerbation of symptoms should have their serum ferritin levels measured and, when appropriate, supplemented with iron sulfate and, when clinically indicated, undergo an evaluation for iron deficiency.[103]

Specific drug therapy for patients with RLS/WED should be entertained for patients who described insomnia, daytime consequences, or poor sleep quality or duration. Prescribers should monitor for treatment-related side effects, and emergence of DA-specific side effects including augmentation, rebound, daytime somnolence, and impulse control behaviors (ICB). Management with DA and alpha-2-delta ligands are the most well studied and may represent the most appropriate first-line option for most patients who present with moderate to severe primary RLS/WED.[100–102] The FDA-approved dopamine agonists include ropinirole, pramipexole, and rotigotine, and the alpha-2-delta ligand gabapentin enacarbil.[104,105]

Specific drug class–associated side effects attributable to dopaminergic agents include nausea, hallucinations, hypotension, and ICB.[106] Augmentation refers to a geographic spread of sensory symptoms to previously unaffected body parts, as well as to onset of RLS/WED symptoms earlier in the day. The rates of these DA-specific side effects can be as high as 70% of patients treated with dopamine precursors (carbidopa, levodopa), especially in doses exceeding 200 mg.[107] Adverse effects of alpha-2-delta ligands generally include hypersomnolence, weight gain, and dizziness.[105] Alpha-2-delta ligands may be appropriate for patients with RLS/WED who have experienced significant comorbid insomnia and anxiety, and for those who have a history of, or report, DA-induced augmentation.

Benzodiazepines, particularly clonazepam, may be efficacious in RLS/WED and may also help patients with bothersome PLMDS, but are limited because of sedation and respiratory depression, which is particularly problematic for older adults.[108] Note that, as of February 2016, there are currently no FDA-approved treatments specifically to address PLMD.

Summary of the Case Presentation

Given that the patient reported frequent episodes of RLS/WED symptoms that affected his QOL, he was placed on a DA on a nightly basis, which completely resolved his symptoms and even reduced the leg jerks noted by his wife. However, a few weeks after initiating therapy, his wife, who was well informed about ICB, noted that he was compulsively shopping online and spending hundreds of dollars each week on nones-sential items. The patient was immediately switched to an alpha-2-delta ligand, which resolved his compulsive shopping and improved his nighttime and daytime symptoms arising from RLS/WED.

CASE F: RAPID EYE MOVEMENT SLEEP BEHAVIOR DISORDER

Patients who present with RBD are generally older men with potentially injurious nocturnal behaviors; these individuals have high rates of phenoconversion to a neuro-degenerative disease.

Case Presentation

A happily married 65-year-old man presents with episodes of dream enactment since 2013 associated with flailing of the arms, kicking of the legs, thrashing, yelling, and screaming. One sleep episode resulted in kicking of his leg as if trying to kick a ball, leading to fracture of his right toe. Another spell involved punching of a thief in his dream, but resulted in punching of his wife, resulting in severe ecchymosis and zygomatic fracture. Since then, he has begun to sleep in a sleeping bag so as to protect himself from hurting himself and his wife. He was seen by his primary care physician who prescribed him clonazepam at night to help calm him down, at a dose of 0.25 mg, which contributed to 80% improvement within 2 weeks of therapy. He is on no other medications besides clonazepam and his general and neurologic examination are normal. His wife is apprehensive because she read on the Internet that people who fight during their dreams may develop Parkinson dis-ease later in life.

Clinical Questions

1. What is RBD?
2. How is RBD diagnosed?
3. What are some specific treatment strategies for RBD?
4. What should your response be regarding the wife's concerns about RBD?

Discussion

Parasomnias are defined as abnormal and undesirable sensory, motor, or verbal phenomena that manifest during sleep or sleep-wake transition. Parasomnias are sub-divided into episodes that occur during NREM sleep, also known as disorders of arousal, which include sleepwalking, sleep terrors, and confusional arousals.[109,110] REM sleep parasomnias consist of isolated sleep paralysis, nightmares, and RBD, for which memory is typically retained for the event on awakening, usually in the form of a dream.[109–111] REM sleep is accompanied by a loss of skeletal muscle tone throughout most of the body. However, in RBD, patients experience pathologic augmentation of skeletal muscle tone during REM sleep along with unusual, often complex, and sometimes vigorous, violent, and potentially injurious motor activity during the dream enactment sequence. The potential for patients to harm themselves and their bed partners, as in the patient described earlier, is high.[112,113]

The prevalence of RBD is about 0.5% of the population.[114] The disorder has a unique gender predilection, affecting male patients by a factor of 9, and is more likely to manifest in older patients, more than age 50 years. The reason for this gender pre-dilection remains unclear.[115–117]

The diagnosis is suspected clinically, but must be confirmed by conducting a sleep study to show abnormal increase of chin or limb muscle tone during REM sleep with synchronous complex motor activity associated with elaborate dream enactment that corresponds and synchronizes with the dream sequence (**Fig. 8**).[112] The spectrum of abnormal behaviors is wide, ranging from unpleasant hallucinatory behaviors to kicking, yelling, punching, and pugilistic or negative dream content often involving experiences of being confronted by an intruder requiring patients to defend or protect themselves.

REM SLEEP BEHAVIOR DISORDER

Patients who lose their ability to be paralyzed during REM sleep begin to act out their dreams and are usually unaware of these occurrences because the episodes occur during sleep. Often the first episodes are observed by the spouses of the patients.

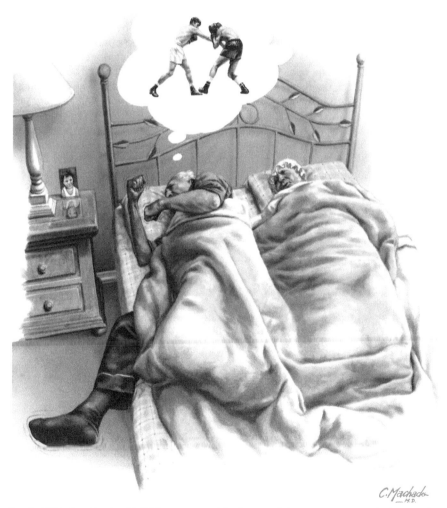

Fig. 8. RBD. A patient with RBD presents with abnormal dreams enactment behavior clinically, as manifested in this illustration of a man who is punching the wall, as in the case presented in the text, as if in a quasi–dream enactment flight/boxing match, with potential for injuries to self and bed partner.

However, many times it is the injury to the patient and the patient's bed partner that brings the patient to the attention of the clinician. When awoken from an episode, some patients have vivid recall and report dream mentation that correlates with the observed behavior. The frequency of RBD spells is variable from infrequent (ie, once a month) to as frequent as nightly. More frequent episodes lead to significant sleep disruption and are more likely to result in sleep fragmentation, hypersomnolence, and increased likelihood to translate to a referral to the specialist.[118] The potential for injury such as facial ecchymosis, skin lacerations, and skull fractures requires these patients to be evaluated and treated quickly. Safety concerns warrant immediate and effective pharmacologic interventions.[118]

RBD exists as 2 distinct phenotypes: an acute and a chronic form. The acute form of RBD is often encountered in younger patients (<50 years of age) and is likely related to antidepressant medication, substance abuse, CNS injury in the REM-generating neuronal network, and metabolic derangements. Common causes of drug-related and substance-related RBD include abrupt withdrawal of sedative-hypnotic agents, introduction of SSRIs, atypical antidepressants, tricyclic antidepressants, monoamine oxidase inhibitors, biperiden, and cholinergic medications.[119–129] Some case reports also link excessive caffeine consumption as a trigger.[130,131] Brainstem lesions caused by cerebrovascular accidents, MS, subarachnoid hemorrhage, and brainstem neoplasm have been all described as causes of the acute form of RBD.[112,117,132–136] The chronic form of RBD is typically seen in older patients (>50 years of age); most cases are idiopathic, and a minority are associated with neurodegenerative disorders.[112] A spectrum of dementias are implicated in RBD and include the alpha-synucleinopathies, including dementia with Lewy bodies with a characteristic alpha-synuclein inclusion in the nerve cell bodies.[137] The underlying mechanism of RBD is presumed to be related to abnormal brainstem control of medullary inhibitory regions.[138] Data from single-photon emission computed tomography neuroimaging reveal a potential mechanism relating to abnormalities in dopaminergic systems showing decreased striatal dopaminergic innervation as well as reduced striatal dopamine transporters.[139–141]

Polysomnographic data show increased and excessive muscle tone during REM sleep. According to the third edition of the ICSD-III, a diagnosis of RBD requires there to be repeated episodes of sleep-related dream enactment behaviors; these episodes can be documented by polysomnography to occur during REM sleep, or can be based on clinical history of dream enactment, which is presumed to occur during REM sleep.[63] Polysomnographic recording shows episodes of REM sleep without atonia, as shown in **Fig. 9**.[142] The last requirement indicates that the disturbance is not better explained by another medical, psychiatric, neurologic, or sleep disorder, or related to a medication or substance use.[63,112]

The differential diagnosis of RBD includes nocturnal frontal lobe seizures, confusional arousals, sleepwalking, sleep terrors, posttraumatic stress disorder, and nightmares.[63,112,143] Patient with RBD are often distinguished based on the complex nature of their episodes, timing later in the night when REM density is highest, and the characteristic patients who are older men.[112]

Patients with RBD should be assessed carefully with particular attention to risk for injury during the nocturnal episodes. The highest level of evidence for therapy calls for ensuring environmental safety (level A evidence), especially in patients (as in the case presentation) who experience injurious spells, displacement from bed, and aggressive behavior.[144]

Suggested level of therapy (level B evidence) lists 2 pharmacologic agents: clonazepam and melatonin.[144] The former is prescribed in typical dosages ranging from 0.25 mg to 1 mg by mouth at bedtime, achieving improvement in most (90%) patients

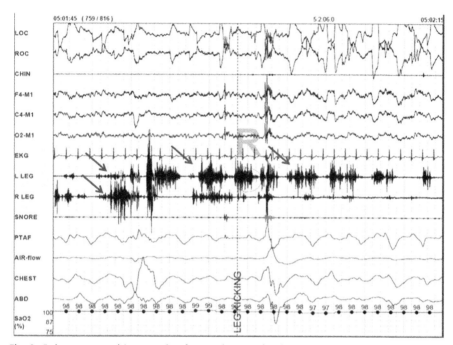

Fig. 9. Polysomnographic example of RBD. The specific abnormality in this 30-second epoch from a patient with RBD includes abnormally sustained muscle activity during REM sleep in which greater than 50% of the epoch reveals REM sleep without atonia, as indicated by the arrows pointing to the augmentation of electromyogram tone in the right and left legs (*blue arrows*). Reference electrodes (F4, C4, O2), referenced to M1 or AVG.

with little evidence of tolerance or abuse in this clinical context.[145–148] Treatment of RBD with melatonin 3 to 12 mg at bedtime is advantageous because it may restore REM sleep atonia and can be as effective as benzodiazepines.[149–151] Clinicians should be aware that melatonin is a dietary supplement, and is currently not approved by the FDA for any indications. Melatonin also has poor regulation in terms of pharmacologic preparation, and side effects have not been widely studied. Other drugs that may have some efficacy for RBD include imipramine (25 mg by mouth at bedtime), carbamazepine (100 mg by mouth 3 times daily) as well as pramipexole and carbidopa-levodopa.[152–154] Recent data from the Minnesota group suggest the use of an innovative alarm to reduce episodes of RBD in patients who may be refractory to traditional pharmacologic agents.[155]

An important prognostic observation is that RBD may precede the emergence of alpha-synucleinopathies by more than a decade.[156–160] Most patients with RBD eventually develop a neurodegenerative disorder from several months to decades after initial diagnosis in a dose-response pattern with a phenoconversion rate of approximately 50% every 10 years.[137,142,161] Given that RBD is an important biomarker of alpha-synucleinopathies, RBD represents a unique and powerful opportunity to screen patients and potentially treat those at risk with novel neuroprotective agents to help delay, if not reverse, the eventual evolution to dementia.[162,163]

Summary of the Case Presentation

The patient was diagnosed with RBD based on the clinical features of his spells and polysomnography showing REM sleep without atonia. Although clonazepam was prescribed in a serendipitous manner to treat aggression, it was the correct therapy. The issue of whether the condition could translate to a neurodegenerative condition later in life deserved closer observation. It is the authors' opinion, as those expressed in recent review of the ethical considerations in RBD, that the potential of risk-associated neurodegeneration should be disclosed and not hidden from patients and families.[164] In the spirit of transparency and disclosure of a diagnosis of RBD as well as disclosure of risk of the potential implications, given the risk, physicians should dedicate time to review the data and the possible emergence of future neuro-degeneration, factor in the educational level of the patient and family, help to uncover potential fears, and clarify that the alpha-synucleinopathies are manageable conditions even if they do eventually manifest themselves.[164]

SUMMARY

As shown by the patients discussed earlier, a variety of sleep disorders are highly prevalent among patients with neurologic diagnoses. Commonly associated conditions are comorbid OSA in the setting of epilepsy, insomnia in individuals with MS, advanced sleep phase circadian rhythm disorder in AD, NT1 in patients with hypothalamic injury, RLS in patients with peripheral neuropathy, and RBD in individuals with Parkinson disease. Often the neurologic condition contributes to the development of the sleep disorder, and if left untreated the sleep disorder may worsen the comorbid neurologic condition, showing a reciprocal relationship. It is therefore important for practitioners to maintain a high index of suspicion for sleep disorders in their patients with neurologic conditions.

REFERENCES

1. Giorelli AS, Passos P, Carnaval T, et al. Excessive daytime sleepiness and epilepsy: a systematic review. Epilepsy Res Treat 2013;2013:629469.
2. Touchon J, Baldy-Moulinier M, Billiard M, et al. Sleep organization and epilepsy. Epilepsy Res Suppl 1991;2:73–81.
3. Maestri M, Giorgi FS, Pizzanelli C, et al. Daytime sleepiness in de novo untreated patients with epilepsy. Epilepsy Behav 2013;29:344–8.
4. Lurie A. Obstructive sleep apnea in adults: epidemiology, clinical presentation, and treatment options. Adv Cardiol 2011;46:1–42.
5. Li P, Ghadersohi S, Jafari B, et al. Characteristics of refractory vs. medically controlled epilepsy patients with obstructive sleep apnea and their response to CPAP treatment. Seizure 2012;21:717–21.
6. Malow BA, Levy K, Maturen K, et al. Obstructive sleep apnea is common in medically refractory epilepsy patients. Neurology 2000;55:1002–7.
7. Devinsky O, Ehrenberg B, Barthlen GM, et al. Epilepsy and sleep apnea syndrome. Neurology 1994;44:2060–4.
8. Al-Abri M, Al-Asmi A, Al-Shukairi A, et al. Frequency of obstructive sleep apnea syndrome among patients with epilepsy attending a tertiary neurology clinic. Oman Med J 2015;30:31–5.
9. Young T, Palta M, Dempsey J, et al. The occurrence of sleep-disordered breathing among middle-aged adults. N Engl J Med 1993;328:1230–5.
10. Chihorek AM, Abou-Khalil B, Malow BA. Obstructive sleep apnea is associated with seizure occurrence in older adults with epilepsy. Neurology 2007;69:1823–7.
11. Nguyen-Michel VH, Pallanca O, Navarro V, et al. How are epileptic events linked to obstructive sleep apneas in epilepsy? Seizure 2015;24:121–3.

12. Pornsriniyom D, Shinlapawittayatorn K, Fong J, et al. Continuous positive airway pressure therapy for obstructive sleep apnea reduces interictal epileptiform discharges in adults with epilepsy. Epilepsy Behav 2014;37:171–4.

13. Lundblad LC, Fatouleh RH, McKenzie DK, et al. Brain stem activity changes associated with restored sympathetic drive following CPAP treatment in OSA subjects: a longitudinal investigation. J Neurophysiol 2015;114:893–901.

14. Dlouhy BJ, Gehlbach BK, Kreple CJ, et al. Breathing inhibited when seizures spread to the amygdala and upon amygdala stimulation. J Neurosci 2015;35: 10281–9.

15. Foldvary-Schaefer N, Stephenson L, Bingaman W. Resolution of obstructive sleep apnea with epilepsy surgery? Expanding the relationship between sleep and epilepsy. Epilepsia 2008;49:1457–9.

16. Vaughn BV, D'Cruz OF. Sleep and epilepsy. Semin Neurol 2004;24:301–13.

17. Jain SV, Glauser TA. Effects of epilepsy treatments on sleep architecture and daytime sleepiness: an evidence-based review of objective sleep metrics. Epilepsia 2014;55:26–37.

18. Romigi A, Izzi F, Placidi F, et al. Effects of zonisamide as add-on therapy on sleep-wake cycle in focal epilepsy: a polysomnographic study. Epilepsy Behav 2013;26:170–4.

19. Bell C, Vanderlinden H, Hiersemenzel R, et al. The effects of levetiracetam on objective and subjective sleep parameters in healthy volunteers and patients with partial epilepsy. J Sleep Res 2002;11:255–63.

20. Viana P, Rodrigues E, Fernandes C, et al. INMS: chronic insomnia disorder in multiple sclerosis - a Portuguese multicentre study on prevalence, subtypes, associated factors and impact on quality of life. Mult Scler Relat Disord 2015;4:477–83.

21. Bamer AM, Johnson KL, Amtmann D, et al. Prevalence of sleep problems in individuals with multiple sclerosis. Mult Scler 2008;14:1127–30.

22. American Academy of Sleep Medicine. The international classification of sleep disorders: diagnostic and coding manual, ICSD-2. 2nd edition. Westchester (IL): American Academy of Sleep Medicine; 2005.

23. Veauthier C, Gaede G, Radbruch H, et al. Sleep disorders reduce health-related quality of life in multiple sclerosis (Nottingham health profile data in patients with multiple sclerosis). Int J Mol Sci 2014;16:16514–28.

24. Vitkova M, Gdovinova Z, Rosenberger J, et al. Factors associated with poor sleep quality in patients with multiple sclerosis differ by disease duration. Disabil Health J 2014;7:466–71.

25. Amtmann D, Askew RL, Kim J, et al. Pain affects depression through anxiety, fatigue, and sleep in multiple sclerosis. Rehabil Psychol 2015;60:81–90.

26. Boe Lunde HM, Aae TF, Indrevag W, et al. Poor sleep in patients with multiple sclerosis. PLoS One 2012;7:e49996.

27. Drewes AM. Pain and sleep disturbances with special reference to fibromyalgia and rheumatoid arthritis. Rheumatology (Oxford) 1999;38:1035–8.

28. Lautenbacher S, Kundermann B, Krieg JC. Sleep deprivation and pain perception. Sleep Med Rev 2006;10:357–69.

29. Valiquette G, Herbert J, Maede-D'Alisera P. Desmopressin in the management of nocturia in patients with multiple sclerosis. A double-blind, crossover trial. Arch Neurol 1996;53:1270–5.

30. Baron KG, Corden M, Jin L, et al. Impact of psychotherapy on insomnia symptoms in patients with depression and multiple sclerosis. J Behav Med 2011;34: 92–101.

31. Sularo C, Bergamaschi II, Hozzani C, et al. Duloxetine is effective in treating depression in multiple sclerosis patients: an open-label multicenter study. Clin Neuropharmacol 2013;36:114–6.

32. Fishbain DA, Hall J, Meyers AL, et al. Does pain mediate the pain interference with sleep problem in chronic pain? Findings from studies for management of diabetic peripheral neuropathic pain with duloxetine. J Pain Symptom Manage 2008;36:639–47.

33. Thorpy MJ. Classification of sleep disorders. Neurotherapeutics 2012;9:687–701.

34. Pigeon WR. Treatment of adult insomnia with cognitive-behavioral therapy. J Clin Psychol 2010;66:1148–60.

35. Jacobs GD, Pace-Schott EF, Stickgold R, et al. Cognitive behavior therapy and pharmacotherapy for insomnia: a randomized controlled trial and direct comparison. Arch Intern Med 2004;164:1888–96.

36. Attarian H, Applebee G, Applebee A, et al. Effect of eszopiclone on sleep disturbances and daytime fatigue in multiple sclerosis patients. Int J MS Care 2011;13:84–90.

37. Foral P, Dewan N, Malesker M. Insomnia: a therapeutic review for pharmacists. Consult Pharm 2011;26:332–41.

38. Yeung WF, Chung KF, Yung KP, et al. Doxepin for insomnia: a systematic review of randomized placebo-controlled trials. Sleep Med Rev 2015;19:75–83.

39. Kishi T, Matsunaga S, Iwata N. Suvorexant for primary insomnia: A systematic review and meta-analysis of randomized placebo-controlled trials. PLoS One 2015;10:e0136910.

40. Marrie RA, Reider N, Cohen J, et al. A systematic review of the incidence and prevalence of sleep disorders and seizure disorders in multiple sclerosis. Mult Scler 2015;21:342–9.

41. Braley TJ, Segal BM, Chervin RD. Obstructive sleep apnea and fatigue in patients with multiple sclerosis. J Clin Sleep Med 2014;10:155–62.

42. Brass SD, Li CS, Auerbach S. The underdiagnosis of sleep disorders in patients with multiple sclerosis. J Clin Sleep Med 2014;10:1025–31.

43. Porter VR, Buxton WG, Avidan AY. Sleep, cognition and dementia. Curr Psychiatry Rep 2015;17:97.

44. Butt M, Quan SF, Pentland AS, et al. Gender differences in real-home sleep of young and older couples. Southwest J Pulm Crit Care 2015;10:289–99.

45. Redline S, Kirchner HL, Quan SF, et al. The effects of age, sex, ethnicity, and sleep-disordered breathing on sleep architecture. Arch Intern Med 2004;164:406–18.

46. Bonakis A, Economou NT, Paparrigopoulos T, et al. Sleep in frontotemporal dementia is equally or possibly more disrupted, and at an earlier stage, when compared to sleep in Alzheimer's disease. J Alzheimers Dis 2014;38:85–91.

47. Auyeung TW, Lee JS, Leung J, et al. Cognitive deficit is associated with phase advance of sleep-wake rhythm, daily napping, and prolonged sleep duration–a cross-sectional study in 2,947 community-dwelling older adults. Age (Dordr) 2013;35:479–86.

48. Musiek ES, Xiong DD, Holtzman DM. Sleep, circadian rhythms, and the pathogenesis of Alzheimer disease. Exp Mol Med 2015;47:e148.

49. Pace-Schott EF, Spencer RM. Sleep-dependent memory consolidation in healthy aging and mild cognitive impairment. Curr Top Behav Neurosci 2015;25:307–30.

50. Guarnieri B, Musicco M, Caffarra P, et al. Recommendations of the sleep study group of the Italian Dementia Research Association (SINDem) on clinical assessment and management of sleep disorders in individuals with mild cognitive impairment and dementia: a clinical review. Neurol Sci 2014;35: 1329–48.

51. Song Y, Blackwell T, Yaffe K, et al. Relationships between sleep stages and changes in cognitive function in older men: The MROS sleep study. Sleep 2015;38:411–21.

52. Tranah GJ, Blackwell T, Stone KL, et al. Circadian activity rhythms and risk of incident dementia and mild cognitive impairment in older women. Ann Neurol 2011;70:722–32.

53. Hahn EA, Wang HX, Andel R, et al. A change in sleep pattern may predict Alzheimer disease. Am J Geriatr Psychiatry 2014;22:1262–71.

54. Lucey BP, Bateman RJ. Amyloid-beta diurnal pattern: possible role of sleep in Alzheimer's disease pathogenesis. Neurobiol Aging 2014;35(Suppl 2): S29–34.

55. Kang JE, Lim MM, Bateman RJ, et al. Amyloid-beta dynamics are regulated by orexin and the sleep-wake cycle. Science 2009;326:1005–7.

56. Rothman SM, Herdener N, Frankola KA, et al. Chronic mild sleep restriction accentuates contextual memory impairments, and accumulations of cortical Aβ and pTau in a mouse model of Alzheimer's disease. Brain Res 2013;1529:200–8.

57. Ooms S, Overeem S, Besse K, et al. Effect of 1 night of total sleep deprivation on cerebrospinal fluid beta-amyloid 42 in healthy middle-aged men: a randomized clinical trial. JAMA Neurol 2014;71:971–7.

58. Mendelsohn AR, Larrick JW. Sleep facilitates clearance of metabolites from the brain: glymphatic function in aging and neurodegenerative diseases. Rejuvenation Res 2013;16:518–23.

59. Sloane PD, Williams CS, Mitchell CM, et al. High-intensity environmental light in dementia: effect on sleep and activity. J Am Geriatr Soc 2007;55:1524–33.

60. Gehrman PR, Connor DJ, Martin JL, et al. Melatonin fails to improve sleep or agitation in double-blind randomized placebo-controlled trial of institutionalized patients with Alzheimer disease. Am J Geriatr Psychiatry 2009;17:166–9.

61. Grippe TC, Goncalves BS, Louzada LL, et al. Circadian rhythm in Alzheimer disease after trazodone use. Chronobiol Int 2015;32(9):1311–4.

62. Mayo MC, Deng JC, Albores J, et al. Hypocretin deficiency associated with narcolepsy type 1 and central hypoventilation syndrome in neurosarcoidosis of the hypothalamus. J Clin Sleep Med 2015;11:1063–5.

63. American Academy of Sleep Medicine. The international classification of sleep disorders, revised: diagnostic and coding manual. 3rd edition. Darien (IL): American Academy of Sleep Medicine; 2014.

64. Thorpy MJ, Dauvilliers Y. Clinical and practical considerations in the pharmacologic management of narcolepsy. Sleep Med 2015;16:9–18.

65. Scammell TE. Narcolepsy. N Engl J Med 2015;373:2654 62.

66. Akintomide GS, Rickards H. Narcolepsy: a review. Neuropsychiatr Dis Treat 2011;7:507–18.

67. Leschziner G. Narcolepsy: a clinical review. Pract Neurol 2014;14:323–31.

68. Dauvilliers Y, Siegel JM, Lopez R, et al. Cataplexy-clinical aspects, pathophysiology and management strategy. Nat Rev Neurol 2014;10(7):386–95.

69. Liblau RS, Vassalli A, Seifinejad A, et al. Hypocretin (orexin) biology and the pathophysiology of narcolepsy with cataplexy. Lancet Neurol 2015;14:318–28.

70. Arango MT, Kivity S, Shoenfeld Y. Is narcolepsy a classical autoimmune disease? Pharmacol Res 2015;92:6–12.
71. De la Herran-Arita AK, Garcia-Garcia F. Narcolepsy as an immune-mediated disease. Sleep Disord 2014;2014:792007.
72. Thorpy MJ. Update on therapy for narcolepsy. Curr Treat Options Neurol 2015; 17:347.
73. Swick TJ. Treatment paradigms for cataplexy in narcolepsy: past, present, and future. Nat Sci Sleep 2015;7:159–69.
74. Yassin W, Sugihara G, Oishi N, et al. Hypothalamic-amygdalar-brainstem volume reduction in a patient with narcolepsy secondary to diffuse axonal injury. J Clin Sleep Med 2015;11:581–2.
75. Sakuta K, Nakamura M, Komada Y, et al. Possible mechanism of secondary narcolepsy with a long sleep time following surgery for craniopharyngioma. Intern Med 2012;51:413–7.
76. Kanbayashi T, Sagawa Y, Takemura F, et al. The pathophysiologic basis of secondary narcolepsy and hypersomnia. Curr Neurol Neurosci Rep 2011;11: 235–41.
77. Watson NF, Doherty MJ, Zunt JR. Secondary narcolepsy following neurocysticercosis infection. J Clin Sleep Med 2005;1:41–2.
78. Marcus CL, Trescher WH, Halbower AC, et al. Secondary narcolepsy in children with brain tumors. Sleep 2002;25:435–9.
79. Rao DG, Singhal BS. Secondary narcolepsy in a case of multiple sclerosis. J Assoc Physicians India 1997;45:321–2.
80. Hening WA, Allen RP, Chaudhuri KR, et al. Clinical significance of RLS. Mov Disord 2007;22(Suppl 18):S395–400.
81. Yee B, Killick R, Wong K. Restless legs syndrome. Aust Fam Physician 2009;38: 296–300.
82. Walters AS, Frauscher B, Allen R, et al. Review of quality of life instruments for the restless legs syndrome/Willis-Ekbom disease (RLS/WED): critique and recommendations. J Clin Sleep Med 2014;10:1351–7.
83. Atkinson MJ, Allen RP, DuChane J, et al. Validation of the restless legs syndrome quality of life instrument (RLS-QLI): findings of a consortium of national experts and the RLS foundation. Qual Life Res 2004;13:679–93.
84. Notcutt W, Price M, Miller R, et al. Initial experiences with medicinal extracts of cannabis for chronic pain: results from 34 'n of 1' studies. Anaesthesia 2004;59: 440–52.
85. Dao TT, Lund JP, Lavigne GJ. Comparison of pain and quality of life in bruxers and patients with myofascial pain of the masticatory muscles. J Orofac Pain 1994;8:350–6.
86. Rothdach AJ, Trenkwalder C, Haberstock J, et al. Prevalence and risk factors of RLS in an elderly population: the memo study. Memory and Morbidity in Augsburg Elderly. Neurology 2000;54:1064–8.
87. Chesson A Jr, Hartse K, Anderson WM, et al. Practice parameters for the evaluation of chronic insomnia. An American Academy of Sleep Medicine report. Standards of practice committee of the American Academy of Sleep Medicine. Sleep 2000;23:237–41.
88. Auger C, Montplaisir J, Duquette P. Increased frequency of restless legs syndrome in a French-Canadian population with multiple sclerosis. Neurology 2005;65:1652–3.
89. Deriu M, Cossu G, Molari A, et al. Restless legs syndrome in multiple sclerosis: a case-control study. Mov Disord 2009;24:697–701.

90. Baier PC, Winkelmann J, Hohne A, et al. Assessment of spontaneously occurring periodic limb movements in sleep in the rat. J Neurol Sci 2002;198:71-7.

91. Picchietti DL, Walters AS. The symptomatology of periodic limb movement disorder. Sleep 1996;19:747-8.

92. Anderson DJ, Hector MP, Linden RW. The effects of unilateral and bilateral chewing, empty clenching and simulated bruxism, on the masticatory-parotid salivary reflex in man. Exp Physiol 1996;81:305-12.

93. Montplaisir J, Boucher S, Poirier G, et al. Clinical, polysomnographic, and genetic characteristics of restless legs syndrome: A study of 133 patients diagnosed with new standard criteria. Mov Disord 1997;12:61-5.

94. Allen RP. Restless leg syndrome/Willis-Ekbom disease pathophysiology. Sleep Med Clin 2015;10:207-14, xi.

95. Hening WA, Allen RP, Washburn M, et al. The four diagnostic criteria for restless legs syndrome are unable to exclude confounding conditions ("mimics"). Sleep Med 2009;10:976-81.

96. Allen RP, Picchietti DL, Garcia-Borreguero D, et al. Restless legs syndrome/ Willis–Ekbom disease diagnostic criteria: Updated International Restless Legs Syndrome Study Group (IRLSSG) consensus criteria – history, rationale, description, and significance. Sleep Med 2014;15:860-73.

97. Ondo WG. Common comorbidities and differential diagnosis of restless legs syndrome. J Clin Psychiatry 2014;75:e06.

98. Hogl B, Zucconi M, Provini F. RLS, PLM, and their differential diagnosis–a video guide. Mov Disord 2007;22(Suppl 18):S414-9.

99. Ferini-Strambi L. RLS-like symptoms: differential diagnosis by history and clinical assessment. Sleep Med 2007;8(Suppl 2):S3-6.

100. Silber MH, Becker PM, Earley C, et al, Medical Advisory Board of the Willis-Ekbom Disease Foundation. Willis-Ekbom Disease Foundation revised consensus statement on the management of restless legs syndrome. Mayo Clin Proc 2013;88:977-86.

101. Picchietti DL, Hensley JG, Bainbridge JL, et al. Consensus clinical practice guidelines for the diagnosis and treatment of restless legs syndrome/Willis-Ekbom disease during pregnancy and lactation. Sleep Med Rev 2015;22:64-77.

102. Garcia-Borreguero D, Kohnen R, Silber MH, et al. The long-term treatment of restless legs syndrome/Willis-Ekbom disease: evidence-based guidelines and clinical consensus best practice guidance: a report from the International Restless Legs Syndrome Study Group. Sleep Med 2013;14:675-84.

103. Daubian-Nose P, Frank MK, Esteves AM. Sleep disorders: a review of the interface between restless legs syndrome and iron metabolism. Sleep Sci 2014;7:234-7.

104. Littner MR, Kushida C, Anderson WM, et al. Practice parameters for the dopaminergic treatment of restless legs syndrome and periodic limb movement disorder. Sleep 2004;27:557-9.

105. Wilt TJ, MacDonald R, Ouellette J, et al. Pharmacologic therapy for primary restless legs syndrome: a systematic review and meta-analysis. JAMA Intern Med 2013;173:496-505.

106. Evans AH, Butzkueven H. Dopamine agonist-induced pathological gambling in restless legs syndrome due to multiple sclerosis. Mov Disord 2007;22:590-1.

107. Allen RP, Earley CJ. Augmentation of the restless legs syndrome with carbidopa/ levodopa. Sleep 1996;19:205-13.

108. Chesson AL Jr, Anderson WM, Littner M, et al. Practice parameters for the nonpharmacologic treatment of chronic insomnia. An American Academy of Sleep

Medicine report. Standards of Practice Committee of the American Academy of Sleep Medicine. Sleep 1999;22:1128–33.

109. Kimble B, Bonitati AE, Millman RP. A review of the adult primary sleep parasomnias. Med Health R I 2002;85:95 8.

110. Howell MJ. Parasomnias: an updated review. Neurotherapeutics 2012;9:753–75.

111. Giglio P, Undevia N, Spire JP. The primary parasomnias. A review for neurologists. Neurologist 2005;11:90–7.

112. Boeve BF. REM sleep behavior disorder: updated review of the core features, the REM sleep behavior disorder-neurodegenerative disease association, evolving concepts, controversies, and future directions. Ann N Y Acad Sci 2010;1184:15–54.

113. Mahowald MW, Schenck CH. The REM sleep behavior disorder odyssey. Sleep Med Rev 2009;13:381–4.

114. Ohayon MM, Caulet M, Priest RG. Violent behavior during sleep. J Clin Psychiatry 1997;58:369–76 [quiz: 377].

115. Abad VC, Guilleminault C. Review of rapid eye movement behavior sleep disorders. Curr Neurol Neurosci Rep 2004;4:157–63.

116. Ozekmekci S, Apaydin H, Kilic E. Clinical features of 35 patients with Parkinson's disease displaying REM behavior disorder. Clin Neurol Neurosurg 2005;107: 306–9.

117. Schenck CH, Bundlie SR, Patterson AL, et al. Rapid eye movement sleep behavior disorder. A treatable parasomnia affecting older adults. JAMA 1987; 257:1786–9.

118. Schenck CH, Mahowald MW. Rem sleep behavior disorder: Clinical, developmental, and neuroscience perspectives 16 years after its formal identification in sleep. Sleep 2002;25:120–38.

119. Tachibana M, Tanaka K, Hishikawa Y, et al. A sleep study of acute psychotic states due to alcohol and meprobamate addiction. Adv Sleep Res 1975;2:177–205.

120. Passouant P, Cadilhac J, Ribstein M. Les privations de sommeil avec mouvements oculaires par les anti-depresseurs. Rev Neurol (Paris) 1972;127:173–92.

121. Guilleminault C, Raynal D, Takahashi S, et al. Evaluation of short-term and long-term treatment of the narcolepsy syndrome with clomipramine hydrochloride. Acta Neurol Scand 1976;54:71–87.

122. Besset A. Effect of antidepressants on human sleep. Adv Biosci 1978;21:141–8.

123. Shimizu T, Ookawa M, Iijuma S, et al. Effect of clomipramine on nocturnal sleep of normal human subjects. Ann Rev Pharmacopsychiat Res Found 1985;16:138.

124. Bental E, Lavie P, Sharf B. Severe hypermotility during sleep in treatment of cataplexy with clomipramine. Isr J Med Sci 1979;15:607–9.

125. Akindele MO, Evans JI, Oswald I. Mono-amine oxidase inhibitors, sleep and mood. Electroencephalogr Clin Neurophysiol 1970;29:47–56.

126. Carlander B, Touchon J, Ondze B, et al. Rem sleep behavior disorder induced by cholinergic treatment in Alzheimer's disease. J Sleep Res 1996;5(suppl. 1):28.

127. Ross JS, Shua-Haim JR. Aricept-induced nightmares in Alzheimer's disease: 2 case reports. J Am Geriatr Soc 1998;46:119–20.

128. Schenck CH, Mahowald MW, Kim SW, et al. Prominent eye movements during NREM sleep and REM sleep behavior disorder associated with fluoxetine treatment of depression and obsessive-compulsive disorder. Sleep 1992;15:226–35.

129. Schutte S, Doghramji K. REM behavior disorder seen with venlafaxine (Effexor). Sleep Res 1996;25:364.

130. Stolz SE, Aldrich MS. REM sleep behavior disorder associated with caffeine abuse. Sleep Res 1991;20:341.

131. Vorona RD, Ware JC. Exacerbation of REM sleep behavior disorder by chocolate ingestion: a case report. Sleep Med 2002;3:365–7.
132. Xi Z, Luning W. REM sleep behavior disorder in a patient with pontine stroke. Sleep Med 2009;10:143–6.
133. Schenck CH, Mahowald MW. Rapid eye movement sleep parasomnias. Neurol Clin 2005;23:1107–26.
134. Plazzi G, Montagna P. Remitting REM sleep behavior disorder as the initial sign of multiple sclerosis. Sleep Med 2002;3:437–9.
135. Postuma RB, Gagnon JF, Tuineaig M, et al. Antidepressants and REM sleep behavior disorder: isolated side effect or neurodegenerative signal? Sleep 2013;36:1579–85.
136. Kolla BP, Mansukhani MP. Antidepressants trigger an early clinical presentation of REM sleep behavior disorder: the jury is still out. Sleep 2014;37:1393.
137. Schenck CH, Boeve BF. The strong presence of REM sleep behavior disorder in PD: clinical and research implications. Neurology 2011;77:1030–2.
138. Mahowald MW, Schenck CH, Bornemann MA. Pathophysiologic mechanisms in REM sleep behavior disorder. Curr Neurol Neurosci Rep 2007;7:167–72.
139. Eisensehr I, Linke R, Noachtar S, et al. Reduced striatal dopamine transporters in idiopathic rapid eye movement sleep behavior disorder. Comparison with Parkinson's disease and controls. Brain 2000;123:1155–60.
140. Eisehsehr I, Linke R, Tatsch K, et al. Increased muscle activity during rapid eye movement sleep correlates with decrease of striatal presynaptic dopamine transporters. IPT and IBZM SPECT imaging in subclinical and clinically manifest idiopathic REM sleep behavior disorder, Parkinson's disease, and controls. Sleep 2003;26:507–12.
141. Albin RL, Koeppe RA, Chervin RD, et al. Decreased striatal dopaminergic innervation in REM sleep behavior disorder. Neurology 2000;55:1410–2.
142. Ferri R, Fantini ML, Schenck CH. The role of REM sleep without atonia in the diagnosis of REM sleep behavior disorder: past errors and new challenges. Sleep Med 2014;15:1007–8.
143. Pressman MR, Mahowald MW, Schenck CH. Sleep terrors/sleepwalking–not REM behavior disorder. Sleep 2005;28:278–9.
144. Aurora RN, Zak RS, Maganti RK, et al. Best practice guide for the treatment of REM sleep behavior disorder (RBD). J Clin Sleep Med 2010;6:85–95.
145. Schenck CH, Mahowald MW. Polysomnographic, neurologic, psychiatric, and clinical outcome report on 70 consecutive cases with REM sleep behavior disorder (RBD): Sustained clonazepam efficacy in 89.5% of 57 treated patients. Cleve Clin J Med 1990;57(Suppl):S9–23.
146. Mahowald MW, Schenck CH. REM sleep behavior disorder. Philadelphia: WB Saunders; 1994.
147. Mahowald MW, Ettinger MG. Things that go bump in the night: the parasomnias revisited. J Clin Neurophysiol 1990;7:119–43.
148. Ferri R, Marelli S, Ferini-Strambi L, et al. An observational clinical and video polysomnographic study of the effects of clonazepam in REM sleep behavior disorder. Sleep Med 2013;14:24–9.
149. Takeuchi N, Uchimura N, Hashizume Y, et al. Melatonin therapy for REM sleep behavior disorder. Psychiatry Clin Neurosci 2001;55:267–9.
150. Boeve B. Melatonin for treatment of REM sleep behavior disorder: response in 8 patients. Sleep 2001;24(suppl):A35.
151. Avidan AY, Zee PC. Handbook of sleep medicine. Philadelphia: Wolters Kluwer Health/Lippincott Williams & Wilkins; 2011.

152. Schmidt MH, Koshal VD, Schmidt HC. Use of pramipexole in REM sleep behavior disorder: Results from a case series. Sleep Med 2006;7:418–23.

153. Fantini ML, Gagnon JF, Filipini D, et al. The effects of pramipexole in REM sleep behavior disorder. Neurology 2003;61:1418–20.

154. Tan A, Salgado M, Fahn S. Rapid eye movement sleep behavior disorder preceding Parkinson's disease with therapeutic response to levodopa. Mov Disord 1996;11:214–6.

155. Howell MJ, Arneson PA, Schenck CH. A novel therapy for REM sleep behavior disorder (RBD). J Clin Sleep Med 2011;7:639–644A.

156. Pareja JA, Caminero AB, Masa JF, et al. A first case of progressive supranuclear palsy and pre-clinical REM sleep behavior disorder presenting as inhibition of speech during wakefulness and somniloquy with phasic muscle twitching during REM sleep. Neurologia 1996;11:304–6.

157. Boeve BF, Silber MH, Ferman JT, et al. Association of REM sleep behavior disorder and neurodegenerative disease may reflect an underlying synucleinopathy. Mov Disord 2001;16:622–30.

158. Boeve BF, Silber MH, Parisi JE, et al. Synucleinopathy pathology often underlies REM sleep behavior disorder and dementia or parkinsonism. Neurology 2003; 61:40–5.

159. Schenck CH, Bundlie SR, Mahowald MW. Delayed emergence of a parkinsonian disorder in 38% of 29 older men initially diagnosed with idiopathic rapid eye movement sleep behavior disorder. Neurology 1996;46:388–93.

160. Montplaisir J, Petit D, Decary A, et al. Sleep and quantitative EEG in patients with progressive supranuclear palsy. Neurology 1997;49:999–1003.

161. Postuma RB. Prodromal Parkinson's disease–using REM sleep behavior disorder as a window. Parkinsonism Relat Disord 2014;20(Suppl 1):S1–4.

162. Schenck CH, Montplaisir JY, Frauscher B, et al. Rapid eye movement sleep behavior disorder: devising controlled active treatment studies for symptomatic and neuroprotective therapy–a consensus statement from the international rapid eye movement sleep behavior disorder study group. Sleep Med 2013;14:795–806.

163. Postuma RB, Gagnon JF, Bertrand JA, et al. Parkinson risk in idiopathic REM sleep behavior disorder: preparing for neuroprotective trials. Neurology 2015; 84:1104–13.

164. Vertrees S, Greenough GP. Ethical considerations in REM sleep behavior disorder. Continuum 2013;19:199–203.

Evaluating and Treating Epilepsy Based on Clinical Subgroups

Elderly Onset Seizure and Medically Resistant Partial-Onset Epilepsy

Emily L. Johnson, MD, Gregory L. Krauss, MD*

KEYWORDS

- Seizure • Convulsive syncope • Epilepsy • Late-onset epilepsy
- Medically refractory epilepsy • Nonmedical therapy

KEY POINTS

- New-onset epilepsy is common in older adults.
- Seizures in the elderly can be missed or mistaken for other causes.
- After seizures, despite trials of 2 or more appropriately chosen antiepileptic drugs, patients should have a detailed evaluation for medically refractory epilepsy.

INTRODUCTION

For optimal treatment, clinicians must recognize key subgroups of patients with epilepsy who have distinctive patterns of seizures, causes, and treatment needs. Particularly important subgroups are (1) patients who develop seizures in their late adult or elderly years and (2) patients with medically resistant epilepsy. Currently the largest age group of patients diagnosed with new-onset epilepsy is older adult and elderly patients; these patients have a rapidly increasing incidence of seizures beginning in the late 50s and represent the graying of America and the influence of vascular risk factors on producing seizures. Clinicians and their elderly patients often do not recognize this pattern along with distinctive clinical presentations and treatment needs of this group. Another key group that is important to recognize is patients with medically resistant epilepsy. The International League Against Epilepsy (ILAE) has recently redefined this as patients with persisting seizures despite adequate trials of 2 appropriately selected

Disclosures. G. L. Krauss has been a consultant for Esai Inc and Acorda and receives research support from UCB Pharma, SK Lifesciences, Upsher Smith, Pfizer and the NIH/NIA (R01AB048349). Department of Neurology, Johns Hopkins School of Medicine, 600 N Wolfe Street, Baltimore, MD 21287, USA
* Corresponding author.
E-mail address: gkrauss@jhmi.edu

Neurol Clin 34 (2016) 595–610
http://dx.doi.org/10.1016/j.ncl.2016.04.004   **neurologic.theclinics.com**

and dosed medications.[1] There are several new medications and stimulation and surgical treatments available to treat patients with medically resistant epilepsy, and it is helpful to review how patient factors can be used to select among these options.[2]

CASE 1: EPILEPSY IN THE ELDERLY

A 60-year-old man presented for evaluation after a reported seizure. Two weeks ago, his wife was woken at around 4 AM by his thrashing movements and found him very confused with mild limb and body stiffening and shaking. She said the stiffening and shaking episode lasted about 2 minutes. He gradually recovered and was able to converse with her after about 20 minutes, when paramedics arrived and placed him in an ambulance. In the local emergency department (ED), he had a normal examination, head computed tomography (CT), and general laboratory test results. He had a history of hypertension, with no history of heavy alcohol use or other obvious seizure risk factors. He was started on levetiracetam 1000 mg twice a day and was discharged. He was scheduled for an outpatient electroencephalogram (EEG) and brain MRI and referred to a neurologist. In his neurology consultation visit, his wife reported that he had been evaluated for 2 brief episodes in the previous 6 months during which he briefly paused in his activities and appeared dazed: one episode occurred while standing on a dock fishing and the other while sitting at dinner. These episodes had been diagnosed as probable syncopal events linked to his hypertension treatment.

What is the Differential Diagnosis for Episodes of Confusion in the Elderly?

Confusional episodes are common causes of physician visits for the elderly (**Box 1**). There are limited numbers of causes, however, for sudden phasic confusional episodes. Seizures and syncope are most common; most other disorders, such as vestibular disorders, concussions, pain reactions, dissociative states, and medication intoxications, can usually be easily identified by patients' history. Although transient ischemic attacks (TIAs) are frequently considered as a cause of episodic confusion, patients rarely develop altered awareness as part of motor or other TIA symptoms. Convulsive syncope is often mistaken for a seizure. Patients often lose consciousness and may have brief myoclonic limb jerks during major hypotensive episodes (usually with blood pressure [BP] <50 mm

---

Box 1
Differential diagnosis for confusional episodes in the elderly

Seizure

Syncope and convulsive syncope

Vestibular causes

Medication intoxication

Infection

Pain reaction

Concussion

Transient ischemic attack

Dissociative episode or other psychiatric causes

Transient global amnesia

Sleep disorders

Hg systolic).[3] Extremely severe hypotension can trigger full major convulsions. Convulsive syncope can usually be picked out by the clinical history; most patients with convulsive syncope initially have typical syncope symptoms of lightheadedness or are observed to have initial passing out with collapsing, limp behavior, and pallor; they then may develop brief myoclonic jerking.[4] Convulsive syncope should not be confused with epileptic seizures because syncope does not benefit from treatment with anticonvulsants. Many patients can have syncope confirmed with simple postural BP checks that identify orthostatic hypotension or histories of hypotension measured by emergency responders; some patients require tilt table testing to confirm this diagnosis.

What Features in This Patient's History Help Distinguish Seizure from Other Causes Such As Syncope?

This patient's episode occurred in bed (not triggered by a change in position) and so was unlikely to be syncope linked to postural hypotension. His wife also did not report typical signs of syncope, such as pallor or limp behavior; she also observed tonic stiffening and then rhythmic clonic shaking, with prolonged confusion, symptoms more typical of a tonic clonic seizure.

A detailed history of patients' episodes, the presence of precipitants, prodromal symptoms, the duration of the episode and recovery, and signs during the episode, usually helps identify seizures and excludes other entities. More than 90% of seizures (not including the postictal recovery phase) have durations less than 4 minutes,[5] and so patients with a several hour amnestic or confused episode are likely to have another type of disorder, such as a psychiatric dissociative episode or transient global amnesia, rather than seizure.

Syncope may be more difficult to distinguish from seizures; however, distinguishing common features of each usually supports an accurate diagnosis from history alone. It is particularly important to interview an observer of the patients' episodes (in this case, the patient's wife). Syncope is usually precipitated by standing or sitting and is often associated with dehydration; confusional episodes occurring while prone are more likely to be seizures.[4] Seizures may be preceded by a brief aura, most commonly autonomic sensory symptoms, such as tingling or rising gastric sensations or by psychic sensations; syncope is more typically preceded by brief lightheadedness and nausea, which is followed by loss of consciousness, collapsing, and loss of body tone. Patients are usually pale and often sweaty. Seizures often involve brief staring and unresponsiveness; patients may have confusion (recently termed "dyscognitive symptoms") and fumbling or mild stiffening and limb shaking during complex partial seizures. Focal seizures can spread bilaterally rapidly and produce major convulsions. Focal seizures with bilateral spread often begin with focal symptoms, such as asymmetric stiffening or head and eye turning, and then may evolve into full tonic (limb and body) stiffening and clonic shaking. Patients often recover awareness rapidly following syncope episodes but as a result of transient hypotension often feel exhausted or washed out; patients with seizures are more likely to have gradual recovery from foggy states that correspond in severity and duration to the severity of the seizure. Patients with full tonic-clonic seizures, for example, usually recover very slowly over 30 minutes or longer; patients often become aware while in an ambulance or ED. Elderly patients can have a more prolonged postictal state of confusion than younger patients.[6] Patients often bite their tongue during tonic-clonic seizures, a sign that is uncommon with syncope episodes.

With questioning, the patient's wife also described features of the previous confusional episodes that had features more typical of seizures than syncope. While sitting at the dinner table, he suddenly appeared dazed, repetitively tapped his left hand on his thigh, and stared forward. When one shouted at him he looked at her but did not respond. *The episode lasted about a minute; he then gradually recovered after about a minute. He had no other abnormal physical signs, such as slumping or paleness. His brief staring, decreased responsiveness, and motor automatisms are typical of a complex partial seizure (recently termed by the ILAE as a focal seizure with dyscognitive features).*[7]

What Clinical Tests are Useful for Evaluating Seizures in This 60-Year-Old Patient?

EEG helps confirm the clinical diagnosis of a seizure and is particularly important in evaluating unobserved unconscious episodes that may have been seizures. This patient's EEG should be used carefully, however, as many older patients have normal variant EEG patterns that are often misread as epileptiform discharges; a normal EEG does not exclude seizures and epilepsy. Common variant EEG patterns found in older patients are brief bursts of slow waves during drowsiness, wicket rhythms –6 to 11 Hz temporal lobe discharges present during drowsiness, and a related pattern of minor sharp and slow waves.[8]

The patient had a normal acute head CT; this can exclude serious conditions, such as a large tumors or hemorrhage, but often misses small lesions that can be detected on brain MRI, especially if coronal and axial fluid-attenuated inversion recovery (FLAIR) MRI sequences are performed.

*This patient had a normal head CT in the ED after his convulsion; his EEG showed left temporal wicket rhythm (a normal variant; **Fig. 1**). After his neurology clinic visit, he received a brain MRI, which showed no focal abnormalities. He had prominent bilateral white matter T2 hyperintensity signals consistent with microvascular disease. In his neurology consultation, the patient and his wife were surprised to learn that seizures can develop later in life, even in the absence of stroke or trauma.*

How Common is New-Onset Epilepsy in Older Adults Such As This Patient, and What are Important Causes of Seizures in the Elderly?

Unprovoked first seizures are more common in adults older than 75 years than in any other age group[9] (**Fig. 2**). Single seizures are common; up to 10% of the population will

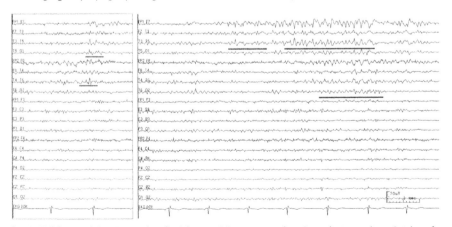

Fig. 1. Wicket activity. Example of wicket activity, a normal variant that may be mistaken for epileptiform activity. Wicket rhythm is underlined. (*From* Krauss GL, Abdallah A, Lesser R, et al. Clinical and EEG features of patients with EEG wicket rhythms misdiagnosed with epilepsy. Neurology 2005;64:1879–83.)

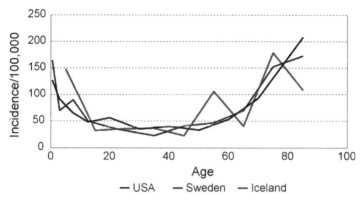

Fig. 2. Incidence of unprovoked seizures in developed countries. (*From* Cloyed, Hauser W, Towne A, et al. Epidemiological and medical aspects of epilepsy in the elderly. Epilepsy Res 2006;68(Suppl 1):39–48.)

have a seizure by 70 years of age.[10] Many acute factors can provoke a single seizure without leading to further seizures: stroke, metabolic disturbances, trauma, alcohol withdrawal, drug exposures, and infection are among the common causes.[11,12] About 60% of people who have a single seizure will not have recurrence and, therefore, do not have epilepsy, which is "a disorder of the brain characterized by an enduring predisposition to generate epileptic seizures."[13] A new "practical clinical definition of epilepsy" includes the concept that patients may be defined as having epilepsy after a single seizure if their recurrence risk is very high, for example, greater than 60%.[14] In practice, however, it is difficult to identify risk factors that increase recurrence risks to these levels. The incidence of new-onset epilepsy has a bimodal distribution, with moderate rates (100 per 100,000 person-years) in the first year of life, low rates (20 per 100,000) between 20 and 60 years of age, and the highest rates (175 per 100,000) after 80 years of age,[9,10] with this increase beginning in the late 50s. The cumulative lifetime incidence of epilepsy also increases significantly in late adulthood, from 1.7% at 50 years of age to 3.4% by 80 years of age.[10]

The patient had a normal head CT and examination and no history of trauma, stroke, or other common causes of seizures. He had signs of subcortical microvascular disease on MRI, which is common in patients with histories of hypertension at this age.

What are the Most Common Causes of New-Onset Seizures in the Elderly?

As with this patient, more than half of elderly patients with seizures have vascular risk factors, which may predispose them to seizures. Major ischemic and hemorrhagic strokes account for up to 38% of first-time seizures in the elderly.[15] After a stroke, the risk of seizures in the next year increases dramatically to 23 times that of the general population.[16]

Dementia (including Alzheimer disease) increases risks for unprovoked seizures 6 times that of the general population.[10] Neurocognitive disorders and dementia account for 10% to 17% of late-onset epilepsy.[17] Patients with mild Alzheimer disease in their 50s have a more than 10-fold increase in seizures compared with those without dementia,[18] and the risk remains elevated in all age groups with Alzheimer disease. One study identified a history of seizures in nearly one-fifth of patients with autopsy-proven Alzheimer disease, with higher rates of seizures in those with an earlier onset of dementia.[18] This patient did not have dementia, though seizures may occur even before clinical dementia is recognized.[20] The incidence is, however, most prevalent late in the disease course.[19] A careful physical examination, including bedside mental status testing, should be done in patients with late-onset seizures to screen for memory problems and dementia.

Other common causes of seizures late in life are cerebral trauma and neoplasms (primary central nervous system [CNS] or metastases). Twenty-two percent of patients with late-onset seizures have a history of cancer.[15]

This patient had no history of trauma, did not have a brain tumor on MRI, and scored 29/30 on bedside mini-mental status testing and so had no evidence of dementia. His medical history was most significant for a history of hypertension, diagnosed at 50 years of age, and treated with lisinopril. His BP in the office was 170/100. The diffuse subcortical microvascular disease seen on his MRI is atypical for normotensive people at his age of 60 years (but is common for patients in their 80s). Hypertension and the microvascular disease seen on MRI are his main seizure risk factors.

How are Seizures Linked to Hypertension and Microvascular Disease?

This patient's seizures may be linked to the hypertension that was diagnosed in his 50s. Patients who develop seizures in later years usually have risk factors that developed much earlier, including hypertension (as in the authors' patient), elevated cholesterol, microvascular disease on imaging, and left ventricular hypertrophy. Medical comorbidities are common in patients with late-onset seizures: 65% have a history of hypertension,[15] which is significantly more common in patients with adult-onset epilepsy than in those without seizures.[21] White matter changes on MRI are a marker of microvascular disease and are significantly more prevalent in patients with late-onset epilepsy than in age-matched controls.[22] Other vascular risk factors, including high cholesterol, left ventricular hypertrophy, and cardiac disease, are also elevated in patients with late-onset epilepsy.[15,23]

The keys to brain aging later in life are found in earlier decades: a cohort study of adults without dementia found that hypertension in midlife was significantly associated with a later decrease in executive function and increase in white matter hyperintensity volume on MRI (a marker for poor vascular cerebral status[24]). In addition, midlife smoking, diabetes, and elevated waist-to-hip ratio were all predictive of worsened structural cerebral measures at later measurements.[24] These structural white matter changes are directly associated with cognitive decline across multiple functional domains, as is hypertension.[25]

In Addition to Blood Pressure Control, What Lifestyle Modifications Would Help This Patient?

Exercise has a beneficial effect in helping control BP but also may stimulate neurogenesis in the adult mammalian brain and help preserve memory during aging. This finding was initially shown in adult mice, as running increased cell proliferation and neurogenesis in the dentate gyrus of the hippocampus.[26] This finding was then shown in humans: moderate exercise increased the size of the hippocampus and improved memory in the elderly.[27] Older adults (in their 60s and 70s) had an increase in total brain volume with 6 months of aerobic exercise compared with those who had toning and stretching exercises only.[28] In another study, older adults (mean age 65 years) had increased white matter fiber bundle thickness associated with improvement in their aerobic fitness after 1 year of an exercise intervention; short-term memory also improved in those with improved aerobic fitness.[29]

This patient had been taking levetiracetam 1000 mg twice daily and had no further seizures. However, his wife complained that he had become very difficult to live with because of irritability.

What Special Considerations Affect the Choice of Antiepileptic Drugs in This Patient and in the Elderly?

Side effects from antiepileptic drugs (AEDs) often occur at lower doses in elderly patients than in younger patients. Elderly patients are particularly vulnerable to CNS-related drug effects. (For example, dizziness, drowsiness, and imbalance are common with AED use.) Elderly patients also often have decreased hepatic and renal clearance of AEDs and increased free concentrations of protein-bound AEDs.[6,30] Levetiracetam is generally well tolerated in elderly patients, but up to 10% of patients have irritability or mood disturbances with treatment; sedation is uncommon with levetiracetam but may occur in elderly patients. Patients should be warned carefully about monitoring for possible AED side effects; often, patients may not be aware of cognition or mood-related side effects that occur because of treatment; obtaining history about possible drug effects from this patient's wife is equally important.

Studies specifically examining side effects in elderly patients have shown most patients tolerate lamotrigine and levetiracetam well. In a multicenter, double-blind study comparing elderly patients treated with carbamazepine or lamotrigine, the dropout rate due to side effects from carbamazepine was more than twice as high as the dropout rate for lamotrigine, whereas rates of seizure freedom were higher for patients treated with lamotrigine.[31] A randomized study of elderly patients at Veterans Affairs' centers in the United States found a higher rate of retention for lamotrigine compared with gabapentin and carbamazepine.[32] A randomized controlled trial in the elderly in Europe showed that the retention rate of elderly patients on levetiracetam is significantly higher than that for carbamazepine. If used, extended-release carbamazepine should be used to improve tolerability compared with immediate-release carbamazepine.[33,34] Similarly, topiramate may impair language and general cognitive function and so should be used cautiously with low doses prescribed for older patients. Because of the reduced circulating albumin, reduced renal clearance, and impaired hepatic metabolism, CNS concentrations of many AEDs are elevated in elderly patients.[30,35] Consequently, elderly patients with seizures should usually be started at AED doses one-third to one-half those of younger adults and titrated slowly to low target ranges.

This patient takes lisinopril, which has no known drug interaction with levetiracetam. Elderly patients often have multiple medical conditions, and it is important to minimize drug interactions with AEDs. Many older AEDs are hepatic cytochrome inducers (phenytoin, carbamazepine, and phenobarbital), are enzyme inhibitors (valproic acid), and may interact with other drugs metabolized by similar hepatic cytochromes. Patients on anticoagulation, with warfarin in particular, need close monitoring and adjustment if taking an enzyme-inducing AED.[36] In general, newer AEDs have fewer drug-drug interactions and, therefore, may be preferred for this reason.[37] A survey of 43 expert adult epileptologists identified lamotrigine and levetiracetam as the most appropriate first-line AED choices for elderly patients.[38]

This patient started lamotrigine and titrated up to 150 mg twice a day over 6 weeks and then discontinued levetiracetam. He and his wife reported mood improvement, and he has had no further seizures.

This patient's presentation and course illustrated many key features of epilepsy in older patients: (1) Patients and physicians are often not aware that epilepsy is increasingly common in the elderly population. (2) Many of the vascular risk factors associated with the onset of epilepsy in later years are present during midlife with increased incidences of seizure beginning in the late 50s/early 60s age group. (3) Patients may present with tonic-clonic seizures but usually have symptomatic forms of seizures with focal onset. Most frequently patients have general vascular risk factors associated with microvascular disease on MRI, often without major strokes; trauma, tumors, and degenerative disorders are also common causes of seizures in older adults. (4) Elderly patients are particularly susceptible to CNS-related effects of AEDs, such as dizziness and sedation, and usually need treatment with slow titration of well-tolerated AEDs to low target ranges.

CASE 2: MEDICALLY RESISTANT EPILEPSY

A 28-year-old right-handed woman with recurring seizures is evaluated in an epilepsy center. She has a history of seizures since 14 years of age and currently has 1 or 2 seizures every month consisting of a warning of an odd feeling in her stomach, followed by staring, chewing, and unresponsiveness. Seizures last about 2 minutes, with confusion resolving over 5 minutes. She has more severe seizures evolving into tonic-clonic convulsions about once per year.

She has no clear cause for her seizures; she has no history of birth complications, such as prematurity, febrile seizures, head trauma, meningitis, or encephalitis, and has no family history of seizures.

At 18 years of age, she had an EEG showing occasional left temporal sharp waves. A brain MRI at 23 years of age was normal, including axial FLAIR images and pre-contrast and postcontrast T1 imaging.

She has been treated with levetiracetam 1500 mg twice a day, with lacosamide 200 mg twice a day added recently for recurrent seizures. In the past, she took oxcarbazepine 300 mg twice a day but stopped due to dizziness.

Does This Patient Have Drug-Resistant Epilepsy?

The ILAE defines medically resistant epilepsy as the failure to achieve seizure freedom after adequate trials of 2 well-tolerated, appropriately chosen, and used AEDs.[1] This patient has seizures despite treatment with 2 AEDs indicated for her focal seizure type, both given at high target doses, and so she is classified as having medically resistant epilepsy. A third AED produced side effects at low doses and so does not count towards seizures persisting on 2 AEDs. Most people with epilepsy will achieve seizure freedom with medications alone.[39] However, a large minority (30%–40%) of patients such as this one has drug-resistant epilepsy, which translates into 20 to 26 million people worldwide.[40] After the failure of 2 or more appropriate AEDs (failure due to seizures rather than intolerable side effects), only 4% of patients will become seizure free with treatment with a third AED; and fourth, fifth, and successive AEDs completely controlled seizures in less than 1%.[39]

This patient has continued seizures despite 2 appropriate AEDs. She, therefore, has medically refractory epilepsy and has a less than 10% chance of becoming seizure free with additional medical treatment using current AEDs.

What are Additional Treatment Options for Her?

Her seizures have not been controlled with monotherapy, and she is a candidate for adjunctive treatment with complementary AEDs.[41] Additional adjunctive treatments she has not tried include carbamazepine, topiramate, zonisamide, perampanel, eslicarbazepine, and lamotrigine. She also may be a candidate to receive treatment with an investigational agent if trials with promising AEDs are available in her region.[2] Her seizures persisted despite 2 first-line AEDs for her seizure types, and she was referred to an epilepsy center for further evaluation. Prolonged video-EEG monitoring would help confirm she has epilepsy (and not psychogenic nonepileptic seizures), characterize her seizures as generalized or focal types, and determine whether she had received appropriate AED treatment (lacosamide is not indicated for generalized epilepsy) (**Table 1**: AEDs for seizure types). Future treatment depends on the patient's individual treatment goals and whether they would consider evaluation for epilepsy surgery. Does the patient strongly wish to drive and potentially reduce or stop AEDs to minimize side effects? Both are feasible goals if she is found to be a good candidate for focal resective surgery. Does she instead want to avoid surgery, for example, her most frequent seizures are not disabling and she does not wish to risk surgery and, therefore, receive additional medication trials? If patients decline surgery, their seizures may improve with some of the newer AEDs.[2]

This Patient's Goal is to Obtain Her Drivers' License and Minimize Disability Associated with Seizures. What are the Next Steps in Management?

This patient's goal is to become seizure free so that she can drive and prevent disability associated with seizures. Additional AED trials may reduce her seizure frequency; however, they are unlikely to bring her seizure freedom,[39] and so she is scheduled for video-EEG to determine whether she is a candidate for surgical treatment. Two randomized controlled trials have found that surgical treatment provides seizure freedom in 60% to 85% of patients with temporal lobe epilepsy who qualify for surgery, whereas continued medical management provided seizure freedom in 0% to 8% of patients.[42,43] Social outcomes, such as employment and quality of life, were significantly improved after successful surgery compared with continued medical management.[42,43]

This patient next had video-EEG monitoring and had 4 left anterior temporal-onset seizures recorded.

Table 1
Commonly used antiepileptic drugs for focal and generalized epilepsies

Focal Epilepsies	Generalized Epilepsies
Carbamazepine	Clobazam
Clobazam	Ethosuximide
Eslicarbazepine	Lamotrigine
Gabapentin	Levetiracetam
Lacosamide	Perampanel
Lamotrigine	Topiramate
Levetiracetam	Valproate
Oxcarbazepine	Zonisamide
Perampanel	
Phenytoin	
Topiramate	
Valproate	
Zonisamide	

What Additional Testing Should be Done on This Patient?

Her MRI should be repeated using an epilepsy protocol with closely spaced coronal FLAIR imaging. The role of MRI for selecting patients for surgery has increased with improvements in imaging quality. Many patients have subtle lesions detected on modern MRI, which may be causes for focal seizures. These lesions include focal cortical dysplasia (found in one-third of children with refractory epilepsy), traumatic contusion injuries (often missed on head CT), and mesial temporal sclerosis (MTS) (atrophy and increased signal in the hippocampus). Lesions that correspond to the area of seizure onset on video-EEG help guide surgical planning (and may obviate intracranial monitoring). Up to 65% of patients with focal epilepsy and normal 1.5-T MRIs finding no abnormalities are found to have focal lesions with a 3-T MRI, which often changes the clinical management.[44]

> She had a 3-T epilepsy protocol MRI, which showed increased T2 FLAIR signal in the left hippocampus compared with the right and mild left hippocampal volume loss in the left hippocampus compared with the right, consistent with left MTS (not previously seen on 1.5-T MRI at 23 years of age; **Fig. 3**).

Is This Patient a Surgical Candidate?

The patient may be a candidate for temporal lobectomy with amygdalohippocampectomy. All of her seizures during epilepsy monitoring unit (EMU) admission were left temporal in onset; her MRI showed evidence of left hippocampal sclerosis, with atrophy and signal increase. In surgical planning, congruent findings help pinpoint the site of seizure onset. For this patient, these findings would be a typical clinical semiology of temporal lobe seizures (confusion and often chewing), left temporal lobe seizure onset on interictal and ictal scalp EEG recordings, and imaging abnormalities and neuropsychology testing showing left temporal dysfunction (mild naming and new verbal learning deficits).[45]

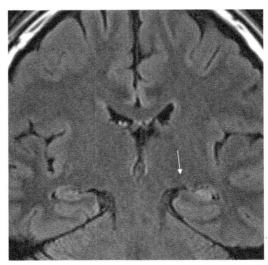

Fig. 3. Left MTS. The left hippocampus (*arrow*) has reduced volume compared with the right with increased signal on FLAIR imaging, consistent with MTS.

Would This Patient Still be a Surgical Candidate if Her MRI was Normal?

If the patient's MRI is normal, functional imaging with PET may help localize her seizures; approximately 40% of patients with epilepsy have localizing PET findings despite normal MRI.[46]

Would This Patient Still be a Surgical Candidate if Her Scalp Electroencephalogram did Not Show a Clear Lateralization?

If she had seizures during her EMU admission without a clear lateralization at onset, she could still benefit from intracranial monitoring. Poorly localized seizures, or seizures apparently arising close to eloquent cortex, may be localized with intracranial recording with subsequent successful resection.[47] Magnetoencephalography (MEG) may help guide placement of intracranial electrodes, especially if EEG localization of patients' seizures is unclear. In one study, MEG localized an interictal dipole source in most patients (78%); when surgical resection included the source identified by MEG, a significantly higher proportion of patients were seizure free after surgery (compared with those whose resection did not include the MEG source).[48]

Patients with clearly independent multifocal seizures or seizures arising from dominant temporal language areas may not be surgical candidates and should consider alternative approaches to treatment (discussed later).

What is This Patient's Expected Seizure Outcome from Left Temporal Lobectomy?

This patient has a very good chance of becoming seizure free with surgery, as she has evidence of MTS on MRI in her left hippocampus and has left temporal seizure onset on EEG. Eighty percent to 90% of patients with unilateral MTS are seizure free after temporal lobe resection that includes medial structures.[49]

Will She Have Any Memory or Speech Impairment After Surgery?

It is important to evaluate and counsel the patient about her risks for cognitive losses with surgery: Her greatest risk is of decreased naming ability and a decrease in new verbal learning following dominant temporal lobe surgery. Between 22% and 65% of patients undergoing left (dominant) anterior temporal lobectomy will have a decline in verbal memory[50]; however, the greatest risk is for patients with normal memory and naming preoperatively and normal imaging of their hippocampus before surgery.

On preoperative neuropsychology testing, this patient has a mild naming deficit and low-average new verbal learning abilities and with evidence of left MTS on MRI has a low risk for major declines in memory abilities with surgery.[50,51]

What if She had Frontal Lobe Epilepsy Rather than Temporal Lobe Epilepsy? Would She Still be a Surgical Candidate?

If this patient had a discrete extratemporal lesion likely causing her seizures, such as a cavernous angioma in a noncritical area, she may be a good candidate for successful surgery.[52] Common extratemporal seizure foci include arteriovenous malformations, neoplasms, and focal cortical dysplasia. In general, the chances of patients becoming seizure freedom following extratemporal resection are lower than those following temporal lobectomy. After resection of extratemporal cortical dysplasia, 55% of patients in one series were seizure free; however, focal MRI findings predicted much better outcomes.[52] Patients with nonlesional extratemporal lobe seizures often have large cortical epileptogenic regions, which may involve critical language, motor, or sensory areas, which cannot be safely resected. Consequently, seizure-free rates for nonlesional extratemporal lobe surgery are about 29% to 38%.[53] Carefully selected patients still may benefit from surgery, though these rates are still higher than for continued medical management.

This Patient Wants to Minimize Her Risks for Cognitive Loss and Minimize Recovery Time after Surgery. Are There Alternatives to Open Temporal Lobe Resection?

She may be a candidate for MRI-guided thermal ablation for selective amygdalohippo-campotomy. This therapy is a new, minimally invasive therapy for mesial temporal lobe epilepsy in which patients have stereotactic laser ablation of the amygdala and hippo-campus.[54] Patients typically recover from their procedure within several days compared with several-week periods of recovery with major craniotomy with anterior temporal resection and amygdalohippocampectomy. She should be warned that the rates of seizure freedom in preliminary series are slightly lower than shown for open resection, around 55% to 60% for temporal lobe seizures.[54,55] Preliminary results suggest risks for cognitive loss following standard resective surgery may be reduced with selective ablation; patients with standard resections in one series, on average, declined in one or more naming or object recognition task, whereas patients with selective laser amyg-dalohippocampotomy had stable performance.[56]

If This Patient had Both Left and Right Temporal Lobe Seizures During Video Electroencephalogram Monitoring, Would She Have Any Options Besides Additional Medications?

Some patients have multifocal epilepsy or have seizure foci not amenable to resection because of involvement of primary motor or language areas. Many seizure causes, such as trauma and encephalitis, may be associated with more than one epileptogenic site or may have broad epileptogenic zones that cannot be removed safely.

Nonsurgical approaches to drug-resistant epilepsy include stimulation therapies and treatment with new generations of AEDs (**Table 2**). Vagus nerve stimulation (VNS) involves implanting a subcutaneous stimulator unit in the upper chest and chronic intermittent stimulation through an electrode clipped to the left vagus nerve in the neck. VNS helps reduce seizures and possibly seizure severity in approximately one-half of patients and so should be viewed as a safe but palliative therapy.[57] Ran-domized controlled studies of VNS use found a 24% to 45% reduction in seizures (compared with 6%–15% reduction in a low-stimulation VNS comparison group), with 31% to 38% of patients experiencing at least a 50% decrease in seizures.[58–60] Seizure reduction seems to improve over time with VNS.[60] Rates of seizure freedom are low, reported in less than 5% of patients.[57] Patients, such as this one, who may be candidates for potentially curative epilepsy surgery, should be evaluated for this before pursuing palliative VNS therapy.

If the patient had 2 seizure foci identified on scalp recordings or had seizures involving critical regions that could not be resected safely (eg, posterior perisylvian areas on the left dominant temporal region), she may be a candidate for responsive neurostimulation (RNS).[61] RNS is a closed-loop system with intracranial electrodes

Table 2 Nonmedical therapies by seizure type	
Focal Epilepsies	**Generalized Epilepsies**
Open resection or thermal ablation	Dietary therapy
Responsive neurostimulation	Vagus nerve stimulation
Dietary therapy	
Vagus nerve stimulation	

placed in seizure-onset zones. The device records ictal EEG and counterstimulates to attempt to interrupt synchronized ictal spread of seizures. Patients with RNS have had an average of 48% to 66% reduction in seizures during 3 to 6 years of follow-up, with 16% of patients seizure free.[62] The response from RNS is often delayed several months during stimulation therapy, suggesting a modulatory effect of responsive stimulation in seizure zones in reducing seizures.[61]

If this patient was not a surgical candidate and has frequent disabling seizures despite multiple trials of AEDs, she may benefit from dietary therapy. The modified Atkins diet is a form of ketogenic diet that is often well tolerated in adults and helps reduced seizures (>50%) in 22% to 67% of patients.[63,64] This intervention can be effective for all seizure types and, although more commonly used in children, has growing use in adults.

This patient underwent MRI-guided thermal ablation of her left amygdala and hippocampus. She has been seizure free for the past year since surgery and had no decrease in her verbal and memory skills. Her case highlights the importance of video-EEG monitoring and imaging testing to investigate possible surgical or other treatments for medically refractory epilepsy. Patients with medically resistant epilepsy can be identified early in their course after failing optimized treatment with 2 or 3 AEDs. Many patients are candidates for potentially curative surgery; others may be candidates for new stimulation treatments or for a diet therapy.

REFERENCES

1. Kwan P, Arzimanoglou A, Berg AT, et al. Definition of drug resistant epilepsy: consensus proposal by the ad hoc Task Force of the ILAE Commission on Therapeutic Strategies. Epilepsia 2010;51:1069–77.
2. Krauss GL, Sperling MR. Treating patients with medially resistant epilepsy. Neurol Clin Pract 2011;1:14–23.
3. Grubb BP, Gerard G, Roush K, et al. Differentiation of convulsive syncope and epilepsy with head-up tilt testing. Ann Intern Med 1991;115:871–6.
4. Sheldon R. How to differentiate syncope from seizure. Cardiol Clin 2015;33: 377–85.
5. Theodore WH, Porter RJ, Penry JK. Complex partial seizures: clinical characteristics and differential diagnosis. Neurology 1983;33:1115–21.
6. Cloyd J, Hauser W, Towne A, et al. Epidemiological and medical aspects of epilepsy in the elderly. Epilepsy Res 2006;68(Suppl 1):S39–48.
7. Berg AT, Berkovi SF, Brodie MJ, et al. Revised terminology and concepts for organization of seizures and epilepsies: report of the ILAE Commission on Classification and Terminology, 2005-2009. Epilepsia 2010;51:676–85.
8. Krauss GL, Abdallah A, Lesser R, et al. Clinical and EEG features of patients with EEG wicket rhythms misdiagnosed with epilepsy. Neurology 2005;64:1879–83.
9. Hauser WA, Annegers JF, Kurland LT. Incidence of epilepsy and unprovoked seizures in Rochester, Minnesota: 1935-1984. Epilepsia 1993;34:453–68.
10. Hesdorffer DC, Logroscino G, Benn EK, et al. Estimating risk for developing epilepsy: a population-based study in Rochester, Minnesota. Neurology 1996; 46:727–30.
11. Krumholz A, Wiebe S, Gronseth G, et al. Practice parameter: evaluating an apparent unprovoked first seizure in adults. Neurology 2007;69:1996–2007.
12. Beghi E, Carpio A, Forsgren L, et al. Recommendation for a definition of acute symptomatic seizure. Epilepsia 2010;51:671–5.

13. Krumholtz A, Uhinner U, Fronch J, et al. Evidence-based guideline management of an unprovoked first seizure in adults. Neurology 2015;85:1526–7.

14. Fisher RS, Acevedo C, Arzimanoglou A, et al. ILAE official report: a practical clinical definition of epilepsy. Epilepsia 2014;55:475–82.

15. Ramsay RE, Pryor F. Epilepsy in the elderly. Neurology 2000;55(5 Suppl 1):S9–14 [discussion: S54–8].

16. So EL, Annegers JF, Hauser WA, et al. Population-based study of seizure disorders after cerebral infarction. Neurology 1996;46:350–5.

17. Hommet C, Mondon K, Camus V, et al. Epilepsy and dementia in the elderly. Dement Geriatr Cogn Disord 2008;25:293–300.

18. Amatniek JC, Hauser WA, DelCastillo-Castaneda C, et al. Incidence and predictors of seizures in patients with Alzheimer's disease. Epilepsia 2006;47:867–72.

19. Mendez MF, Catanzaro P, Doss RC, et al. Seizures in Alzheimer's disease: a clinicopathologic study. J Geriatr Psychiatry Neurol 1994;7:230–3.

20. Picco A, Archetti S, Ferrara M, et al. Seizures can precede cognitive symptoms in late-onset Alzheimer's disease. J Alzheimers Dis 2011;27:737–42.

21. Ng SK, Hauser WA, Brust JC, et al. Hypertension and the risk of new-onset unprovoked seizures. Neurology 1993;43:425–8.

22. Maxwell H, Hanby M, Parkes LM, et al. Prevalence and subtypes of radiological cerebrovascular disease in late-onset isolated seizures and epilepsy. Clin Neurol Neurosurg 2013;115:591–6.

23. Li X, Breteler MM, de Bruyne MC, et al. Vascular determinants of epilepsy: the Rotterdam Study. Epilepsia 1997;38:1216–20.

24. Debbette S, Seshadri S, Beiser A, et al. Midlife vascular risk factor exposure accelerates structural brain aging and cognitive decline. Neurology 2011;77:461–8.

25. Ylikoski R, Ylikoski A, Raininko R, et al. Cardiovascular diseases, health status, brain imaging findings and neuropsychological functioning in neurologically healthy elderly individuals. Arch Gerontol Geriatr 2000;30:115–30.

26. Van Praag H, Kempermann G, Gage FH. Running increases cell proliferation and neurogenesis in the adult mouse dentate gyrus. Nat Neurosci 1999;2:266–70.

27. Erickson KI, Voss MW, Prakash RS, et al. Exercise training increases size of hippocampus and improves memory. Proc Natl Acad Sci U S A 2011;108:3017–22.

28. Colcombe SJ, Erickson KI, Scalf PE, et al. Aerobic exercise training increases brain volume in aging humans. J Gerontol A Biol Sci Med Sci 2006;11:1166–70.

29. Voss MW, Heo S, Prakash RS, et al. The influence of aerobic fitness on cerebral white matter integrity and cognitive function in older adults: results of a one-year exercise intervention. Hum Brain Mapp 2013;34:2972–85.

30. Kirmani BF, Robinson DM, Kikam A, et al. Selection of antiepileptic drugs in older people. Curr Treat Options Neurol 2014;16:295.

31. Brodie MJ, Overstall PW, Giorgi L. Multicentre, double-blind, randomized comparison between lamotrigine and carbamazepine in elderly patients with newly diagnosed epilepsy. Epilepsy Res 1999;37:81–7.

32. Rowan AJ, Ramsay RE, Collins JF, et al. New onset geriatric epilepsy: a randomized study of gabapentin, lamotrigine, and carbamazepine. Neurology 2005;64:1868–73.

33. Ficker DM, Privitera M, Krauss G, et al. Improved tolerability and efficacy in epilepsy patients with extended-release carbamazepine. Neurology 2005;65:593–5.

34. Werhahn KJ, Trinka E, Dobesberger J, et al. A randomized, double-blind comparison of antiepileptic drug treatment in the elderly with new-onset focal epilepsy. Epilepsia 2015;56(3):450–9.

35. Johannessen Landmark C, Baftiu A, Tysse I, et al. Pharmacokinetic variability of four newer antiepileptic drugs: lamotrigine, levetiracetam, oxcarbazepine, and topiramate: a comparison of the impact of age and comedication. Ther Drug Monit 2012;34:440–5.

36. Patsolos PN, Froscher W, Pisani F, et al. The importance of drug interactions in epilepsy therapy. Epilepsia 2002;43:365–85.

37. Patsalos PN. Drug interactions with the newer AEDs. Clin Pharmacokinet 2013; 52:1045–61.

38. Karceski S, Morrell M, Carpenter D. Treatment of epilepsy in adults: expert opinion. Epilepsy Behav 2005;7:S1–64.

39. Brodie MJ, Barry SJ, Bamagous GA, et al. Patterns of treatment response in newly diagnosed epilepsy. Neurology 2012;78:1548–54.

40. Moshe SL, Perucca E, Ryvlin P, et al. Epilepsy: new advances. Lancet 2015;385: 884–98.

41. Kwan P, Brodie MJ. Combination therapy in epilepsy. Drugs 2006;66:1817–29.

42. Weibe S, Blume WT, Girvin JP, et al, the Effectiveness and Efficiency of Surgery for Temporal Lobe Epilepsy Study Group. A randomized, controlled trial of surgery for temporal-lobe epilepsy. N Engl J Med 2001;345:311–8.

43. Engel J Jr, McDermott MP, Wiebe S, et al. Early surgical therapy for drug-resistant temporal lobe epilepsy: a randomized trial. JAMA 2012;207(9):922–30.

44. Knake S, Triantafyllou C, Wald LL, et al. 3T phased array MRI improves the pre-surgical evaluation in focal epilepsies. Neurology 2005;65:1026–31.

45. Engel J, McDermott MP, Wiebe S, et al. Design considerations for a multicenter randomized controlled trial of early surgery for mesial temporal lobe epilepsy. Epilepsia 2010;51:1978–86.

46. Menon RN, Radhakrishnan A, Parameswaran R, et al. Does F-18 FDG-PET substantially alter the surgical decision-making in drug-resistant partial epilepsy? Epilepsy Behav 2015;51:133–9.

47. Weinand ME, Wyler AR, Richey ET, et al. Long-term ictal monitoring with subdural strip electrodes: prognostic factors for selecting temporal lobectomy candidates. J Neurosurg 1992;77:20–8.

48. Englot DJ, Nagarajan SS, Imber BS, et al. Epileptogenic zone localization using magnetoencephalography predicts seizure freedom in epilepsy surgery. Epilepsia 2015;56:949–58.

49. Cascino GD. Surgical treatment for epilepsy. Epilepsy Res 2004;60:179–86.

50. Dulay MF, Busch RM. Prediction of neuropsychological outcome after resection of temporal and extratemporal seizure foci. Neurosurg Focus 2012;32:E4.

51. Chelune GJ, Naugle RI, Luders H, et al. Prediction of cognitive change as a function of preoperative ability status among temporal lobectomy patients seen at 6-month follow up. Neurology 1991;41:399–404.

52. Xue H, Cai L, Dong S, et al. Clinical characteristics and post-surgical outcomes of focal cortical dysplasia subtypes. J Clin Neurosci 2016;23:68–72.

53. Noe K, Sulc V, Wong-Kisiel L, et al. Long-term outcomes after nonlesional extra-temporal lobe epilepsy surgery. JAMA Neurol 2013;70:1003–8.

54. Willie JT, Laxpati NG, Drane DL, et al. Real-time magnetic resonance-guided stereotactic laser amygdalohippocampotomy for mesial temporal lobe epilepsy. Neurosurgery 2014;74:584–5.

55. Waseem H, Osborn K, Schoenberg M, et al. Laser ablation therapy: an alternative treatment for medically resistant mesial temporal lobe epilepsy after age 50. Epilepsy Behav 2015;51:152–7.

56. Drane DL, Loring DW, Voets NL, et al. Better object recognition and naming outcome with MRI-guided stereotactic laser amygdalohippocampotomy for temporal lobe epilepsy. Epilepsia 2015;56:101–13.

57. Englot DJ, Chang EF, Auguste KI. VNS for epilepsy: a meta analysis of efficacy and predictors of response. J Neurosurg 2011;115:1248–55.

58. Vagus Nerve Stimulation Study Group. A randomized controlled trial of chronic vagus nerve stimulation for treatment of medically intractable seizures. Neurology 1995;45:224–30.

59. Handsforth A, DeGiorgio C, Schachter S, et al. Vagus nerve stimulation therapy for partial-onset seizures: a randomized active-control trial. Neurology 1998;51:48–55.

60. DeGiorgio C, Schachter S, Handforth A, et al. Prospective long-term study of vagus nerve stimulation for the treatment of refractory seizures. Epilepsia 2000;41: 1195–200.

61. Ben-Menachem E, Krauss GL. Epilepsy: responsive neurostimulation – modulating the epileptic brain. Nat Rev Neurol 2014;10:247–8.

62. Bergey GK, Morrell MJ, Mizrahi EM, et al. Long-term treatment with responsive brain stimulation in adults with refractory partial seizures. Neurology 2015; 84(8):810–7.

63. Sirven J, Whedon B, Caplan D, et al. The ketogenic diet for intractable epilepsy in adults: preliminary results. Epilepsia 1999;40:1721–6.

64. Kossoff EH, Henry BJ, Cervenka MC. Efficacy of dietary therapy for juvenile myoclonic epilepsy. Epilepsy Behav 2013;26:162–4.

Neuro-Ophthalmology Cases for the Neurologist

Stacy V. Smith, MD[a], Alec L. Amram, MD[b], Elsa M. Rodarte, MD[c], Andrew G. Lee, MD[a,b,d,e,f,g,h],*

KEYWORDS

- Giant cell arteritis • Arterial dissection • Intracranial aneurysm
- Pituitary adenoma and apoplexy • Mucormycosis

KEY POINTS

- Neurologists should be aware of specific urgent and emergent neuro-ophthalmic conditions, including giant cell arteritis, arterial dissection, intracranial aneurysm, pituitary apoplexy, and invasive sino-orbital fungal infection (eg, mucormycosis).
- Early recognition and treatment of these disorders can greatly impact patient morbidity and mortality, including the preservation of both vision and life.
- Neurologists should be cognizant of the key and differentiating clinical and radiographic features for these presentations.

INTRODUCTION

Neurologists may be the first point of medical contact for patients with neuro-ophthalmic disorders, which can threaten life or vision. This article presents the key clinical and radiographic features for the following neuro-ophthalmic emergencies: (1) giant cell arteritis (GCA), (2) sino-orbital mucormycosis, (3) pituitary apoplexy, (4) pupil-involving third nerve palsy due to aneurysm, and (5) carotid dissection with

Disclosures: None of the authors have any disclosures.
[a] Department of Ophthalmology, Blanton Eye Institute, Houston Methodist Hospital, 6560 Fannin Street, Scurlock 450, Houston, TX 77030, USA; [b] Department of Ophthalmology, University of Texas Medical Branch, 301 University Boulevard, Galveston, TX 77555, USA; [c] Department of Neurobiology and Anatomy, University of Texas Health Science Center at Houston, 6431 Fannin Street, MSB 7.420, Houston, TX 77030, USA; [d] Department of Ophthalmology, Baylor College of Medicine, One Baylor Plaza, Houston, TX 77030, USA; [e] Department of Ophthalmology, Weill Cornell Medicine, 1300 York Avenue, New York, NY 10065, USA; [f] Department of Neurology, Weill Cornell Medicine, 1300 York Avenue, New York, NY 10065, USA; [g] Department of Neurosurgery, Weill Cornell Medicine, 1300 York Avenue, New York, NY 10065, USA; [h] Section of Ophthalmology, UT MD Anderson Cancer Center, 1515 Holcombe Boulevard, Houston, TX 77030, USA
* Corresponding author. Department of Ophthalmology, Blanton Eye Institute, Houston Methodist Hospital, 6560 Fannin Street, Scurlock 450, Houston, TX 77030.
E-mail address: AGLee@HoustonMethodist.org

Horner syndrome. Representative, composite case-based examples are used to illustrate specific points.

CASE 1: GIANT CELL ARTERITIS

An 80-year-old man presented to the emergency room with new onset, severe, temporal headaches, and 2 transient visual loss episodes in the right eye (oculus dexter; OD). He also experienced 3 episodes of transient binocular horizontal diplopia over the course of the last week. He was seen by an outside ophthalmologist and had a normal eye examination and was referred to a neurologist. His past medical history was significant for well-controlled hypertension on amlodipine. Visual acuity was 20/20 in both eyes (oculus utro; OU) and the remainder of the eye and neurologic examinations were normal. The patient was admitted to an outside hospital for work-up of transient ischemic attack (TIA). A carotid ultrasound, electrocardiogram, echocardiogram, and MRI of the brain and magnetic resonance angiography (MRA) of the head and neck were normal. The episodes were attributed to migraines and TIA and the patient was started on aspirin 81 mg per day and discharged. Three days later, however, the patient again presented to the emergency room but now with complete vision loss OD. Neuro-ophthalmology examination showed a vision of no light perception (NLP) OD and 20/20 in the left eye (OS). The right pupil was nonreactive and amaurotic with a relative afferent pupillary defect OD. Fundoscopic examination demonstrated pallid optic disc edema OD (**Fig. 1**). The remainder of the eye examination was normal OU. The left fundus showed a normal optic nerve but the cup to disc ratio was 0.4 OS. Palpation over the right temple elicited localized pain and tenderness. Laboratory tests showed an elevated C-reactive protein (CRP) of 2.3 mg/dL (normal 0.8 mg/dL or less) and erythrocyte sedimentation rate (ESR) of 75 mm/h (normal for a man aged 80 years = 40 mm/h). The platelet count was elevated at 550 per uL (normal <450 per uL). Due to concern for GCA the patient was immediately started on 1000 mg of intravenous (IV) methylprednisolone for 3 days and then continued on oral prednisone at 1 mg/kg. A temporal artery biopsy confirmed the diagnosis of GCA. The patient continued on high-dose oral steroid therapy but the vision remained NLP OD.

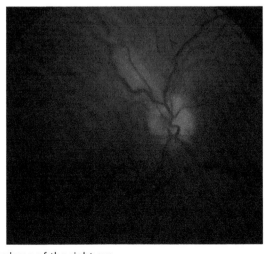

Fig. 1. Pallid disc edema of the right eye.

Clinical Questions

1. What are the common presenting symptoms and signs of GCA?
2. What is the recommended treatment protocol for GCA?
3. What is the prognosis for visual changes due to GCA?

Discussion

GCA (also known as temporal arteritis) is a medium and large vessel vasculitis that almost exclusively affects people older than the age of 50 years.[1] Transmural inflammation and intimal hyperplasia cause occlusion of predominantly extracranial branches of the aorta, resulting in end-organ ischemia.[1] The most worrisome complication of GCA, irreversible loss of vision, is typically due to ischemic infarction of the optic nerve (arteritic ischemic optic neuropathy).[2,3]

The most common presenting symptoms of GCA include new onset headache, scalp tenderness, visual complaints, and jaw and tongue claudication. Visual complaints may include permanent or transient vision loss, diplopia, and eye pain. Constitutional symptoms such as fever, weight loss, and proximal joint pain and weakness (ie, polymyalgia rheumatic) are also common.[3–5] **Table 1** (adapted from Paraskevas and colleagues[3] and Hellman[4]) lists the common features of GCA. Machado and colleagues[6] investigated the clinical manifestations of temporal arteritis in residents of Olmsted County, Minnesota, from 1950 to 1985. They found that headache was present more than 50% of the time,[6] transient vision loss was present in 5% to 6%, blindness was present in 12%, and diplopia was present 12% to 13%.[6] In a meta-analysis, Shmerling and Smetana[5] looked at 14 common presenting symptoms of GCA and found that only jaw claudication and diplopia (positive likelihood ratios of 4.2 and 3.4) significantly increased the chances for GCA. However, the sensitivities of diplopia and jaw claudication were only 9% and 34%, respectively.[5]

Immediate high-dose systemic corticosteroids is the treatment of choice for GCA but the exact route, frequency, route, type, and dosage of corticosteroid remains somewhat controversial.[2,7] Many investigators recommend an initial high-dose (1000 mg for example) of IV methylprednisolone for patients with visual loss and there is some evidence that this regimen allows for more rapid tapering of oral glucocorticoids and it may allow a greater number of patients to experience sustained remission

Table 1
Symptoms and signs of giant cell arteritis

Ocular	Oral	Other or Systemic
Amaurosis fugax	Jaw claudication	Headache
Blindness	Trismus	Fever
Diplopia	Odontogenic pain	Proximal joint (shoulder, hip girdle)
Ophthalmoplegia	Dysphagia	pain and weakness
Ptosis	Dysarthria	Fever
Miosis	Submandibular mass	Dry cough
Eye pain	Chin hypoaesthesia	Hoarseness or change in voice
	Macroglossia	Anorexia
	Glossitis	Weight loss
	Lip necrosis	Tinnitus
	Tongue necrosis	Scalp tenderness
	Tongue claudication	Palpable temporal artery

From Hellmann DB. Temporal arteritis: a cough, toothache, and tongue infarction. JAMA 2002;287:2996–3000; and Paraskevas KI, Boumpas DT, Vrentzos GE, et al. Oral and ocular/orbital manifestations of temporal arteritis: a disease with deceptive clinical symptoms and devastating consequences. Clin Rheumatol 2007;26:1044–8.

from GCA.[9] Other Investigators recommend 1 to 1.5 mg/kg of oral prednisone (espe
cially for cases without visual loss).[2,7] Although there has been no head to head randomized clinical trial to demonstrate superior efficacy and safety of high-dose IV
steroid compared with oral steroids in GCA, the authors generally recommend IV
treatment in GCA with acute visual loss. Regardless of whether or not the loading
dose is used, in our practice 1 to 1.5 mg/kg of oral prednisone is typically maintained
for at least 4 weeks because patients are at particularly high risk for vision loss within
the first several days to weeks after initial presentation.[2,7] The length of time patients
must stay on corticosteroids varies based on individual patient response and,
although most patients can discontinue the steroids after 1 to 2 years, others might
require prolonged or even lifelong low-dose maintenance steroid therapy.[2,7] The authors generally recommend a slow tapering schedule to the minimal dose of corticosteroids that will prevent an increase in ESR and CRP. Return of symptoms and the
decision to taper should be balanced against the corticosteroid-related side effects.[2,7]
We typically coordinate the steroid dose and monitoring of side effects with the primary care physician and/or rheumatology. In patients who are intolerant of steroid
therapy, other immunosuppressive or immunomodulating agents (eg, methotrexate
or biologics) have been used in GCA. However, results have been variable and inconclusive and corticosteroids remain first-line therapy.[2,9]

If a patient has already developed changes in his or her vision on initial presentation,
the visual prognosis is guarded. Although there are anecdotal reports of vision
improvement in affected eyes after starting steroid therapy the most commonly
accepted rationale for steroid treatment is the prevention of fellow eye involvement
or complications of systemic vasculitis.[10–14] The odds of regaining vision can be
improved if the diagnosis is made and treatment is started early in the disease
course.[11,12]

Neurologists should consider GCA in the differential diagnosis of every elderly patient with neuro-ophthalmic symptoms or signs, including transient visual loss or
diplopia that can mimic TIA from other causes. Although an ESR and/or CRP are suggestive of GCA, they may be normal. Likewise, the classic symptoms of GCA,
including headache, temporal pain, or scalp tenderness, may be minimal or absent
in some cases (ie, occult GCA). High-dose corticosteroids should be initiated immediately if there is clinical suspicion for GCA and the temporal artery biopsy (TAB) remains
the gold standard for diagnosis. Steroid treatment should not be delayed while await-
ing the performance and results of a TAB.

CASE 2: MUCORMYCOSIS

A 56-year-old Hispanic man with uncontrolled diabetes presented with a 3-week history of recurrent high-grade fever, throbbing headache, unilateral facial pain, and
proptosis. One week later, the patient developed a loss of visual acuity OD and facial
swelling of the nasal, infraorbital, and orbital regions. These lesions then ulcerated and
produced a foul smelling mucopurulent discharge. On examination, the patient
appeared ill, weak, and disoriented. The vision measured no light perception OD
and the right pupil was dilated and unresponsive to light or near stimulus. There
was a complete ophthalmoplegia OD. The remainder of the examination was normal
OU. Computerized tomography (CT) of the orbit and sinuses showed obliteration of
the right maxillary sinus and soft tissue edema in infiltration in to the right orbit.
Head and neck endoscopic examination of the nasal cavity and hard palate revealed
areas of black necrotic tissue. Endoscopic biopsy and debridement showed fungal
hyphae. Aggressive metabolic control of the diabetic hyperglycemia was initiated

along with initial broad spectrum antibiotic coverage followed by liposomal amphotericin B. The final pathologic testing confirmed *Rhizopus arrhizus*. Despite prolonged inpatient and outpatient antifungal therapy, the vision did not recover OD.

Clinical Questions

1. What are the common presentations of invasive fungal disease?
2. What risk factors predispose patients to mucormycosis?
3. What is the recommended treatment of invasive fungal disease?

Discussion

Mucormycosis is a rare fungal infection that can affect different parts of the body. The most common form of mucormycosis is cerebro-rhino-orbital mucormycosis.[15] Although mucormycosis is rare, special attention is warranted due to its overly aggressive behavior. Rapid recognition and accurate diagnosis, correction of risk factors, surgical debridement, and initiation of antifungal therapy are critical.[16]

A high clinical suspicion, followed by appropriate directed laboratory investigations, urgent imaging studies, and debridement or biopsy, is important to make the proper diagnosis of *Mucor*. Early diagnosis and initiation of therapy results in better clinical outcomes.[17,18] Chamilos and colleagues[19] reported that if treatment was initiated within 5 days of diagnosis, survival was markedly improved compared with initiation of polyene therapy at 6 or more days after diagnosis (83% vs 49% survival). CT imaging of the sinuses can show the typical sinus disease, bony invasion, and sino-orbital extension. Although MRI for most neuro-ophthalmic conditions is generally more sensitive, in an acutely ill patient in whom *Mucor* is suspected, CT scanning is faster, provides better bone and sinus detail, and is a better initial study than MRI in most settings of *Mucor* (**Fig. 2**).

Most cases of *Mucor* occur in immunocompromised patients but up to 20% of cases have no identifiable risk factor.[20] The most common risk factor associated with rhinocerebral mucormycosis is diabetes mellitus but multiple other risk factors have been identified (**Table 2**).[18,20–28] Control of underlying systemic disease (eg, medical control of diabetes and ketoacidosis) and discontinuation of potentially exacerbating medical therapy (eg, glucocorticosteroid) is important in the initial management of *Mucor*.[28] Aggressive surgical debridement of infected tissues and systemic antifungal therapy is critical in these cases. The debridement process and removal of necrotic tissue may improve systemic antifungal penetration of drug.[29] Radical

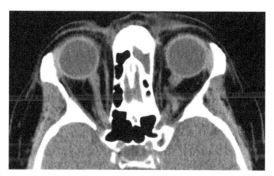

Fig. 2. CT of the sinuses shows hyperdense material in the sinuses. Left orbital involvement is evidenced by vascular congestion (left ophthalmic artery is enlarged), fat stranding at the orbital apex, and mild proptosis.

Table 2		
Underlying disorders, medical therapies, and local conditions associated with *Mucor*		
Underlying Systemic Disease	Result of Therapy	Local Conditions
Diabetes mellitus (Type I and II)	Antibiotics	Burns
Leukemia	Deferoxamine	Trauma
Lymphoma	Corticosteroids	—
Acute renal failure	—	—
Neutropenia	—	—
Metabolic ketoacidosis	—	—

surgical debridement of infected tissues usually results in higher rates of survival but benefit for intracranial disease remains in doubt.[30]

Liposomal amphotericin B has also been shown to be more effective than earlier regimens for treatment of *Mucor*.[31] Posaconazole has shown some efficacy in treating mucormycosis cases that are refractory to polyene therapy.[18,32] Posaconazole also has been used for primary prophylaxis for some high-risk patients (eg, acute myelogenous leukemia).[18] This regimen has been shown to successfully reduce incidence rates.[33–35]

Neurologists should be aware of the risk factors for *Mucor* (eg, diabetic ketoacidosis, deferoxamine use). Early clinical recognition, prompt CT imaging and biopsy, aggressive surgical debridement, control of systemic and local risk factors, and intensive antifungal therapy may save vision, eye, or life in these patients.

CASE 3: PITUITARY APOPLEXY

A 52-year-old woman presented with increasing headaches and loss of her peripheral vision in OU over the previous 2 days. She reported increased fatigue, weight gain, and polyuria. The rest of her medical and family history was unremarkable. The visual acuity was 20/20 OU. Automated perimetry (Humphrey visual field 24-2) revealed a bitemporal hemianopia (**Fig. 3**). The remainder of the examination was normal except for mild optic disc atrophy OU. Gadolinium-enhanced MRI of the brain showed a large intrasellar mass with suprasellar extension and compression of the optic chiasm consistent with pituitary macroadenoma (**Fig. 4**). She was referred by the outside ophthalmologist to neurosurgery but 2 days before her scheduled outpatient appointment, she developed the acute onset of the worst headache of her life and new binocular horizontal diplopia. Examination showed a left partial third nerve palsy. Noncontrast head CT scan in the emergency room revealed an acute hemorrhage within the previously described suprasellar mass. Emergent transsphenoidal but subtotal resection of the mass was performed. The pathologic result was pituitary adenoma with hemorrhage consistent with pituitary apoplexy. Endocrinologic evaluation during her hospitalization showed panhypopituitarism for which she started hormone replacement therapy. On follow-up, the diplopia and third nerve palsy had resolved, the visual acuity was 20/20 OU, and she had partial improvement in her previously seen bitemporal hemianopia.

Clinical Questions

1. What are the clinical manifestations of pituitary adenoma?
2. What is the differential diagnosis for a suprasellar mass?
3. What is the approach to treatment of pituitary adenomas, and does it vary depending on tumor type?

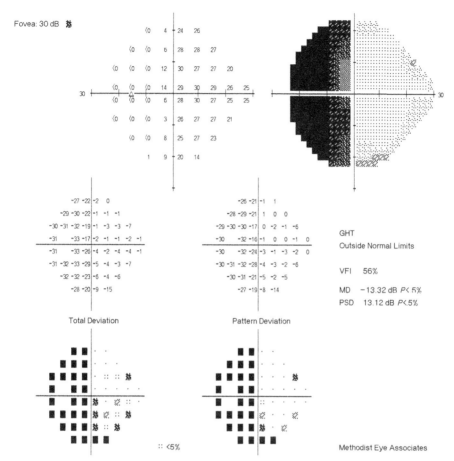

Fig. 3. Temporal field deficits bilaterally, each respecting the vertical midline. GHT, glaucoma hemifield test; MD, mean deviation; PMD, pattern standard deviation; VFI, visual field index.

Discussion

Pituitary adenomas are tumors derived from the adenohypophysis and typically produce slowly progressive neuro-ophthalmology symptoms or signs. Pituitary adenomas, however, can also bleed and present acutely as endocrinologic and neurosurgical emergencies. Pathogenic oncogene and tumor suppressor mutations lead to deregulation of mitosis, apoptosis, autophagy, and immune-targeting[36] and, because these are not restricted to the pituitary gland, 13% of patients have additional primary tumors.[37] Plotting the Surveillance, Epidemiology, and End Results (SEER) database demographics on benign adenoma incidence and median size shows a female biphasic and increasing incidence for benign tumors peaking at 30 to 34 and 70 to 74 years with a two-fold increase in median size with menopause. Male pituitary adenoma incidence also increases with age, and median size increases in the third and fourth decades. By 50 years of age, both genders have a median size around 2 cm.[38] Functional tumors typically present earlier due to the systemic symptoms, whereas nonfunctional tumors may not present until they have grown to size sufficient to compress adjacent structures (**Table 3**). Whereas prolactinomas are the most common type of functional pituitary adenoma, elevated prolactin levels alone do not

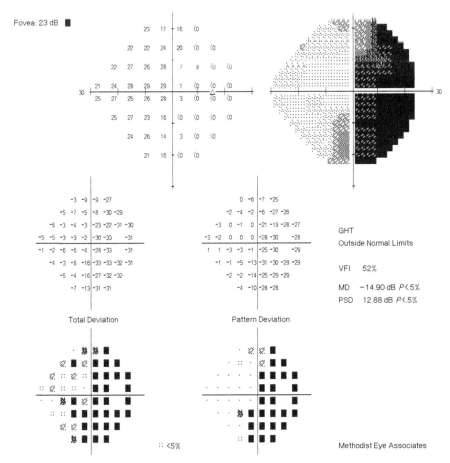

Fig. 3. (*continued*)

necessarily indicate a prolactin-secreting tumor because compression of the pituitary stalk by any mass lesion will disrupt dopamine input to the anterior pituitary and result in loss of inhibition of prolactin secretion. In general, the levels of prolactin from this stalk effect are lower than the prolactin levels of prolactinoma (eg, <150–200 ng/mL).

Although only 0.2% of the pituitary tumors are associated with metastases (eg, pituitary carcinoma), as many as 42% of pituitary adenomas are invasive, causing dysfunction of the suprasellar structures and thus requiring gross or subtotal resection because extent of disease adversely correlates with survival.[41] The patient presented with fatigue from secondary hypothyroidism, obesity from growth hormone (GH) deficiency, normoprolactinemia from lactotroph insufficiency, and diabetes insipidus (DI) from longstanding pressure on the ventromedial axons.[42] DI due to apoplexy alone is rare because of compensation by the inferior hypophyseal arteries.

Although around 50% to 60% of patients with sellar masses present with visual symptoms, 75% of patients with pituitary apoplexy will present with visual symptoms. Concerning for pituitary apoplexy are those with acute presentations, and those with cavernous sinus and brainstem involvement. Cavernous sinus involvement can cause third, fourth, and sixth cranial nerve palsies, and often present with diplopia and extraocular muscle dysfunction. The patient discussed previously presented with diplopia

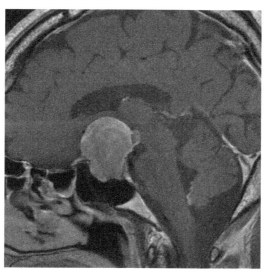

Fig. 4. The postcontrast MRI T1-weighted sequences demonstrate a large sellar and supra-sellar mass creating mass-effect on the optic chiasm, as well as the third ventricle.

Table 3 Pituitary adenomas	
Functional Tumors	
Lactotroph tumors (prolactin-secreting)	• 26.3% of the resected functional adenomas • Syndrome: amenorrhea, galactorrhea, gynecomastia, and loss of libido • Laboratory: prolactin, β-human chorionic gonadotropin, thyroid-stimulating hormone, free thyroxine (FT4)
Somatotroph tumors (growth hormone–secreting)	• Second most common functional tumor • Syndromes: acromegaly or gigantism • Laboratory: insulinlike growth factor-1, oral glucose challenge test • Assess: blood pressure, EKG, and sleep studies[59]
Corticotroph tumors (adrenocorticotropic hormone [ACTH]-secreting)	• 80% of nonexogenous Cushing syndromes • Laboratory: ACTH, cortisol
Gonadotroph tumors (luteinizing hormone and follicle-stimulating hormone–secreting)	Tend to be clinically silent beyond puberty
Thyrotroph tumors (thyroid-stimulating hormone–secreting)	• Least common • Laboratory: thyroid stimulating hormone, FT4
Nonfunctional	
Null-cell (nonreactive on immunocytochemistry)	• 33% of the pituitary adenomas[40] • Usually present late as macroadenomas (>1 cm) • Common syndrome: bitemporal inferior quadrantanopia or hemianopia with early loss of red vision

due to a phenomenon known as hemifield slide. A dense bitemporal hemianopia re sults in a lack of overlap between the fields of the left and right eye and, therefore, difficulty fusing the 2 images in the central nervous system. However, once bleeding compressed the cavernous sinus, she experienced horizontal diplopia due to a third nerve palsy.

The optic chiasm is located 1 cm above the sella in 90% of the population. Because the orientation of the fibers from the retina is conserved, the inferior nasal fibers will be the first affected by a sellar mass whose pressure vector is directed superiorly. Thus, the earliest visual field changes will occur in the superior temporal quadrants before progressing to bitemporal hemianopia.[43] Visual acuity may not be compromised because of retinal nerve fiber redundancy for the central degrees of vision. Thinning of the retinal nerve fiber layer on optical coherence tomography and clinical visualization of optic nerve atrophy has been used as a prognostic test for postsurgical reversibility of the visual symptoms.[43] The loss of nasal fibers correlates with a temporal pattern of atrophy commonly described as band or bowtie atrophy.

Versions and the 3-step test have to be assessed to diagnose third, fourth, and sixth nerve palsies. A suprasellar mass may also cause a Horner's syndrome since the sympathetic plexus covers the cavernous portion of the carotid artery. Hydrocephalus and a dorsal midbrain syndrome may also be present in the setting of a giant lesion or subarachnoid hemorrhage.[43]

In the setting of apoplexy, a change in mental status or acute compressive symptoms should prompt imaging (noncontrast head CT scan) and surgical decompression before diagnosis. Immunocytochemistry for hormone fractions and transcription factor expression have replaced color and pH-based staining for tumor diagnosis. Numerous other sellar and suprasellar lesions can occur, and must remain on the differential (**Table 4**).

The treatment approach is dictated by the patient's clinical presentation and pathologic diagnosis.[46–48] In the acute setting, neurosurgical referral and transsphenoidal decompression are indicated for changes in mental status, compressive signs, and bleeding on noncontrast CT. Transsphenoidal resection remains first-line treatment of adenomas but has been replaced in some instances. Dopamine agonists mimic

Table 4	
The differential diagnosis of sellar and suprasellar lesions	
Neoplastic[44]	• Anterior hypophyseal tumors (pituitary carcinoma, spindle cell oncocytoma) • Posterior hypophyseal tumors (pituicytoma, gangliocytoma, granular cell tumor) • Nonpituitary tumors (meningioma, glioma, metastasis, dysgerminoma)
Congenital[45]	• Cysts (Rathke cleft, arachnoid, and epidermoidal cyst) • Craniopharyngioma
Idiopathic	Empty sella turcica
Inflammatory[45]	• Lymphocytic hypophysitis • Granulomatous: sarcoidosis, tuberculosis, Langerhans cell histiocytosis
Vascular	• Intrasellar carotid artery aneurysms • Pituitary apoplexy • Subarachnoid hemorrhage • Skull base trauma
Infectious	• Tuberculosis • Abscess

the physiologic hypothalamic inhibition on the lactotrophs and usually decrease tumor size, even in the presence of chiasmatic syndrome. Nonfunctioning adenomas can undergo a dopamine agonist trial (lactotroph insufficiency may follow the stalk effect). Somatostatin or GH-receptor antagonist may be offered to patients with acromegaly. Radiotherapy can be offered for subtotal resection, tumor recurrence, or persistence of hormone secretion. Many patients also require replacement hormone therapy for hypopituitarism following treatment of the adenoma. The histologic grade determines the prognosis. Around 75% of patients with pituitary microadenomas are cured but 60% of macroadenomas will recur within 5 years of surgery.[47]

Neurologists should be aware of the possible acute presentations of pituitary adenoma, including hemorrhagic or necrotic apoplexy. Patients with pituitary apoplexy may present with acute, painful loss of vision in 1 or both eyes (eg, bitemporal or homonymous hemianopia), diplopia from ophthalmoplegia, ptosis, or anisocoria (eg, Horner syndrome or third nerve palsy). Early recognition, prompt sellar neuroimaging, and endocrinologic evaluation and hormonal replacement may be necessary. Neurosurgical treatment (eg, transsphenoidal decompression) may be necessary in the acute setting and patients may develop apoplexy with or without a known primary pituitary adenoma.

CASE 4: THIRD NERVE PALSY

A 61-year-old woman presented to the emergency room with blurry vision and drooping of her left eyelid. She denied double vision but did note that her typical migraine headaches seemed worse recently. Her father died at the age of 36 from a ruptured intracranial aneurysm. The rest of her medical history was significant only for hypertension controlled with amlodipine. On clinical examination, the visual acuity was 20/20 OU with correction. The right pupil was 4 mm in the dark and 2 mm in the light, whereas the left pupil was 7 mm in dark and poorly constricted to light. There was no relative afferent pupillary defect. In primary position, the left eye was down and out with a 20 prism diopter exotropia and 7 prism diopter left hypotropia. The left lid had 3 mm of ptosis. There were no other cranial nerve deficits and the rest of the neurologic and ophthalmologic examinations were normal. An urgent CT in the emergency department showed no abnormalities, so she was admitted for further evaluation, including an MRI and CT angiogram (CTA), which suggested a posterior communicating artery aneurysm on the left. Diagnostic catheter angiogram confirmed the aneurysm and she underwent endovascular coil embolization the following day. Follow-up evaluation 3 months later showed complete resolution of the pupil-involving third nerve palsy and angiographic confirmation of complete obliteration of the aneurysm.

Clinical Questions

1. What is the differential diagnosis for a third nerve palsy?
2. What work-up should be considered for new-onset third nerve palsy?

Discussion

A third nerve palsy is typically characterized by some degree of ipsilateral ptosis and ophthalmoplegia involving the extraocular muscles innervated by the oculomotor nerve (eg, deficits in supraduction, adduction, and infraduction), as demonstrated in **Fig. 5**.[49] There may or may not be pupil involvement and anisocoria (greater in the light). Depending on the extent of the nerve lesion, the ptosis and motility deficits may demonstrate a complete or partial third nerve palsy.[49] A partial third nerve palsy

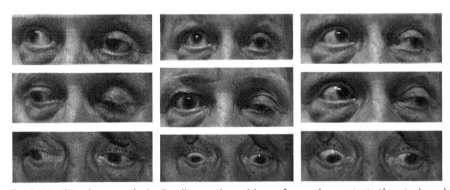

Fig. 5. Motility photographs in the diagnostic positions of gaze demonstrate the ptosis and impaired supraduction, adduction, and infraduction of a left third nerve palsy. The pictured patient did not have pupil involvement but, if present, would appear as a larger pupil on the ipsilateral side as the ptosis and ophthalmoplegia.

may consist of milder symptoms of ptosis and motility dysfunction, or may involve significant impairment in the distribution of a single division of the third nerve. Anisocoria characterized by a large, poorly reactive pupil on the ipsilateral side may or may not be present, and is a key differentiating sign between a compressive versus ischemic vascular cause of the complete third nerve palsy in most cases.[49,50] The parasympathetic fibers which provide innervation to the sphincter muscle for pupillary constriction travel on the superficial surface of the oculomotor nerve, and thus are more susceptible to compressive injury than the internally located motor fibers.[49,51] In fact, ipsilateral pupil enlargement may be the first and only sign of the third nerve palsy. The most worrisome cause of a pupil-involving third nerve palsy is compression by an aneurysm of the posterior communicating artery in the subarachnoid space (**Fig. 6**).

Any pupil-involving third nerve palsy should be considered a neurologic emergency due to the possibility of an unstable aneurysm (typically posterior communicating but also basilar artery aneurysms). CT with CTA of the brain is the typical first-line evaluation for possible aneurysm-producing third nerve palsy especially in the acute setting. If the CT-CTA is negative then an MRI of the brain and orbit with and without

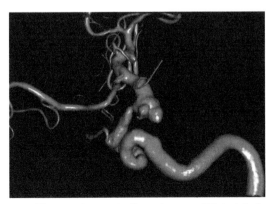

Fig. 6. CTA reconstructed images demonstrating a large multilobulated posterior communicating artery aneurysm.

contrast is probably still required because of nonaneurysmal causes of third nerve palsy. Although the combined sensitivity of a CTA with MRI and MRA approaches 95% to 100%,[49] standard catheter angiography remains the gold standard for diagnosis and, if there remains high clinical suspicion for an aneurysm, should be considered even if CTA and/or MRA is negative.[52] It is not the first imaging study performed due to the invasive nature of the test and small risk of neurologic morbidity and mortality (1%–2% in the literature but may be much lower in certain care centers and if the patient baseline risk of cerebrovascular event is removed).[49,53,54] However, it is more sensitive for detecting small aneurysms and can also rule out aneurysm in cases of false-positive MRA-CTA.[54] Catheter cerebral angiogram is also the next step in assessment and possibly the treatment of an aneurysm once identified. A neurosurgeon or interventional radiologist will determine the most appropriate treatment, which may include a combination of intravascular coiling, liquid embolic agents, and stenting or surgical clipping.[52] Medical therapy includes hypertension control, smoking cessation, and follow-up angiographic imaging.[52] Until the aneurysm is secured, the patient remains at risk for spontaneous rupture and significant neurologic morbidity or mortality, especially in aneurysms greater than 5 mm.[52]

A complete third nerve palsy that spares the pupil is most likely due to microvascular ischemia.[49,51,55] Work-up and treatment is typically directed at identification and management of vascular risk factors such as hypertension, diabetes mellitus, hyperlipidemia, obstructive sleep apnea, and tobacco use. A patient with multiple vascular risk factors who presents with a pupil-sparing complete third nerve palsy can be observed for clinical improvement over the next 4 to 8 weeks.[49,51,56] However, if the patient does not have significant known vascular risk factors and/or the third nerve palsy is partial, consider immediate neuroimaging. In a partial third nerve palsy, pupil involvement may be present but undetectable clinically or the pupil fibers may not yet be involved, depending on the exact point of compression. In cases of compressive neuropathy, the anisocoria may develop within a few days if not present on initial examination.[49] Thus, a partial third nerve palsy is often worked-up acutely (eg, CT-CTA and possible MRI-MRA if negative) regardless of whether pupil involvement is seen clinically.[49,51]

The prognosis for a third nerve palsy is variable and depends on underlying cause. Ischemic third nerve palsies often spontaneously improve without additional treatment. If due to aneurysmal compression, most patients experience improvement in oculomotor function after surgical or endovascular treatment. Gu and colleagues[57] reported 47% of patients had complete resolution and 42% of patients demonstrated incomplete recovery.

Neurologists should be aware that third nerve palsy with or without pain or pupil involvement can be the first or only sign of intracranial aneurysm. Cranial CT-CTA is the usual first-line imaging study in the acute setting followed by cranial MRI-MRA for other nonaneurysmal causes of third nerve palsy. Standard catheter angiography may still be necessary even with negative CT-MR angiography if the clinical suspicion for aneurysm is high or if the quality of the noninvasive imaging is not sufficient to exclude aneurysm.

CASE 5: CAROTID ARTERY DISSECTION

A 28-year-old man presented with new-onset headache to the emergency department following a head injury while playing basketball. He denied dizziness, weakness, numbness, tingling, decreased visual or auditory acuity, diplopia, dysphagia, dysarthria, nausea, vomiting, and seizures. Neurologic examination was significant for right-sided ptosis and miosis (Fig. 7). The remainder of the eye and neurologic exam ination were normal. Topical apraclonidine testing confirms a Horner syndrome OD. Head and neck MRI-MRA demonstrated a dissection of the right internal carotid artery (ie, crescent sign). Further evaluation with a catheter angiogram confirmed the cervical carotid dissection (**Fig. 8**). The patient was discharged on oral aspirin and had no new symptoms at the time of his follow-up appointment 3 months later.

Clinical Questions

1. What is the clinical presentation of Horner syndrome?
2. What is the ocular sympathetic pupil pathway?
3. What neurologic emergency can present with new-onset Horner syndrome?

Discussion

Horner syndrome, or damage to the ocular sympathetic palsy, is characterized by the triad of unilateral ptosis, miosis (pupillary constriction), and anhidrosis (absent sweating). The evaluation of any patient presenting acutely with anisocoria and ptosis should involve measurement of pupil size in both light and dark; this will help to establish if the involved pupil is not dilating (eg, Horner syndrome) versus not constricting (eg, parasympathetic or oculomotor nerve palsy or iris abnormality) properly. Horner syndrome can result from disruption of oculosympathetic outflow at any point along its path. The sympathetic signal originates in the hypothalamus, descends caudally within the brainstem to synapse in the ciliospinal center of Budge (spinal cord level C8 to T2). The second-order neuron exits the spinal cord to travel with the sympathetic trunk over the lung apex to the superior cervical ganglion, where it synapses near the bifurcation of the common carotid artery. The third-order neuron ascends within the adventitia of the internal carotid artery through the cavernous sinus, then travels for a short course on cranial nerve VI before joining the first division of the trigeminal nerve to pass through the superior orbital fissure to innervate the Müller muscle (responsible for upper lid elevation) and the iris dilator. Given this anatomy, disruption of the sympathetic signal at any 1 of several locations can result in Horner syndrome, including the hypothalamus, brainstem, cervical spinal cord, lung apex, carotid artery, cavernous sinus, and orbit. As such, MRI-MRA or CT-CTA should be ordered to include the orbit, brain, brainstem, and cervical and thoracic spine to the level of T2.

Pharmacologic testing for the Horner syndrome includes indirect sympathomimetic agents (eg, cocaine or hydroxyamphetamine) or more commonly now, topical apraclonidine. Apraclonidine is a direct, nonspecific alpha-agonist with a predominant alpha-2 effect and weak alpha-1 effect.[58] Horner syndrome results in denervation hypersensitivity with upregulation of postsynaptic alpha-1 receptors.[59] Apraclonidine can cause reversal of the anisocoria (or dilation of the affected miotic pupil) in the Horner syndrome because the relative predominance of alpha-1 receptors leads to

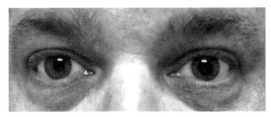

Fig. 7. Note the subtle ptosis and smaller pupil in a patient with a right-sided Horner syndrome.

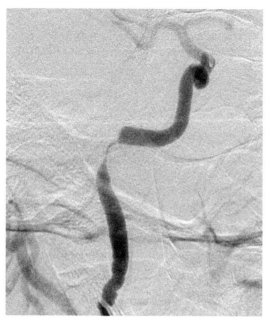

Fig. 8. Right internal CAD resulting in a high degree of stenosis (carotid string sign).

pupil dilation in the affected eye, as well as improvement in the ptosis. The normal alpha-2 action in the fellow eye leads to pupil constriction. This reversal of anisocoria on bilateral apraclonidine drop administration is diagnostic for Horner syndrome with high sensitivity and specificity.[60] In the acute setting where the clinical findings of the Horner syndrome are obvious, topical testing can be deferred and neuroimaging of the ocular sympathetic axis from head to T2 in the chest (eg, CT-CTA of head and neck) can be performed urgently.

Carotid artery dissection (CAD) occurs when an intimal tear leads to the formation of an intramural hematoma and can occur spontaneously or secondary to trauma.[61] CAD has an incidence of approximately 2.6 per 100,000 in the United States.[59] Horner syndrome develops in around 25% of patients with CAD.[62] Pain is the most common presenting complaint for CAD, occurring in 70% to 80% of cases, and may localize to the face, head, or neck ipsilateral to the dissection.[62,63] Treatment of CAD is controversial given the relative paucity of randomized clinical trials, but the recent Cervical Artery Dissection in Stroke Study (CADISS) trial demonstrated a low prevalence of stroke in patients with symptomatic CAD and no difference in efficacy of antiplatelet versus anticoagulant medications at preventing stroke and death.[64] Follow-up imaging is generally recommended to establish whether a dissection has healed.[65] Clinical outcome is good for most patients, with recanalization or resolution in up to 80% of dissections.[66]

Neurologists should be aware of the Horner syndrome as a presenting sign of CAD because this may be the only clinical abnormality initially and there is risk of downstream ischemic events including monocular vision loss and hemispheric stroke if the dissection goes untreated. Familiarity with apraclonidine testing is important because patients may have undergone this testing in neuro-ophthalmology clinic (with temporary reversal of the clinical signs of Horner syndrome) before being directed to the emergency department for urgent evaluation.

SUMMARY

Neurologists should be aware of specific clinical and radiographic presentations of neuro ophthalmic emergencies including GCA, arterial dissection, intracranial aneurysm, pituitary apoplexy, and invasive sino-orbital fungal infection (eg, mucormycosis). Early recognition and treatment of these disorders can greatly impact patient morbidity and mortality, including the preservation of both vision and life.

ACKNOWLEDGMENTS

We wish to acknowledge our medical student contributors, Mr. Tyler Boulter and Mr. Earnest Pucket who researched and compiled two of the example, composite cases and added substantively to this report in terms of content, manuscript review, and preparation for publication.

REFERENCES

1. Weyand CM, Goronzy JJ. Medium- and large-vessel vasculitis. N Engl J Med 2003;349:160–9.
2. Chew SSL, Kerr NM, Danesh-Meyer HV. Giant cell arteritis. J Clin Neurosci 2009; 16:1263–8.
3. Paraskevas KI, Boumpas DT, Vrentzos GE, et al. Oral and ocular/orbital manifestations of temporal arteritis: a disease with deceptive clinical symptoms and devastating consequences. Clin Rheumatol 2007;26:1044–8.
4. Hellmann DB. Temporal arteritis: a cough, toothache, and tongue infarction. JAMA 2002;287:2996–3000.
5. Shmerling RH, Smetana GW. Does this patient have temporal arteritis? JAMA 2002;287:92–101.
6. Machado EB, Michet CJ, Ballard DJ, et al. Trends in incidence and clinical presentation of temporal arteritis in Olmsted County, Minnesota, 1950-1985. Arthritis Rheum 1988;31:745–9.
7. Hayreh SS, Zimmerman B. Management of giant cell arteritis. Our 27-year clinical study: new light on old controversies. Ophthalmologica 2003;217:239.
8. Mazlumzadeh M, Hunder GG, Easley KA, et al. Treatment of giant cell arteritis using induction therapy with high-dose glucocorticoids: a double-blind, placebo-controlled, randomized prospective clinical trial. Arthritis Rheum 2006;54:3310–8.
9. Ostrowski RA, Bussey MR, Tehrani R, et al. Biologic therapy for the treatment of giant cell arteritis. Neuroophthalmol 2014;38:107–12.
10. Danesh-Meyer H, Savino PJ, Gamble GG. Poor prognosis of visual outcome after visual loss from giant cell arteritis. Ophthalmology 2005;112:1098–103.
11. Hayreh SS, Zimmerman B, Kardon RH. Visual improvement with corticosteroid therapy in giant cell arteritis. Report of a large study and review of literature. Acta Ophthalmol Scand 2002;80:355–67.
12. Liu GT, Glaser JS, Schatz NJ, et al. Visual morbidity in giant cell arteritis. Clinical characteristics and prognosis for vision. Ophthalmology 1994;101:1779.
13. Ezeonyeji AN, Borg FA, Dasgupta B. Delays in recognition and management of giant cell arteritis: results from a retrospective audit. Clin Rheumatol 2011;30: 259–62.
14. Font C, Cid MC, Coll-Vinent B, et al. Clinical features in patients with permanent visual loss due to biopsy-proven giant cell arteritis. Br J Rheumatol 1997;36:251.
15. Pinto ME, Manrique HA, Guevara X, et al. Hyperglycemic hyperosmolar state and rhino-orbital mucormycosis. Diabetes Res Clin Pract 2011;91:e37–9.

16. Wali U, Balkhair A, Al-Mujaini A. Cerebro-rhino orbital mucormycosis: an update. J Infect Public Health 2012;5(2):116–26.
17. Spellberg B, Ibrahim A. Recent advances in the treatment of mucormycosis. Curr Infect Dis Rep 2010;12:423–9.
18. Cornely OA, Arikan-akdagli S, Dannaoui E, et al. ESCMID and ECMM joint clinical guidelines for the diagnosis and management of mucormycosis 2013. Clin Microbiol Infect 2014;20:5–26.
19. Chamilos G, Lewis RE, Kontoyiannis DP. Delaying amphotericin B-based frontline therapy significantly increases mortality among patients with hematologic malignancy who have zygomycosis. Clin Infect Dis 2008;47:503–9.
20. Roden MM, Zaoutis TE, Buchanan WL, et al. Epidemiology and outcome of zygomycosis: a review of 929 reported cases. Clin Infect Dis 2005;41:634–53.
21. Mignogna MD, Fortuna G, Leuci S, et al. Mucormycosis in immunocompetent patients: a case-series of patients with maxillary sinus involvement and a critical review of the literature. Int J Infect Dis 2011;15:e533–40.
22. Spellberg B, Edwards J, Ibrahim A. Novel perspectives on mucormycosis: pathophysiology, presentation, and management. Clin Microbiol Rev 2005;18:556–69.
23. Ibrahim AS, Gebermariam T, Fu Y, et al. The iron chelator deferasirox protects mice from mucormycosis through iron starvation. J Clin Invest 2007;117:2649–57.
24. Kontoyiannis DP, Lionakis MS, Lewis RE, et al. Zygomycosis in a tertiary-care cancer center in the era of Aspergillus-active antifungal therapy: a case–control observational study of 27 recent cases. J Infect Dis 2005;191:1350–60.
25. Bagdade JD, Nielson K, Root R, et al. Host defense in diabetes mellitus: the feckless phagocyte during poor control and ketoacidosis. Diabetes 1970;19:364–6.
26. Ferguson BJ, Mitchell TG, Moon R, et al. Adjunctive hyperbaric oxygen for treatment of rhinocerebral mucormycosis. Rev Infect Dis 1988;10:551–9.
27. Artis WM, Fountain JA, Delcher HK, et al. A mechanism of susceptibility to mucormycosis in diabetic ketoacidosis: transferring and iron availability. Diabetes 1982;31:109–14.
28. Lionakis MS, Kontoyiannis DP. Glucocorticoids and invasive fungal infections. Lancet 2003;362:1828–38.
29. Blitzer A, Lawson M, Meyers BR, et al. Patient survival factors in paranasal sinus mucormycosis. Laryngoscope 1980;90:635–48.
30. Abedi E, Sismanis A, Choi K, et al. Twenty five years' experience treating cerebro-rhino-orbital mucormycosis. Laryngoscope 1984;94:1060–2.
31. Singh N, Aguado JM, Bonatti H, et al. Zygomycosis in solid organ transplant recipients: a prospective, matched case–control study to assess risks for disease and outcome. J Infect Dis 2009;200:1002–11.
32. Ivan Burik JA, Hare RS, Solomon HF, et al. Posaconazole is effective as salvage therapy in zygomycosis: a retrospective summary of 91 cases. Clin Infect Dis 2006;42:e61–5.
33. Greenberg RN, Mullane K, van Burik JA, et al. Posaconazole as salvage therapy for zygomycosis. Antimicrob Agents Chemother 2006;50:126–33.
34. Cornely OA, Maertens J, Winston DJ, et al. Posaconazole vs. fluconazole or itraconazole prophylaxis in patients with neutropenia. N Engl J Med 2007;356:348–59.
35. Ullmann AJ, Lipton JH, Vesole DH, et al. Posaconazole or fluconazole for prophylaxis in severe graft-versus-host disease. N Engl J Med 2007;356:335–47.
36. Hanahan D, Weinberg RA. The hallmarks of cancer: the next generation. Cell 2011;144(5):646–74.
37. Couldwell WT, Cannon-Albright LA. Co-prevalence of other tumors in patients harboring pituitary tumors. J Neurosurg 2014;121(6):1474–7.

38. McDowell BD, Wallace RB, Carnahan RM, et al. Demographic differences in incidence for pituitary adenoma. Pituitary 2011;14(1):23–30.

39. Orosz A, Csajbók É, Czékus C, et al. Increased short-term beat-to-beat variability of QT interval in patients with acromegaly. PLoS One 2015;10(4):e0125639.

40. Terada T, Kovacs K, Stefaneanu L, et al. Incidence, pathology, and recurrence of pituitary adenomas: study of 647 unselected surgical cases. Endocr Pathol 1995; 6(4):301–10.

41. Hansen TM, Sachin B, Lim M, et al. Invasive adenoma and pituitary carcinoma: a SEER database analysis. Neurosurg Rev 2014;37(2):279–86.

42. Bergsneider M, Mirsadraei L, Yong WH, et al. The pituitary stalk effect: is it a passing phenomenon? J Neurooncol 2014;117(3):477–84.

43. Abouaf L, Vighetto A, Lebas M. Neuro-ophthalmologic exploration in nonfunctioning pituitary adenoma. Ann Endocrinol (Paris) 2015;76(3):210–9.

44. Louis DN, Ohgaki H, Wiestler OD, et al. The 2007 WHO classification of tumours of the central nervous system. Acta Neuropathol 2007;114(2):97–109.

45. Young WF, Machado CAG, Netter FH. The netter collection of medical illustrations. In: Young WF, editor. The endocrine system, vol. 2, 2nd edition. Philadelphia: Saunders Elsevier; 2011. p. 3–33.

46. Chanson P, Salenave S. Diagnosis and treatment of pituitary adenomas. Minerva Endocrinol 2004;4:241–75.

47. Heaney AP, Melmed S. Molecular targets in pituitary tumours. Nat Rev Cancer 2004;4(4):285–95.

48. Bergsneider M, Heaney AP, Lee JYK. Editorial: pituitary tumors. J Neurooncol 2014;117(3):377–8.

49. Bruce BB, Biousse V, Newman NJ. Third nerve palsies. Semin Neurol 2007;27(3): 257–68.

50. Jacobson DM. Pupil involvement in patients with diabetes associated oculomotor nerve palsy. Arch Ophthalmol 1998;116(6):723–7.

51. Lee AG, Hayman LA, Brazis PW. The evaluation of isolated third nerve palsy revisited: an update on the evolving role of magnetic resonance, computed tomography, and catheter angiography. Surv Ophthalmol 2002;47(2):137–57.

52. Jeong HW, Seo JH, Kim ST, et al. Clinical practice guideline for the management of intracranial aneurysms. Neurointervention 2014;9(2):63–71.

53. Jacobson DM, Trobe JD. The emerging role of magnetic resonance angiography in the management of patients with third cranial nerve palsy. Am J Ophthalmol 1999;128(1):94–6.

54. Rustemi O, Alarai A, Shakur SF, et al. Detection of unruptured intracranial aneurysms on noninvasive imaging. Is there still a role for digital subtraction angiography? Surg Neurol Int 2015;6:175.

55. Murchison AP, Gilbert ME, Savino PJ. Neuroimaging and acute ocular motor mononeuropathies: a prospective study. Arch Ophthalmol 2011;129(3):301–5.

56. Capo H, Warren F, Kupersmith MJ. Evolution of oculomotor nerve palsies. J Clin Neuroophthalmol 1992;12(1):21–5.

57. Gu DQ, Luo B, Zhang X, et al. Recovery of posterior communicating artery aneurysm-induced oculomotor nerve paresis after endovascular treatment. Clin Neurol Neurosurg 2012;114(9):1238–42.

58. Abrams DA, Robin AL, Pollack IP, et al. The safety and efficacy of topical 1% ALO 2145 (p-aminoclonidine hydrochloride) in normal volunteers. Arch Ophthalmol 1987;105(9):1205–7.

59. Moodley AA, Spooner RB. Apraclonidine in the diagnosis of Horner's syndrome. S Afr Med J 2007;97(7):506–7.

60. Koc F, Kavuncu S, Kansu T, et al. The sensitivity and specificity of 0.5% apraclonidine in the diagnosis of oculosympathetic paresis. Br J Ophthalmol 2005; 89(11):1442–4.
61. Patel RR, Adam R, Maldjian C, et al. Cervical carotid artery dissection: current review of diagnosis and treatment. Cardiol Rev 2012;20(3):145–52.
62. Lee VH, Brown RD, Mandrekar JN, et al. Incidence and outcome of cervical artery dissection: a population-based study. Neurology 2006;67(10):1809–12.
63. Silbert PL, Mokri B, Schievink WI. Headache and neck pain in spontaneous internal carotid and vertebral artery dissections. Neurology 1995;45(8):1517–22.
64. Markus HS, Hayter E, Levi C, et al. Antiplatelet treatment compared with anticoagulation treatment for cervical artery dissection (CADISS): a randomised trial. Lancet Neurol 2015;14(4):361–7.
65. Goyal MS, Derdeyn CP. The diagnosis and management of supraaortic arterial dissections. Curr Opin Neurol 2009;22(1):80–9.
66. Pelkonen O, Tikkakoski T, Leinonen S, et al. Extracranial internal carotid and vertebral artery dissections: angiographic spectrum, course and prognosis. Neuroradiology 2003;45(2):71–7.

Case Studies of Uncommon and Rare Headache Disorders

Randolph W. Evans, MD

KEYWORDS

- Status migrainosus • Cervical artery dissection
- Spontaneous intracranial hypotension • Hemicrania continua • Migraine with aura
- Limb pain and migraine • Cluster headache • Trigeminal neuralgia

KEY POINTS

- Status migrainosus often lasts a few weeks and may not respond to emergency department treatment.
- Cervical artery dissection can mimic migraine and present with headache and/or neck pain only.
- Spontaneous intracranial hypotension can present with a variety of headaches and be difficult to diagnose.
- Hemicrania continua and cluster headaches are commonly misdiagnosed.
- There are a diverse number of migraine auras.
- Migraine can cause limb pain with or without headache.

About 20% of the practice of the general neurologist consists of seeing patients with headaches, most of whom have primary headache disorders, mainly migraine. These case studies may be of benefit when the uncommon or rare headache disorder presents.

CASE 1. A 12-DAY MIGRAINE WITH RECURRING AURA?

Case 1 is a 60-year-old man with a history of migraine with and without aura since his 40s up to 25 days per month, decreased to about 5 per month on gabapentin 600 mg 3 times a day previously followed for 3 years. The headaches could be at the back of the head or generalized or occasionally with bitemporal pressure with an intensity of 3 to 10/10 associated with light and noise sensitivity but no vomiting relieved by eletriptan

Disclosures: Speaker's Bureau, Allergan, Depomed, Avanir and Pernix, Teva; advisory board, Lilly; royalties or editorial fees from Elsevier, Lippincott Williams & Wilkins; Medlink Neurology; Oxford; Practical Neurology, and UptoDate.
Department of Neurology, Baylor College of Medicine, 1200 Binz #1370, Houston, TX 77004, USA
E-mail address: revansmd@gmail.com

Neurol Clin 34 (2016) 631–650
http://dx.doi.org/10.1016/j.ncl.2016.04.006
0733-8619/16/$ – see front matter © 2016 Elsevier Inc. All rights reserved.
neurologic.theclinics.com

in 2 hours. He would occasionally have a visual aura of flashing lights in both eyes for 20 minutes before the headache.

He presented with a 12-day history of a right temporal, behind the right eye and occasionally right back of the head, sharp pain with an intensity of 4/10 at onset and 7 to 9/10 since associated with nausea, light, and noise sensitivity but no vomiting on a daily basis lasting 2 to 8 hours with ibuprofen or eletriptan. He reported blurred vision with things missing in the right eye intermittently for 3 to 5 hours daily from the day of onset of the headache for 10 days. He had no fever. His primary care physician had placed him on a methylprednisolone dose pack without help. Examination by an ophthalmologist was normal. Neurologic examination was normal.

Question: What is your diagnosis?

Perhaps he has migraine status, which is migraine lasting longer than 72 hours. The headache is different than prior migraines but seems to fit migraine criteria: the headache is unilateral associated with nausea, light, and noise sensitivity. In addition, he has been having daily episodes of blurred vision in the right eye, which may be a migraine aura.

The prevalence of migraine status is uncertain but is probably rare. In a retrospective French study of 25 patients with status migrainosus seen in a tertiary care center (of 8821 migraineurs over 11 years), the demographics were as follows: mean age at first episode, 39 years; male:female ratio, 4:21; duration 4.8 weeks (3–10); relapse of status migrainosus, 32%; and delay of relapse, 61.5 months.[1] Precipitating factors included the following: stress/anxiety, 69%; menses, 31%; and lack of sleep, 6.3%. The great majority of patients had the same attack frequency before and after the status, and most cases occurred in those with low-frequency migraine attacks.

Question: What treatments are effective for migraine status in the emergency department?

Adequate IV hydration is important as indicated, and nonopioids are preferred because the emergency department (ED) visit may be longer than with use of nonopioids[2] and risk of habituation and abuse. Medication use may be guided by comorbidities, which are contraindications to use (such as cardiovascular, cerebrovascular or cerebrovascular disease, history of gastrointestinal bleeding, and pregnancy), prior response to medications, and medications taken before the ED visit. There are a variety of potential adverse events with the medications, including movement disorders with dopamine receptor antagonists.[3]

Little has been published on treatment of migraine status in the ED. Rozen[4] reviewed ED and inpatient management of migraine status.

The Canadian Headache Society performed a systemic review of 44 studies of acute treatment of migraine in the ED and found many were of poor quality and lacking in comparator trials.[5] The Society strongly recommended the use of prochlorperazine IV, metoclopramide IV, sumatriptan subcutaneous, and ketorolac intramuscular. The Society recommended strongly against the use of dexamethasone IV and haloperidol IV.

Persistent or recurrence of migraine without status is common after the ED visit. In a study of 186 migraineurs who presented for treatment to the ED with headaches present with a median duration of 24 hours (12–72 hours), 31% had moderate or severe headache present within 24 hours of ED discharge.[6] Although no data are available, ED treatment of migraine status may not be adequate, and some patients may need to be admitted for longer treatment. In the French study of 25 patients with status migrainosus, 60% required hospitalization for a mean of 6 days and were given IV amitriptyline (not available in the United States). Dihydroergotamine with an antiemetic is commonly used in the United States when there are no contraindications.[1]

However, because migraine is a diagnosis of exclusion and the headache was different than his prior migraines, a migraine mimic or secondary cause needed to be excluded, including temporal arteritis and cervical arterial dissection.[7]

Neuroimaging

Erythrocyte sedimentation rate was 2 mm/h. MRI scan of the brain on the day of the office visit showed small acute/subacute mid and anterior right centrum semiovale white matter infarcts. Magnetic resonance angiography (MRA) of the brain and neck showed a right internal carotid artery dissection (ICAD) extending from distal to the right carotid bulb to the proximal petrous segment with about 60% stenosis.

Questions: How often is headache and/or neck pain the only manifestation of cervical artery dissection? What are the incidence, factors associated, and other symptoms and signs with dissection?

Headache and neck pain were the only symptoms of spontaneous cervical artery dissection (CAD) in 8% in a prospective French series of 247 patients[8] and 20% in a prospective Russian series of 161 patients[9] and can mimic migraine with and without aura and migraine status (**Box 1**). The headache has a thunderclap onset in about 20% of cases. Two percent of all ischemic strokes are due to CAD, but occur in 8% to 25% of strokes in those less than 45 years of age.[10] The mean age is 44 to 46 years affecting men and women equally.

Box 1
Features of headaches due to cervical artery dissection

Carotid artery

Initial manifestation in 47% and present in 60% to 95% of cases

Ipsilateral pain in 91% of cases

Most commonly frontotemporal, occasionally hemicranial or occipital

50% with facial, dental, or orbital pain

25% with unilateral upper anterolateral neck pain

Can have nausea and vomiting

Partial Horner in 25% with ptosis and miosis

Median duration is 3 days with a range of 1 hour to 4 years (90% resolve within 1 week)

Median interval from onset of pain to neurologic symptoms is on average 9 days (range, 1–90 days)

Vertebral artery

Presenting symptom in 70% of cases and present in 88% of cases

Typically a severe ipsilateral occipital or posterior neck throbbing or steady and sharp pain but

Can be bilateral

Rarely frontal or generalized with rare nausea, vomiting, light and noise sensitivity

Mean duration 8.3 days (range 2–35 days)

Median interval from onset of pain to other symptoms is about 2 weeks (range 0.5 hour to 30 days)

Easily and often misdiagnosed as musculoskeletal pain or tension headache

There are numerous factors associated with CAD, including the following major and minor cervical trauma; arterial hypertension; young age; current use of oral contraceptives; migraine; fibromuscular dysplasia; ultrastructural connective tissue abnormalities; vascular subtype of Ehlers-Danlos syndrome; Marfan syndrome; Turner syndrome; Williams syndrome; familial cases; hereditary hemochromatosis; osteogenesis imperfect type I; α1-antitrypsin deficiency; 677T genotype MTHFR; hyperhomocysteinemia; cystic medial necrosis of intracranial vessels; styloid process length; autosomal-dominant polycystic kidney disease; infections; Moyamoya disease; lentiginosis; and vessel redundancies (coils, kinks, loops), especially if bilateral.[11] Migraineurs such as this patient have a 2-fold increased risk of CAD, which does not appear to significantly differ by migraine aura status or gender.[12]

The incidence of spontaneous cervical ICAD is about 2.6/100,000 per year. Headache is the initial manifestation in 47% and occurs in 60% to 95% of those with ICAD preceding other neurologic symptoms and/or signs by a mean time of 4 days. The pain of ICAD, which is ipsilateral in 91% of cases, is typically unilateral frontemporal, facial, dental, or orbital area, 25% one side of the anterolateral neck, and occasionally hemicranial or occipital and is more often aching than throbbing.[13] ICAD can have migraine features, including nausea and vomiting. The median duration of the headache is 3 days with a range of 1 hour to 4 years with 90% resolving within 1 week.

ICAD can mimic migraine with aura with a visual aura only or a march of symptoms (such as visual then sensory then dysphasia) associated with a migraine-like headache.[14,15] In occasional cases where migraine with aura criteria are met in those with a prior history of migraine, the dissection could be incidental or could be a trigger for the migraine with aura episode.

This patient had asymptomatic acute/subacute right hemisphere infarcts on MRI and was also having daily ischemic visual episodes of the right eye. After the onset of pain, the median time to the appearance of neurologic symptoms is on average 9 days (range, 1–90 days).[13] Cerebral or retinal ischemic symptoms have been reported in 50% to 95% of patients in the past, although the frequency has decreased over the years.[16] Rarely, permanent blindness occurs as a result of ischemic optic neuropathy or central retinal artery occlusion.

A partial Horner syndrome occurs in about 25% of cases with ptosis and miosis. About 12% of patients with ICAD have cranial nerve palsies, most commonly involving the lower cranial nerves, especially the hypoglossal, although the oculomotor, trigeminal, and facial nerves may be involved.[17] Twenty-five percent report pulsatile tinnitus.

CASE 2. A MIGRAINEUR WITH A NEW CONSTANT HEADACHE FOR 1 MONTH

Case 2 is a 35-year-old woman with a history of occasional migraine with visual aura as a teen, and migraine without aura since her 20s occurring 1 to 2 times per month, described as a bifrontal aching with light and noise sensitivity relieved with ibuprofen.

One month before, she looked behind the seat in the car and developed a mild crick in her neck. A few hours later, she developed a constant nuchal-occipital and generalized pressure and throbbing without associated symptoms with an intensity of 9 to 10/10. Her primary care physician gave her sumatriptan tablets and an isometheptene mucate, dichloralphenazone, and acetaminophen combination, which helped a little. Over a couple of weeks, the headaches were only bifrontal. After 1 month, the headaches were still constant, bifrontal and right temporal, with an intensity of 3 to 10/10. Neurologic examination was normal.

Question: Does she have migraine status?

Just as in case 1, suspicion is raised because the headache is different than prior migraines, and migraine-associated features are not present, so testing was performed.

Neuroimaging and Follow-up

MRI of the brain showed no ischemic lesions. MRA of the neck suggested a dissection of the proximal to mid left vertebral artery. Computerized tomographic angiography was also suggestive but not diagnostic of a left vertebral dissection. A cerebral arteriogram showed a left vertebral artery aneurysm at the C6 level with a pseudoaneurysm just distal to the narrowing with 50% stenosis.

She was treated with heparin and then warfarin for 3 months. A repeat MRA showed recanalization, and she was placed on daily aspirin. The headache persisted daily with an intensity of 3 to 10/10 and lasting most of the day. The headaches persisted fairly constantly for 7 months as a bifrontal and sometimes nuchal-occipital aching and pressure and occasional throbbing with light and noise sensitivity but no nausea or aura with an intensity ranging from 4 to 10/10 with an average intensity of 5/10. She was placed on topiramate titrated up to 100 mg daily and given bilateral greater occipital nerve blocks with 1% lidocaine, and the headaches decreased to every 1 to 2 days, lasting 30 minutes to 2 hours and not requiring medication after 3 months. After 4 months, the headaches increased to 5 days a week and lasted all day. She was placed on desvenlafaxine 50 mg daily; topiramate was discontinued, and the headaches decreased to 2 to 3 monthly. Three years later, on desvenlafaxine, the headaches were occurring about once a month, lasting a few hours with acetaminophen.

Questions: How often are headaches associated with cervical vertebral artery dissection, and where is the headache in vertebral artery dissection? Can dissection cause new daily persistent headache? How often is the imaging indeterminate in diagnosing dissection? Is antiplatelet or anticoagulation treatment preferred?

Headache is a presenting symptom in about 70% of cases, is reported in 88% of cases, and is typically a severe ipsilateral occipital or posterior neck throbbing or steady and sharp pain but can be bilateral and rarely frontal or generalized (see **Box 1**).[18] The headache is rarely associated with migraine features, such as nausea, vomiting, photophobia or phonophobia, and visual aura.[19,20] The pain can easily be and is often misdiagnosed as being of musculoskeletal origin when the pain is in the back of the neck or a tension headache when in the back of the head and neck. The mean duration of the headache is 8.3 days (range 2-35 days).[13]

As this case illustrates, cervical arterial dissection is a rare secondary cause of new daily persistent headache, which is more common after ICAD.[21]

Transient ischemic attack (TIA) has been variably reported as occurring in 7% to 75% of cases and stroke in 10% to 89% of cases.[22] Rarely, cervical radiculopathy (most often at the C5-6 level), spinal epidural hematoma, and cervical spinal cord ischemia can occur. The median interval from the onset to pain onset to other symptoms is about 2 weeks (range 5 hours to 30 days)[13]

The incidence of spontaneous cervical vertebral artery dissection is about 1.5/100,000 per year. As discussed in case 1, there are numerous factors associated with cervical dissection, including prior mild or trivial trauma estimated to be antecedent in 12% to 36% of cases.[23] In this case, did she develop the dissection from looking in the back seat (unlikely) or did she recall the initial pain from the dissection (the crick in her neck) after the unrelated movement?

Seemingly forever (although the first description of spontaneous CAD was 100 years ago),[24] neurologists have debated the best medication treatment for cervical dissections (the jury is still out on the benefit of endovascular therapy). Now we may have the best answer that we may have for many decades.

The Cervical Artery Dissection in Stroke Study was a randomized trial at hospitals with specialized stroke or neurology services (30 in the United Kingdom and 7 in Australia) of 250 patients with 118 extracranial carotid or 132 extracranial vertebral dissections with onset of symptoms within the prior 7 days with a mean age of 49 years (range 18–87).[25] Presenting symptoms in the 250 patients were as follows: ischemic stroke, 195; TIA, 29; headache, 22; neck pain, 22; Horner syndrome, 4. Patients were randomly assigned to antiplatelet (aspirin, dipyridamole, or clopidogrel alone or in combination) or anticoagulant drugs (unfractionated heparin or low-molecular-weight heparin followed by warfarin aiming for an international normalized ratio of 2–3) for 3 months with the specific treatment decided by the local clinician. In the antiplatelet group, 22% received aspirin alone; 33% received clopidogrel alone; 1% received dipyridamole alone; 28% received aspirin and clopidogrel; and 16% received dipyradomole. In the anticoagulant group, 90% received heparin and warfarin and 10% received warfarin alone.

The diagnosis of dissection could not be confirmed on central imaging review in about 20% of participants despite evidence of dissection on angiographic imaging or cross-sectional imaging through the vessel wall. In some cases, imaging was of poor quality. In others, alternative diagnoses were suggested, including atherosclerosis with an atretic artery, a narrowed artery, or adherent thrombus without dissection.

Excluding patients wherein dissection could not be confirmed, ipsilateral stroke or death occurred in 3 of 101 patients in the antiplatelet group (3%) versus 1 of 96 patients (1%) in the anticoagulant group (odds ratio 0.346, 95% confidence interval 0.006–4.390; $P = 0.66$). There was one subarachnoid hemorrhage in the anticoagulant group. All stroke events occurred in the first 10 days after randomization. There were no deaths in the total population. In the intention-to-treat population, ipsilateral TIA occurred in 1% of the antiplatelet group versus 3% of the anticoagulant group.

There was no difference in efficacy of antiplatelet and anticoagulant drugs and preventing stroke and death. The overall risk of stroke was low.

The study might not have enrolled a small high-risk group, those with early recurrent strokes.[26] Any future trials of newer oral anticoagulants and to detect small effect size may require 5000 participants and require 500 sites and 10 years to complete recruitment.

CASE 3. AN ORTHOSTATIC HEADACHE

Case 3 is a 41-year-old man with no prior headache history with a 2-month history of fairly constant daily back-of-the-head throbbing pain with an intensity of 9 to 10/10 when upright and 1/10 when supine associated with intermittent nausea and occasional vomiting. Past medical history was negative. No history of trauma. Neurologic examination was normal.

Question: What are the causes of orthostatic headaches? What tests should be ordered?

The most common cause of an orthostatic headache is a cerebrospinal fluid (CSF) leak, most commonly iatrogenic after a dural puncture. Other than iatrogenic, CSF leaks can be traumatic or spontaneous (**Box 2**).

Spontaneous intracranial hypotension (SIH) has an estimated annual incidence of 5/100,000 with a female-to-male ratio of 2:1. The peak incidence is around the age of 40 years. SIH is usually due to a spontaneous CSF leak into the epidural space through

---

Box 2
Cause of cerebrospinal fluid hypovolemia or cerebrospinal fluid leaks

- True hypovolemic state, when total body water (including CSF) is reduced
- Overdraining CSF shunts
- Traumatic CSF leaks
  - Obvious major injuries (eg, from motor vehicle accidents, sports injuries)
  - Brachial plexus injuries (eg, nerve root sleeve tears, avulsions)
  - Iatrogenic (eg, following dural punctures or epidural catheterizations)
  - Postsurgical (eg, after cranial, spinal, sinus, or ear surgeries)
- Spontaneous CSF leaks (major etiologic challenge)
  - Unknown cause
  - Pre-existing dural sac weakness, supported by one or more of the following:
    - Presence of meningeal diverticula, often, but not always, multiple
    - Ectasia of dural sac
    - Surgical anatomic observations of attenuated to near-absent dural zones
    - Clinical stigmata of disorders of the connective tissue matrix
      - Marfan syndrome or marfanoid features
      - Joint hypermobility
      - Retinal detachment at young age
      - Abnormalities of elastin/fibrillin in dermal fibroblast cultures
      - Familial occurrence of the leaks
      - Personal or family history of arterial dissections, aneurysms, or nonrheumatic valvular heart disease, such as bicuspid aortic valve
  - Trivial trauma (perhaps becoming relevant in the setting of a pre-existing dural weakness)
- Herniated discs or spondylotic spurs piercing or weakening the dura[13,14]

Data from Mokri B. Spontaneous intracranial hypotension. Continuum (Minneap Minn) 2015;21(4 Headache):1086–108, 1088; and Mokri B. Spontaneous CSF leaks: low CSF volume syndromes. Neurol Clin 2014;32(2):397–422.

---

a defect in the thecal sac at the thoracic or cervicothoracic junction due to spontaneous dural dehiscence and dural tears caused by degenerative causes.

An MRI of the brain with contrast may demonstrate diffuse pachymeningeal enhancement in 80% of cases.[27] Other abnormal abnormalities may include subdural fluid collections, engorgement of venous structures, pituitary hyperemia, and sagging of the brain (including descent of the cerebellar tonsils). An MRI of the spine without contrast may detect the leak. If the study is negative, an MRI myelogram with gadolinium may find the leak.[28]

Routine lumbar puncture may not be helpful. In a series of 106 patients with SIH, the lumbar puncture opening pressure was normal in 61%.[29] In some cases, the location of the leak cannot be located despite extensive spine imaging.[30]

There are other causes of orthostatic headaches.[31] Orthostatic headache can be the most prominent feature of postural orthostatic tachycardia syndrome.[32] Occasionally following decompressive surgery for Chiari malformation, an orthostatic headache may occur with a CSF leak.

Following large decompressive craniectomies for life-threatening cerebral edema, orthostatic headaches may occur that can improve with cranioplasty.[33] Individuals with increased compliance of the dural sac (especially with large lumbar dural sacs and stigmata of connective tissue disease) may develop orthostatic headaches.[34] Finally, orthostatic headaches can be present with colloid cysts of the third ventricle[35] and a supratentorial meningioma.[36]

Neuroimaging Results

An MRI of the brain showed diffuse pachymeningeal enhancement. MRI of the spine without contrast showed a small ventral epidural CSF collection at the C8-T1 level.

Question: What types of headaches occur in spontaneous intracranial hypotension?

The most common headache and clinical manifestation of SIH is an orthostatic headache, which may appear with the upright position or be relieved with recumbency within a few minutes but may be longer.[37] The headache is usually but not always bilateral and may be frontal, fronto-occipital, generalized, or occipital and is often throbbing but may be a pressure with an intensity ranging from mild to severe. In some chronic cases, the orthostatic features may disappear. Associated symptoms may include neck and/or interscapular pain, nausea, vomiting, diplopia, tinnitus, dizziness, change in hearing, cognitive symptoms, and unsteady gait.

Other headaches that may occur with SIH include the following: nonorthostatic headaches from the start; exertional (and Valsalva induced) headaches; acute thunderclap onset of orthostatic headaches; second-half-of-the-day headaches (often with some orthostatic features); paradoxic orthostatic headaches (present in recumbency, relieved when upright); intermittent headaches associated with intermittent leaks; and acephalgic or no headaches presenting with other clinical manifestations.[38]

Questions: Are patients with spontaneous intracranial hypotension without Ehlers-Danlos or Marfan at risk for vascular abnormalities?

Schievink and Deline[39] recommend screening for 2 vascular abnormalities, which occur with a higher frequency in those with SIH than in the general population: intracranial saccular aneurysm and aortic root dilatation, based on single studies.

MRA scans of the brain were performed in 93 patients (mean age 42.2 years, 70% women) with SIH finding 8.6% intracranial saccular aneurysm (mean age 51.4 years).[40] None of the patients with aneurysms had a recognized systemic connective tissue disorder or family history of aneurysm. In a control population of 291 patients (mean age 54.8 years, 56% women), 1% had intracranial aneurysms. Study limitations included not obtaining MRA scans on all patients with SIH and not matching study and control patients for important risk factors.

In a study of 50 consecutive patients with SIH aged 12 to 67 years,[41] 9 had cardiovascular abnormalities with dilatation of the aortic root in 6. The investigators recommend that patients with SIH without a connective tissue disorder may benefit from baseline echocardiographic screening. For those with evidence of a dilated thoracic aorta, they suggest a yearly follow-up for the first 3 to 4 years to determine the risk of progression and rupture. For those with an initial normal study, follow-up examinations in 2- and 5-year intervals are recommended. They also recommend confirmation of their findings in larger cohorts.

CASE 4. A UNILATERAL HEADACHE

Case 4 is a 48-year-old woman seen for a third opinion with a 20-year history of only menstrual headaches always preceded by a visual aura followed by a generalized throbbing with an intensity of 5 to 6/10 associated with light and noise sensitivity but no nausea. The headache would last 2 to 3 days with ibuprofen.

For 3.5 months, she had a daily constant headache, daily since onset, described as a left-sided pressure or throbbing with an intensity ranging from 1 to 10/10 with an average of 6/10 associated with light and noise sensitivity but no nausea, aura, or cranial autonomic symptoms (CAS). She had no triggers.

She had seen 2 headache specialists previously. She had tried sumatriptan orally and subcutaneously, diclofenac powder, ketorolac orally and intramuscularly, and dihydroergotamine nasal spray, and had an occipital nerve block without benefit. Gabapentin and pregabalin did not help. She was placed on indomethacin 75 mg sustained release once a day for 8 days without benefit. Prednisone 60 mg daily for 10 days did not help. An IV dihydroergotamine regimen for 5 days did not help.

An MRI scan and MRA of the brain and cervical spine and magnetic resonance venogram of the brain were negative. Blood tests were normal. She had a past medical history of asthma. Neurologic examination was normal.

The author placed her on an increasing dose of indomethacin to 75 mg 3 times a day with omeprazole, and she became pain free. She has been followed for almost 3 years. The pain resolved for 9 months without medication and then recurred and has been controlled with indomethacin 75 mg daily.[7]

Question: What is the diagnosis, and why might the case be misdiagnosed?

The diagnosis is hemicrania continua (HC), which is an easy diagnosis to miss as in this case because of the similarity to migraine and to new daily persistent headache, which can be unilateral in 11% of cases. She did not have CAS, which are absent in about 25% of cases of HC but are also present in about 50% of migraineurs.

In a study of 52 patients with HC, 52% were misdiagnosed with migraine and 40% met migraine criteria during HC exacerbations.[42] The mean time until correct diagnosis was 5 years. Other studies have reported a delay until diagnosis of 86.1 months to 12 years[43] and up to 70% meeting migraine criteria during exacerbations.[44] The average number of physicians seen before the correct diagnosis was 4.6 with misdiagnoses by a variety of specialists including neurologists and headache specialists. Indomethacin may be underdosed during an indomethacin challenge, which can also lead to misdiagnosis. Patients with HC also may undergo unnecessary dental extractions, temporomandibular disorder, or sinus surgery.

HC is a rare disorder that may have a prevalence of up to 1% of the population. HC is more common in women than men, 1.6:1. The onset is often during the third decade of life with a range from the first to seventh decade.

The pain is almost always unilateral, although occasionally the pain can switch sides, and rare bilateral cases have been reported.[45] The pain is throbbing in 69%, and exacerbations of pain have the following triggers: stress, 51%; alcohol, 38%; irregular sleep, 38%; bright lights, 36%; exercise, 31%; warm environment, 28%; skipping a meal, 23%; strong smell, 15%; weather change, 13%; tiredness, 13%; and period, 10%.[46] Similar to chronic migraine, 75% have exacerbations of severe throbbing or stabbing pain lasting 20 minutes to several days, which can be associated with photophobia (59%), phonophobia which is often unilateral (60%), nausea (53%), and vomiting and pain awakening in one-third (24%). A visual aura can rarely occur.[47]

Cranial autonomic features are present in up to 75% with tearing and then conjunctival injection the most common complaints compared with 56% of migraineurs. A prior history of migraine is common. Primary stabbing headache or jabs and jolts are reported by 41% especially in exacerbations and about 40% of migraineurs.

HC can be labeled unremitting when daily and continuous for at least 1 year without remission periods of at least 1 day and remitting when the pain is not daily or continuous but is interrupted by remission periods of at least 1 day without treatment. In one series, 82% of cases had chronic (unremitting) HC, which was chronic from the onset in 69%.[8] Evolution from the episodic form occurred in 28% after a latency of 7.9 years (range of 2 weeks to 26 years). Some of the patients with the initial episodic form had headaches that were not daily initially, and one patient had about 10 headache days per month. Fifteen percent of patients had the episodic form, which was episodic from the onset in 33% and evolved from the chronic form in 66%.

Indomethacin responsiveness defines HC during an indomethacin trial with complete headache freedom in divided doses from 50 to 300 mg daily, usually 150 mg/d or less. There are rare reports of response at 300 mg daily. Most patients will respond to an indomethacin trial of increasing the dose if not completely headache free on follows: 25 mg 3 times a day for 3 days, 50 mg 3 times a day for 3 days, 75 mg 3 times a day for 3 days,[48] and 100 mg 3 times a day for 3 days.[49] Charlson and Robbins[50] recommend titrating up from 75 mg daily to 150 mg daily to 225 mg daily with each dose tried for 5 days.

The lowest effective dose of indomethacin should be used because of the risk of side effects, including abdominal pain, dizziness, nausea and/or vomiting, diarrhea, ulcer disease, renal impairment, and association with adverse cardiovascular thrombotic events. Some patients may respond to doses as low as 25 to 50 mg daily. One study found benefit from a median dose of 61 mg daily when the patients were asked to taper the doses down to lowest effective dose after 6 months of treatment.[51] Because of the risk of gastroduodenal mucosal injury, indomethacin is typically taken with a proton pump inhibitor.

For patients who respond to indomethacin but have tolerability issues or have contraindications to indomethacin, there are other options that, unfortunately, are not nearly as effective. In one series, greater occipital nerve block and IV dihydroergotamine were effective as a short-term treatment in 35% and 33%, respectively, and topiramate was effective in 41% for prevention,[8] with 100 to 200 mg daily used in different reports. Melatonin 9 to 15 mg at bedtime, ibuprofen 1600 to 2400 mg daily, celecoxib 200 mg twice a day, onabotulinumtoxinA, verapamil 120 to 480 mg daily, gabapentin 600 to 3600 mg daily, pregabalin 150 mg daily, IV methylprednisolone, Boswellia serrata extract 750 mg to 3375 mg daily divided into 3 doses,[52] occipital nerve stimulation, radiofrequency ablation of the C2 ventral ramus, C2 dorsal root ganglion, or sphenopalatine ganglion have been reported as effective in case reports.[11,53]

CASE 5. MIGRAINE WITH AURA AND LIMB PAIN WITHOUT HEADACHE

Case 5 is a 25-year-old woman with a history of headaches since childhood occurring about twice a week described as a left-sided throbbing with an intensity of 6 to 8/10 associated with nausea, light and noise sensitivity but no vomiting relieved in about 2 to 3 hours with an acetaminophen, aspirin, and caffeine combination. For 6 months, she had episodes about once a month; she sees heat waves in the left field for about 30 minutes followed by a typical headache. On 2 occasions, the visual symptoms were followed by mixing up her words for about 10 minutes. On one occasion, she had the visual symptoms followed by numbness of the right arm and then right face and then trouble mixing up words all lasting about 45 minutes followed by a typical headache.

For the last 3 months, she has had episodes about twice a month of tingling and throbbing pain with an intensity of 5/10 of the right upper extremity, which spreads to the right lower extremity without visual symptoms, dysphasia or dysarthria, paresis, or headache lasting about 2 hours. Past medical history is negative. Neurologic examination is normal. She was only taking the combination pain medication.

She saw an ophthalmologist with a normal examination. She saw a vascular neurologist and had normal testing including an MRI of the brain and cervical spine, MRA of the head and neck, 2-dimensional echocardiogram, Holter monitor, and extensive blood tests, including for vasculitis and coagulopathy. An electroencephalogram was normal. Propranolol and amitriptyline were not effective for prevention of the headaches.

Question: What are the manifestations and how common are the various types of migraine with aura? How often does the aura have onset during the headache?

Case 5 has a history of migraine without aura since childhood and a 6-month history of migraine with visual aura and migraine with visual aura and dysphasia and migraine with a visual and sensory aura and dysphasia.

In the United States, the 1-year period of prevalence of migraine with aura is 5.3% in women (30.8% of female migraineurs) and 1.9% in men (32% of male migraineurs).[54] Up to 81% of those with migraine with aura also have attacks of migraine without aura.[55]

The reported age of onset ranges from a mean of 11.9 years (range 4–17)[56] to a mean of 21 years old (range 5–77).[57] In one study, 54.9% of patients suffered from less than one attack per month and 9.7% suffered from more than 3 attacks per month.[58] In another study, the mean of migraine with aura episodes per year per patient was reported to be 29 (ranging from less than one to 156).[59]

In a study of 362 patients with migraine with aura with a mean age of 46 years (range 12–90), at least in some attacks, 99% of patients had a visual aura, 54% had a sensory aura, and 32% had an aphasic aura.[60] Most patients had a combination of aura symptoms as follows: 28% had a visual and sensory aura; 25% had a visual, sensory, and an aphasic aura; 6% had a visual and aphasic aura; and 39% had a visual aura exclusively. When more than one aura symptom occurred, they occurred in succession in 96% and simultaneously in 4% of patients, and 91% had a gradual onset of visual aura symptoms.

The "classic" visual aura is the fortification (looks like a fortified town as viewed from above) spectra or teichopsia ("seeing fortifications"), which is a jagged figure with fortification lines arranged at right angles to one another beginning from a paracentral area, which usually spreads outward leaving visual loss behind. There are often scintillations that may be white, gray, or have colors similar to a kaleidoscope in a semicircle or C-shape surrounding the scotoma or area of visual loss. Scintillating scotomas are typically in one hemifield with visual field defects beginning around fixation and spreading outward. The symptoms reported by patients may be quite variable, however.

Approximately 50% of patients report that the visual auras begin in the periphery and 50% in or adjacent to the center of the visual field. In a series of 122 clinic patients,[61] the laterality of the visual auras was reported as follows: always on the same side of vision (right or left), 22.1%; one sided, but not always on the same side, 23.8%; always on both sides of vision, 23.8%; and sometimes on one side, sometimes on both sides, 29.5%.[17] The color of the visual auras was reported as follows: always black-and-white, 30.3%; always black-and-silver, 20.5%; always colorful, 18.0%; both black-and-white and colorful, 22.2%; and have no color, 9.0%. The visual phenomena were described with the following characteristics and percentages of patients: blurred vision, 54.1%; small bright dots, 47.5%; zigzag lines, 41.8%; flashes of bright light, 38.5%; "blind spots", 33.6%; flickering light, 30.3%; "like looking through heat waves or water", 24.6%; blindness in half of a visual field, 23.0%; white spots, 22.1%; colored dots/spots of light, 19.7%; curved or circular lines, 18.9%; small black dots, 17.2%; beanlike forms, like a crescent or C-shaped, 16.4%; black spots, 14.8%; and tunnel vision, 9.8%. Less common and rare visual auras include corona phenomena, palinopsia,[62] metamorphopsia, macropsia, micropsia, telescopic vision, teleopsia, mosaic vision, and multiple images.

According to the International Classification of Headache Disorders, 3rd edition, beta edition criteria (ICHD-3),[63] migraine aura is considered to be of typical duration when lasting between 5 and 60 minutes. The criteria label aura as lasting longer than an hour and less than a week as probable migraine with aura. Visual aura has been reported as lasting more than 1 hour in 6% to 10% of patients.[64] Other aura symptoms can also last more than 1 hour as follows: somatosensory aura in 14% to 27% and aphasic aura in 17% to 60% of patients.

A sensory aura consists of numbness, tingling, or a pins-and-needles sensation. The aura, which is usually unilateral, commonly affects the hand and then the face, or it may affect either one alone.[65] Paresthesia of one side of the tongue is typical. Less often, the leg and trunk may be involved. A true motor aura is rare, but sensory ataxia or a heavy feeling is often misinterpreted as weakness. Patients often report a speech disturbance when the spreading paresthesias reach the face or tongue. Slurred speech may be present. With involvement of the dominant hemisphere, para-phasic errors and other types of impaired language production and comprehension may occur. Rarely, other aura symptoms may be described, including déjà vu and ol-factory and gustatory hallucinations.

Migraine aura is considered by many to be a distinct phase of the migraine attack preceding the headache. However, in a prospective study of 861 attacks of migraine with aura from 201 patients, during the aura phase, 73% of attacks were associated with headaches with 54% of the headaches fulfilling migraine criteria during the first 15 minutes within the onset of aura.[66] Aura follows headache in about 3% to 8% of cases.[16] The headache may be contralateral to the side of the visual aura, ipsilateral in up to 62% of patients for some attacks,[17] or bilateral.

Question: How do you distinguish migraine aura from cerebral ischemia and seizures?

Unlike symptoms due to cerebral ischemia, migraine visual or sensory auras typi-cally have a slow spreading quality whereby symptoms slowly spread across the vi-sual field or body part followed by a gradual return to normal function in the areas first affected after 20 to 60 minutes.[67] Cerebral ischemic events typically have a sud-den onset with an equal distribution in the relevant vascular territory, although the affected area can expand stepwise if blood flow drops in additional vessels.[68] The pro-gression in partial seizures is typically much more rapid. The return of function in areas first affected while symptoms are occurring in newly affected areas occurs in migraine aura but not in ischemia or seizures. As noted, when more than one aura type occurs, the auras almost always are reported as occurring one after the other, in contrast to cerebral ischemia wherein multiple neurologic symptoms typically occur at the same time. Finally, migraine aura often begins with positive phenomena, such as shimmering lights, zigzags in the vision, or tingling and then followed in minutes by negative symptoms, such as scotoma, numbness, or loss of sensation, which can also occur during seizures but with a typically faster progression of symptoms. This progression from positive to negative symptoms is not typical of cerebral ischemia.

Question: How common are late-life migraine accompaniments and migraine aura without headache?

Fisher[69] reported new onset "late life migrainous accompaniments" in 85 patients ages 40 to 73 years with episodes resembling TIAs similar to the 120 patients he had previously described.[70] Most had visual symptoms occurring alone (44/205) or combined with other aura symptoms. Headache was associated with the episodes in 40% of cases. Subsequent studies have found that accompaniments are not rare, with visual symptoms the most common, followed by sensory, aphasic, and mo-tor auras.[71] There are no randomized controlled studies for prevention. The usual migraine drugs are used for prevention as indicated.

In the Framingham study, visual migrainous symptoms were reported by 1.23% of subjects (1.33% of women and 1.08% of men) with onset after age 50 years in 77%

with the following characteristics: stereotyped in 65%; never accompanied by head-aches in 58%; the number of episodes ranging from 1 to 500 with 10 or more in 69% of subjects; and lasting 15 to 60 minutes in 50%.[72] In a study of 1000 patients presenting for a comprehensive eye examination in Alabama,[73] 6.5% reported visual symptoms consistent with migraine aura without headache, 8.6% women, and 2.9% men with risk factors, including female gender, a history of migraine headaches, and a history of childhood motion sickness.

A retrospective study of 100 aura patients[74] compared those with onset at ages of 45 years or older with those with onset before age 45 and found no differences in gender distribution, family or personal history of migraine without aura, type of aura symptoms, or imaging findings. Aura symptoms were mostly visual. The aura duration was similar in both groups with duration in those with late onset aura as follows: less than 20 minutes, 47.8%; 20 to 60 minutes, 39.1%; greater than 60 minutes, 13%. Headaches were associated with auras less often in those with older onset. The pa-tients with onset age 65 or older were similar to those with onset age 45 or older.

Question: What are the features of migraine with brainstem aura?

Migraine with brainstem aura is the term now used rather than basilar-type migraine because involvement of the basilar artery is unlikely. Migraine with brainstem aura is a rare disorder that usually occurs from ages 7 to 20 years and rarely presents in pa-tients older than 50 years.[75] In one study, the following aura symptoms were reported: vertigo, 61%; dysarthria, 53%; tinnitus, 45%; diplopia, 45%; bilateral visual symp-toms, 40%; bilateral paresthesias, 24%; decreased level of consciousness, 24%, and hypacusis, 21%. Visual symptoms, which usually take the form of blurred vision, shimmering colored lights accompanied by blank spots in the visual field, scintillating scotoma, and graying of vision, may start in one visual field and then spread to become bilateral. The median duration of aura was 60 minutes (range of 2 minutes to 72 hours) with 2 or more aura symptoms always occurring.

Question: What are the features of retinal migraine?

Retinal migraine is rare with a mean age at onset of 25 years presenting with fully reversible monocular positive and/or negative visual phenomena lasting less than 1 hour (**Box 3** provides the criteria).[76] Typically, patients report flashing rays of light and zigzag lightning and less often, bright-colored streaks, halos, or diagonal lines. Negative phenomena may be blurring, "gray-outs," and "blackouts" causing partial or complete blindness. Elementary forms of scotoma are perceived as blank areas, black dots, or spots in the field of vision. Visual field defects can be altitudinal, quad-rantic, central, or arcuate. The headache is usually ipsilateral to the visual loss. Almost 50% have a history of migraine with visual aura. Some patients who report monocular visual disturbance have hemianopsia, which they are not aware of because they do not do a cover/uncover test. This diagnosis is a diagnosis of exclusion of other causes of transient monocular blindness. Retinal migraine can lead to permanent monocular visual loss.

Question: What is Alice in Wonderland syndrome?

Alice in Wonderland syndrome, a term coined by Todd in 1955,[77] is a rare migraine aura where patients usually experience distortion in body image characterized by enlargement, diminution, or distortion of part of or the whole body, which they know is not real. The syndrome can occur at any age but is more common in children. The cause may be migrainous ischemia of the nondominant posterior parietal lobule. Other causes include medications (topiramate,[78] cough syrup with dihydrocodeine phosphate, and DL-methylephredrine hydrochloride), Epstein-Barr virus and other in-fections,[79] depression, seizures, and a right medial temporal lobe stroke.

Question: What is persistent visual aura and visual snow?

Box 3
International Classification of Headache Disorders, 3rd edition (beta version) criteria for retinal migraine

A. At least 2 attacks fulfilling criteria B and C

B. Aura consisting of fully reversible monocular positive and/or negative visual phenomena (eg, scintillations, scotomata, or blindness) confirmed during an attack by either or both of the following:
   1. Clinical visual field examination
   2. The patient's drawing (made after clear instruction) of a monocular field defect

C. At least 2 of the following 3 characteristics
   1. The aura spreads gradually over 5 minutes
   2. Aura symptoms last 5 to 60 minutes
   3. The aura is accompanied, or followed within 60 minutes, by headache

D. Not better accounted for by another ICHD-3 diagnosis, and other causes of amaurosis fugax have been excluded.

From Headache Classification Committee of the International Headache Society (IHS). The International Classification of Headache Disorders, 3rd edition (beta version). Cephalalgia 2013;33:629–808.

Rarely, migraineurs may have persistent visual aura.[80,81] This aura usually consists of simple, unformed hallucinations in the entire visual field of both eyes with a persistent typical migraine aura with oscillation, scotoma, and fortification in one hemifield. ICHD-3 describes persistent aura without infarction as aura symptoms persisting for 1 week or more without evidence of infarction on neuroimaging.

Visual snow is a rare distinct entity whereby patients complain of uncountable flickering tiny dots in the entire visual field of both eyes akin to television snow with often continuous symptoms that can persist for years.[82] Patients also have 2 of the following 4: palinopsia; enhanced entoptic phenomena; photophobia; and impaired night vision. Visual snow occurs more often in migraineurs but also occurs in nonmigraineurs.

Question: What is the cause of the limb pain in the patient presented?

The patient reported episodes twice a month of tingling and throbbing pain of the right upper extremity that spread to the right lower extremity without headache or other symptoms lasting about 2 hours. In 1873, Liveing[83] reported limb pain associated with migraine. Paresthesias and pain of the upper and lower extremity as well as the face have been reported in pediatric and adult migraineurs with and without headache lasting seconds to 4 days.[84–86] Autosomal-dominant familial limb pain associated with migraine has been reported occurring with or without headache.[87] The pain may be due to upregulation of central convergent pathways in the brainstem, cervical cord, thalamus, and cortex.

The pain occurs more often in the upper extremity alone than the in upper and lower extremity than in the lower extremity alone and can be described as throbbing, shooting, stabbing, burning, tearing, or pressing of variable intensity. The frequency can range from daily to occasional. Typical migraine triggers may be reported. The diagnosis is one of exclusion. Migraine-preventive medications may be effective and triptans might be effective acutely. Similar limb pain has also been reported in cluster headache.[88]

CASE 6. NOCTURNAL HEADACHES

Case 6 is a 52-year-old woman with a 5-year history of facial pain that only occurs at night awakening her from sleep about 2 in the morning. She describes a burning or pressure pain in the right upper teeth with an intensity of 10/10, which then spreads to the entire right face associated with nausea, vomiting once, light and noise sensitivity, but no eye redness or tearing, nares congestion or drainage, ptosis or miosis. The pain lasts about 20 to 30 minutes. During an attack, she feels like she cannot lie down and has to get up and move around. The pain may recur a second time within a 2-hour span. The pain may occur daily for 6 to 8 weeks and then go away for about 6 to 9 months before recurring. She saw a neurologist and was diagnosed with trigeminal neuralgia before seeking another opinion.

Question: What is the diagnosis?

There are many primary (cluster, chronic, and episodic paroxysmal hemicrania, hypnic, migraine, and short-lasting unilateral neuralgiform headache attacks with conjunctival injection and tearing) and secondary headaches (medication overuse, nocturnal seizures with postictal headache, obstructive sleep apnea with headache, nocturnal hypertension, pheochromocytoma, temporal arteritis, primary or secondary tumor, subdural hematoma, communicating hydrocephalus, and elevated intracranial intracranial pressure) that can cause nocturnal headaches.

This patient has episodic cluster headache (at least 2 cluster periods lasting from 7 days to 1 year [when untreated] and separated by pain-free remission periods of $\geq$1 month). Cluster headache is misdiagnosed more than 80% of the time when first seeing a physician and even when seeing a neurologist especially in a case like this where there are atypical features.[89]

The duration of each headache (untreated, cluster has a duration of 15–180 minutes), nocturnal awakening, and duration of the bouts are all typical of cluster.

In one study, migrainous symptoms of light and noise sensitivity were reported by 70% and vomiting or nausea in more than 20%.[90] Perhaps 14% of cluster patients report an aura including visual and paresthesia.[47] Gaul and colleagues[90] found headaches occurring between 1 to 6 AM in about 75% of patients.

There are 2 less common features in this case. She does not have associated CAS. In a series of 95 cluster headache patients, 95% had CAS with the following: conjunctival injection and/or lacrimation, 95%; conjunctival injection, 62%; lacrimation, 95%; nasal congestion and/or rhinorrhea, 77%; nasal congestion, 45%; rhinorrhea, 65%; eyelid edema, 21%; and forehead/facial sweating, 57%.[91] Gaul and colleagues' study of 209 consecutive patients with episodic and chronic cluster headaches found at least one CAS in 99.5%.

The ICHD-3 beta criteria[64] for cluster require either or both of at least one CAS or a sense of restlessness or agitation. Gaul and colleagues found restlessnoos in 80% of cases as in this case.

Question: And the distribution of pain?

Gaul and colleagues found periorbital pain location reported by more than 75% of patients followed by occipital neck region and orofacial pain. They note that the orofacial localization and some patients reporting toothache-like pain (40%) may lead to unnecessary dental treatments, including extractions. Based on other series, the pain is behind the eye in about 90%, over the temple in 70%, and over the maxilla in 50%.[92] The pain is often described as sharp, stabbing, piercing, burning, or pulsating. About 15% report that the pain shifts sides between bouts of attacks and, less often, during a bout, but never during a single attack.

Question: What are the features of trigeminal neuralgia?

By ICHD-3 beta criteria, the duration of each paroxysm of pain has a duration of a fraction of a second to 2 minutes. In a prospective series of 158 patients with classical trigeminal neuralgia, the average age of onset was 52.9 years with 60% women affecting the right side of the face in 56%, left side 41%, and bilateral 3%.[93] Pain was reported in the following distributions: V1, 40%; V2, 17%; V3, 19%; V1+V2, 10%; V2+V3, 33%; and V1+V2+V3, 13%. Thirteen percent had a duller persistent pain at the onset of the disorder ("pretrigeminal neuralgia"), while 87% had stabbing paroxysmal pain. The paroxysmal pain was rated on average 10/10 by 50% of the patients. Forty-nine percent of the cohort reported concomitant persistent pain along with the paroxysmal pain.

Forty percent suffered from more than 10 paroxysms of pain per day. Painful awakening at night because of pain attacks at least occasionally was reported by 49%. Trigger factors were reported by 91%, including the following: chewing, 73%; touch, 69%; brushing teeth, 66%; eating, 59%; talking, 58%; and cold wind, 50%. During attacks of pain, 31% experienced ipsilateral autonomic symptoms, most commonly conjunctival tearing or injection. Of the surgery-naïve patients, 29% had sensory abnormalities on examination, most commonly hypesthesia confined to the painful area of the face. Most patients (63%) had periods of remission with the average number per year of disease of 44 with 37% having months of remission and 63% experiencing years of remission.

Question: What is the significance of neurovascular contact in trigeminal neuralgia?

A consecutive series of 135 patients (61% women) with unilateral classical trigeminal neuralgia underwent 3.0 T MRI scans.[94] Neurovascular contact was prevalent on both the symptomatic and the asymptomatic side (89% vs 78%), usually the root entry zone, while severe neurovascular contact was much more prevalent on the symptomatic side compared with the asymptomatic side (53% vs 13%). Severe neurovascular contact that causes displacement or atrophy of the trigeminal nerve is caused by arteries in 98%. Severe neurovascular contact is more common in men (75%) than women (38%) and the odds in favor of being on the symptomatic side are 5.1 times higher in men compared with women.[95]

REFERENCES

1. Beltramone M, Donnet A. Status migrainosus and migraine aura status in a French tertiary-care center: an 11-year retrospective analysis. Cephalalgia 2014;34(8):633–7.

2. Tornabene SV, Deutsch R, Davis DP, et al. Evaluating the use and timing of opioids for the treatment of migraine headaches in the emergency department. J Emerg Med 2009;36(4):333–7.

3. Wijemanne S, Jankovic J, Evans RW. Movement disorders from the use of metoclopramide and other antiemetics in the treatment of migraine. Headache 2016; 25(1):153–61.

4. Rozen TD. Emergency department and inpatient management of status migrainosus and intractable headache. Continuum (Minneap Minn) 2015;21(4 Headache): 1004–17.

5. Orr SL, Aube M, Becker WJ, et al. Canadian Headache Society systematic review and recommendations on the treatment of migraine pain in emergency settings. Cephalalgia 2015;35(3):271–84.

6. Friedman BW, Hochberg ML, Esses D, et al. Recurrence of primary headache disorders after emergency department discharge: frequency and predictors of poor pain and functional outcomes. Ann Emerg Med 2008;52(6):696–704.

7. Evans RW. Migraine mimics. Headache 2015;55(2):313–22.

8. Arnold M, Cumurciuc R, Stapf C, et al. Pain as the only symptom of cervical artery dissection. J Neurol Neurosurg Psychiatry 2006;77(9):1021–4.

9. Kalashnikova LA, Dobrinina LA, Dreval MV, et al. Neck pain and headache as the only manifestation of cervical artery dissection. Zh Nevrol Psikhiatr Im S S Korsakova 2015;115(3):9–16 [in Russian].

10. Schwartz NE, Vertinsky AT, Hirsch KG, et al. Clinical and radiographic natural history of cervical artery dissections. J Stroke Cerebrovasc Dis 2009;18:416–23.

11. Biller J, Sacco RL, Albuquerque FC, et al. American Heart Association Stroke Council. Cervical arterial dissections and association with cervical manipulative therapy: a statement for healthcare professionals from the American Heart Association/American Stroke Association. Stroke 2014;45(10):3155–74.

12. Rist PM, Diener HC, Kurth T, et al. Migraine, migraine aura, and cervical artery dissection: a systematic review and meta-analysis. Cephalalgia 2011;31(8): 886–96.

13. Silbert PL, Mokri B, Schievink WI. Headache and neck pain in spontaneous internal carotid and vertebral artery dissections. Neurology 1995;45:1517–22.

14. Ramadan NM, Tietjen GE, Levine SR, et al. Scintillating scotomata associated with internal carotid artery dissection: report of three cases. Neurology 1991; 41:1084–7.

15. Silverman IE, Wityk RJ. Transient migraine-like symptoms with internal carotid artery dissection. Clin Neurol Neurosurg 1998;100:116–20.

16. Biller J, Sacco RL, Albuquerque FC, et al. Cervical arterial dissections and association with cervical manipulative therapy: a statement for healthcare professionals from the American Heart Association/American Stroke Association. Stroke 2014;45:3155–74.

17. Mokri B, Silbert PL, Schievink WI, et al. Cranial nerve palsy in spontaneous dissection of the extracranial internal carotid artery. Neurology 1996;46:356–9.

18. Arnold M, Bousser MG. Clinical manifestations of vertebral artery dissection. Front Neurol Neurosci 2005;20:77–86.

19. Morelli N, Mancuso M, Gori S, et al. Vertebral artery dissection onset mimics migraine with aura in a graphic designer. Headache 2008;48(4):621–4.

20. Teodoro T, Ferreira J, Franco A, et al. Vertebral artery dissection mimicking status migrainosus. Am J Emerg Med 2013;31(12):1721.e3–5.

21. Mokri B. Headache in cervical artery dissections. Curr Pain Headache Rep 2002; 6:209–16.

22. Gottesman RF, Sharma P, Robinson KA, et al. Clinical characteristics of symptomatic vertebral artery dissection: a systematic review. Neurologist 2012;18(5): 245–54.

23. Engelter ST, Grond-Ginsbach C, Metso TM, et al, Cervical Artery Dissection and Ischemic Stroke Patients Study Group. Cervical artery dissection: trauma and other potential mechanical trigger events. Neurology 2013;80(21):1950–7.

24. Turnball HM. Alterations in arterial structure and their relation to syphilis. Q J Med 1915;8:201–54.

25. CADISS trial investigators. Antiplatelet treatment compared with anticoagulation treatment for cervical artery dissection (CADISS): a randomized trial. Lancet Neurol 2015;14(4):361–7.

26. Kasner SE. CADISS: a feasibility trial that answered its question. Lancet Neurol 2015;14(4):342–3.

27. Steenerson K, Halker R. A practical approach to the diagnosis of spontaneous intracranial hypotension. Curr Pain Headache Rep 2015;19(8):35.

28. Starling A, Hernandez F, Hoxworth JM, et al. Sensitivity of MRI of the spine compared with CT myelography in orthostatic headache with CSF leak. Neurology 2013;81:1789–92.

29. Kranz PG, Tanpitukpongse TP, Choudhury KR, et al. How common is normal cerebrospinal fluid pressure in spontaneous intracranial hypotension? Cephalalgia 2015. [Epub ahead of print].

30. Kranz PG, Luetmer PH, Diehn FE, et al. Myelographic techniques for the detection of spinal CSF leaks in spontaneous intracranial hypotension. AJR Am J Roentgenol 2016;206(1):8–19.

31. Mokri B. Spontaneous low pressure, low CSF volume headaches: spontaneous CSF leaks. Headache 2013;53(7):1034–53.

32. Mokri B, Low PA. Orthostatic headaches without CSF leak in postural tachycardia syndrome. Neurology 2003;61:980–2.

33. Mokri B. Orthostatic headaches in the syndrome of the trephined: resolution following cranioplasty. Headache 2010;50:1206–11.

34. Leep Hunderfund AN, Mokri B. Orthostatic headache without CSF leak. Neurology 2008;71:1902–6.

35. Spears RC. Colloid cyst headache. Curr Pain Headache Rep 2004;8:297–300.

36. Smith RM, Robertson CE, Garza I. Orthostatic headache from supratentorial meningioma. Cephalalgia 2015;35:1214.

37. Mokri B. Spontaneous intracranial hypotension. Continuum (Minneap Minn) 2015; 21(4 Headache):1086–108.

38. Mokri B. Spontaneous CSF leaks: low CSF volume syndromes. Neurol Clin 2014; 32:397–422.

39. Schievink WI, Deline CR. Headache secondary to intracranial hypotension. Curr Pain Headache Rep 2014;18(11):457.

40. Schievink WI, Maya MM. Frequency of intracranial aneurysms in patients with spontaneous intracranial hypotension. J Neurosurg 2011;115:113–5.

41. Pimienta AL, Rimoin DL, Pariani M, et al. Echocardiographic findings in patients with spontaneous CSF leak. J Neurol 2014;261:1957.

42. Rossi P, Faroni J, Tassorelli C, et al. Diagnostic delay and suboptimal management in a referral population with hemicrania continua. Headache 2009;49(2): 227–34.

43. Viana M, Tassorelli C, Allena M, et al. Diagnostic and therapeutic errors in trigeminal autonomic cephalalgias and hemicranias continua: a systematic review. J Headache Pain 2013;14(1):14.

44. Peres M, Silberstein SD, Nahmias S. Hemicrania continua is not that rare. Neurology 2001;57:948–51.

45. Southerland AM, Login IS. Rigorously defined hemicrania continua presenting bilaterally. Cephalalgia 2011;31(14):1490–2.

46. Cittadini E, Goadsby PJ. Hemicrania continua: a clinical study of 39 patients with diagnostic implications. Brain 2010;133(Pt 7):1973–86.

47. Evans RW, Krymchantowski AV. Cluster and other nonmigraine primary headaches with aura. Headache 2011;51(4):604–8.

48. Rozen TD. Trigeminal autonomic cephalalgias. Neurol Clin 2009;27(2):537–56.

49. Prakash S, Golwala P. A proposal for revision of hemicrania continua diagnostic criteria based on critical analysis of 62 patients. Cephalalgia 2012;32(11):860–8.

50. Charlson RW, Robbins MS. Hemicrania continua. Curr Neurol Neurosci Rep 2014; 14(3):436.

51. Pareja JA, Caminero AB, Franco E, et al. Dose, efficacy and tolerability of long-term indomethacin treatment of chronic paroxysmal hemicrania and hemicrania continua. Cephalalgia 2001;21:906–10.

52. Eross EJ. The efficacy of gliacin™, a specialized Boswellia serrata extract, on indomethacin responsive headache syndromes. Headache 2011;51(Suppl 1): 75–6.
53. Beams JL, Kline MT, Rozen TD. Treatment of hemicrania continua with radiofrequency ablation and long-term follow-up. Cephalalgia 2015;35:1208–13.
54. Lipton RB, Scher AI, Kolodner K, et al. Migraine in the United States: epidemiology and patterns of health care use. Neurology 2002;58:885–94.
55. Queiroz LP, Rapoport AM, Weeks RE, et al. Characteristics of migraine visual aura. Headache 1997;37:137–41.
56. Lanzi G, Balottin U, Borgatti R. A prospective study of juvenile migraine with aura. Headache 1994;34:275–8.
57. Eriksen MK, Thomsen LL, Andersen I, et al. Clinical characteristics of 362 patients with familial migraine with aura. Cephalalgia 2004;24:564–75.
58. Manzoni GC, Farina S, Lanfranchi M, et al. Classic migraine—clinical findings in 164 patients. Eur Neurol 1985;24:163–9.
59. Crotogino J, Feindel A, Wilkinson F. Perceived scintillation rate of migraine aura. Headache 2001;41:40–8.
60. Eriksen MK, Thomsen LL, Olesen J. Sensitivity and specificity of the new international diagnostic criteria for migraine with aura. J Neurol Neurosurg Psychiatry 2005;76:212–7.
61. Queiroz LP, Friedman DI, Rapoport AM, et al. Characteristics of migraine visual aura in Southern Brazil and Northern USA. Cephalalgia 2011;31:1652–8.
62. Belcastro V, Cupini LM, Corbelli I, et al. Palinopsia in patients with migraine: a case-control study. Cephalalgia 2011;31:999–1004.
63. Headache Classification Committee of the International Headache Society (IHS). The International Classification of Headache disorders, 2nd edition. Cephalalgia 2004;24:25–36.
64. Viana M, Sprenger T, Andelova M, et al. The typical duration of migraine aura: a systematic review. Cephalalgia 2013;33:483–90.
65. Russell MB, Olesen J. A nosographic analysis of the migraine aura in a general population. Brain 1996;119:335–61.
66. Hansen JM, Lipton RB, Dodick DW, et al. Migraine headache is present in the aura phase: a prospective study. Neurology 2012;79:2044–9.
67. Foroozan R, Cutrer FM. Transient neurologic dysfunction in migraine. Neurol Clin 2009;27:361–78.
68. Cutrer FM, Huerter K. Migraine aura. Neurologist 2007;13:118–25.
69. Fisher CM. Late-life migraine accompaniments–further experience. Stroke 1986; 17:1033–42.
70. Fisher CM. Late-life migraine accompaniments as a cause of unexplained transient ischemic attacks. Can J Neurol Sci 1980;7:9–17.
71. Vongvaivanich K, Lertakyamanee P, Silberstein SD, et al. Late-life migraine accompaniments: a narrative review. Cephalalgia 2015;35(10):894–911.
72. Wijman CA, Wolf PA, Kase CS, et al. Migrainous visual accompaniments are not rare in late life: the Framingham Study. Stroke 1998;29:1539–43.
73. Fleming JB, Amos AJ, Desmond RA. Migraine aura without headache: prevalence and risk factors in a primary eye care population. Optometry 2000;71: 381–9.
74. Martins IP, Goucha T, Mares I, et al. Late onset and early onset aura: the same disorder. J Headache Pain 2012;13:243–5.
75. Kirchmann M, Thomsen LL, Olesen J. Basilar-type migraine: clinical, epidemiologic, and genetic features. Neurology 2006;66:880–6.

76. Evans RW, Grosberg BM. Retinal migraine: migraine associated with monocular visual symptoms. Headache 2008;48:142–5.
77. Todd J. The syndrome of Alice in Wonderland. Can Med Assoc J 1955;73:701–4.
78. Evans RW. Reversible palinopsia and the Alice in Wonderland syndrome associated with topiramate use in migraineurs. Headache 2006;46(5):815–8.
79. Lanska JR, Lanska DJ. Alice in Wonderland syndrome: somesthetic vs visual perceptual disturbance. Neurology 2013;80:1262–4.
80. Evans RW, Aurora SK. Migraine with persistent visual aura. Headache 2012;52: 494–501.
81. Thissen S, Vos IG, Schreuder TH, et al. Persistent migraine aura: new cases, a literature review, and ideas about pathophysiology. Headache 2014;54: 1290–309.
82. Schankin CJ, Goadsby PJ. Visual snow–persistent positive visual phenomenon distinct from migraine aura. Curr Pain Headache Rep 2015;19(6):23.
83. Liveing E. On Megrim, sick-headache and allied disorders. A contribution to the pathology of nerve-storms. London: Churchill; 1873.
84. Guiloff RJ, Fruns M. Limb pain in migraine and cluster headache. J Neurol Neurosurg Psychiatry 1988;51:1022–31.
85. Prakash S, Shah ND, Dholakia SY. Recurrent limb pain and migraine: case reports and a clinical review. Cephalalgia 2009;29(8):898–905.
86. Cuadrado ML, Young WB, Fernández-de-las-Peñas C, et al. Migrainous corpalgia: body pain and allodynia associated with migraine attacks. Cephalalgia 2008;28:87–91.
87. Angus-Leppan H, Guiloff RJ. Familial limb pain and migraine: 8-year follow-up of four generations. Cephalalgia 2015. [Epub ahead of print].
88. Riederer F, Selekler H, Sándor PS, et al. Cutaneous allodynia during cluster headache attacks. Cephalalgia 2009;29:796–8.
89. May A, Evans RW. The sexagenarian woman with new-onset cluster headaches. Headache 2011;51:995–8.
90. Gaul C, Christmann N, Schröder D, et al. Differences in clinical characteristics and frequency of accompanying migraine features in episodic and chronic cluster headache. Cephalalgia 2012;32:571–7.
91. Lai TH, Fuh JL, Wang SJ. Cranial autonomic symptoms in migraine: characteristics and comparison with cluster headache. J Neurol Neurosurg Psychiatry 2009; 80:1116–9.
92. Nesbitt AD, Goadsby PJ. Cluster headache. BMJ 2012;344:e2407.
93. Maarbjerg S, Gozalov A, Olesen J, et al. Trigeminal neuralgia–a prospective systematic study of clinical characteristics in 158 patients. Headache 2014;54: 1574–82.
94. Maarbjerg S, Wolfram F, Gozalov A, et al. Significance of neurovascular contact in classical trigeminal neuralgia. Brain 2015;138(Pt2):311–9.
95. Maarbjerg S, Wolfram F, Gozalov A, et al. Association between neurovascular contact and clinical characteristics in classical trigeminal neuralgia: a prospective clinical study using 3.0 Tesla MRI. Cephalalgia 2015;35:1077–84.

Case Studies in Tremor

Vicki L. Shanker, MD

KEYWORDS

- Tremor • Parkinson's disease • Essential tremor • Dystonia • FXTAS
- Functional tremor

KEY POINTS

- A detailed tremor history is essential and will guide the clinician's physical examination.
- Specific attention should be made to assessing the tremor at rest, posture, and action. When there is an action tremor, multiple tasks, such as writing and pouring, should be introduced into the examination.
- Significant tremor in all modalities is rare and should prompt a differential of less-common tremor causes, such as psychogenic tremor. Clinicians should familiarize themselves with red flags in the history and pearls to the examination to identify functional tremors.
- Fragile X–associated tremor/ataxia syndrome commonly causes action tremor with an intention component and may cause a parkinsonian tremor as well. Identification of the clinical and radiological features will help determine who should be genetically tested.

 Video content accompanies this article at http://www.neurologic.theclinics. com.

CASE 1: TREMOR IN A WOMAN WITH BIPOLAR DISEASE
Case Presentation

A 70-year-old teacher with bipolar disorder presents to the office with hand tremors. Three years before presentation, she had a manic episode and was placed on lithium, quetiapine, and lamotrigine. Within 2 months of the initiation of these medications, she developed tremors in both hands. Tremors are most noticeable when she is lecturing and holding her laser pointer. Her handwriting is sloppier. The tremors are never present at rest. She performs activities of daily living (ADL) independently. She can drink holding a cup with one hand. She is able to pour liquids without spilling. She denies tremor in her voice or neck. She does not feel slower and has not had impairment of her gait or balance. She drinks 1 to 2 glasses of wine daily and is unsure if tremors improve after alcohol consumption. There is no family history of tremor.

The author has nothing to disclose.
Neurology, Icahn School of Medicine at Mount Sinai, 10 Union Square East, Suite 5H, New York, NY 10003, USA
E-mail address: vshanker@chpnet.org

What Are the Key Features of the History Which Will Help Achieve the Diagnosis?

As with any neurologic complaint, a detailed history will help establish a diagnosis. Key features of tremor history include tremor onset, occurrence (ie, continuous, paroxysmal), quality (ie, resting, postural, action), severity (ie, ability to perform ADLs), associated symptoms, and exacerbating and alleviating factors.

Common causes of hand tremor in older patients include an enhanced physiologic tremor, essential tremor (ET), and Parkinson disease (PD). These conditions have key disease features that can guide the clinical examination and diagnosis as highlighted in **Table 1**.

The other components of the history are also useful in tremor assessment. There should be specific inquiry regarding the presence of other medical conditions as well as a detailed medication history. Tremor can be due to not only current medication but also medications recently discontinued as part of a withdrawal or tardive phenomenon. Social history should include exposure to alcohol and other toxic substances. Occupational exposures should be queried. Family history should include specific investigation of tremor or other movement disorders in the family.

In this case, the tremor has an acute-subacute onset and is present in both hands. Aside from the hands, the patient has not noted tremor in other body locations. The tremor is most noticeable when arms are outstretched (ie, holding a laser pointer) and possibly during action. Although tremor is bothersome, it has not interfered with ADL. It is unclear if alcohol improves symptoms. The medication history could be important in this case. The nature of the description suggests an enhanced physiologic tremor; however, an ET cannot be excluded.

What Features of the Examination Will Help to Achieve the Diagnosis?

The movement disorder examination is an essential component of tremor assessment. It is important to examine hand tremor during rest, action, and posture. As the history

Table 1
Distinguishing clinical features in common hand tremor conditions

	Enhanced Physiologic Tremor	ET	Parkinson Tremor
Disease onset/ progression	Acute-subacute/static	Subacute-chronic/ progressive	Subacute-chronic/ progressive
Other common tremor locations	Uncommon	Voice, neck	Tongue, jaw, leg
Prominent tremor modality	Posture most common	Action most common	Rest most common
Hand involvement	Bilateral, usually symmetric	Bilateral, mildly asymmetric	Unilateral
Alleviating factors	Removal of underlying cause (ie, decreased caffeine consumption)	Alcohol	Activity
Other complaints	Nonspecific—often related to underlying cause	Difficulty performing ADLs, such as pouring, drinking from a cup, using a spoon, handwriting changes	Slowness, gait or balance changes, "frozen shoulder," changes in voice

is suggestive of a kinetic tremor, specific focus should be paid to tremor in posture and action. When assessing tremor, it is helpful to note the amplitude and frequency of the tremor. Characteristically, the frequency of limb tremor in ET is 4 to 10 Hz. As tremor progresses over time, there may be an increase in amplitude and a slowing of frequency. Patients may initially only have tremors with action. Over time, an intention component may be observed. A physiologic tremor is a high-frequency (8–12 Hz), low-amplitude tremor that is present in neurologically healthy individuals and may not be easily visible. The tremor can be increased, or "enhanced," in amplitude, from a variety of causes ranging from emotional status to metabolic derangements.

Tremor is best tested in the sitting position. To evaluate postural tremor, the patient is asked to extend the arms in front of the body with the palms facing downward and the fingers spread apart. Then, the patient is instructed to place the arms in a wing position with the hands facing inward, but not touching each other. The patient should sustain these postures for a few seconds. Tremor that presents immediately in posture is more often associated with physiologic tremor and ET, whereas tremor that re-emerges after several seconds is more consistent with a Parkinson tremor.[1]

A thorough neurologic examination, including a movement examination focused on muscle tone, movement quality, and gait, should be performed. The amplitude and speed of the tremor should be observed throughout examination of the tremor. It is ideal to test for action tremor in multiple settings. An initial test has the patient use the index finger to touch the examiner's finger and then return to the patient's nose (or patient's chin with high-amplitude tremors). The examiner's finger should be at a distance such that the patient must move the arm to a full extension to reach the target, allowing the physician to assess for an intention component to the tremor.

A writing sample is useful. A patient is asked to draw Archimedes spirals without resting the arm on the paper in an effort to steady the hand. The patient can be asked to draw continuous loops (or cursive "Ls") across a page, trying not to break when drawing the loops. The patient could also be asked to draw a line connecting dots. Patients with ET will often draw large spirals where periodic intrusion of the tremor may be seen, as demonstrated in **Fig. 1**. If the patient has an intention component, the examiner will observe difficulty placing the pen to the paper and initiating the spiral.

Other helpful tasks that can be performed in the office include pouring water between 2 cups over a sink, drinking water from a cup with one hand, or using a spoon to scoop water from a cup and then place it in the mouth. Through these tasks, the quality and severity of the kinetic tremor can be assessed.

In this case, the motor examination showed a fine, fast postural tremor of both arms. Occasionally, with outstretched legs, a brief low-amplitude high-frequency postural tremor was noted. There was a very mild action tremor of her arms, less prominent than the postural tremor. She did not have resting tremor. Her spiral drawings were not tremulous, and there was no hand tremor while pouring. Her tone was normal. Her rapid alternating movements of her arms and feet were normal and symmetric. She was able to rise unassisted from a chair, and her gait was normal. The remaining neurologic examination was normal. The examination was consistent with an enhanced physiologic tremor.

Is Additional Testing Necessary?

When the clinical picture is suggestive of physiologic tremor and there are no other abnormal findings other than tremor on the examination, imaging is not necessary.

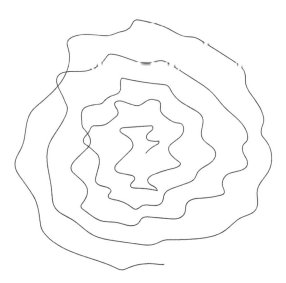

Essential tremor

Fig. 1. Archimedes spiral in a patient with essential tremor.

A routine serum screen for common metabolic causes of enhanced physiologic tremor, such as thyroid and glucose dysfunction (thyroid stimulating hormone [TSH], glycosylated hemoglobin, type A1C), can be checked. It is unnecessary to test for heavy metals unless the history is suggestive of exposure. In this case, a lithium level should be obtained.

The timing of the tremor shortly after the initiation of these 3 drugs raises suspicion that these medications are the source of the tremor. The incidence of lithium-associated tremor ranges from 4% to 65%.[2] Tremor can occur any time during treatment but commonly presents during titration.[3] Tremor is related to lithium serum levels or total lithium dose. Any patient taking lithium who develops tremor should be assessed for lithium toxicity. Lithium has a narrow therapeutic window, and tremor is present in more than half of cases of lithium toxicity. Video 1 shows an example of a woman who developed an enhanced physiologic tremor after starting lithium. Severe lithium toxicity occurs when levels are greater than 3.0 mEq/L. However, elderly patients may have toxicity even at normal levels. The tremor seen in toxicity is typically generalized, coarser in presentation, and associated with other neurologic signs such as mental status changes. Lamotrigine is also associated with postural tremor, and older patients may be more susceptible to this effect.[4] Less commonly, tremor is an adverse reaction to quetiapine.

What Is the Treatment and How Do I Counsel the Patient?

The primary role of the neurologist is to provide reassurance of the relatively benign nature of the condition. Coordination with this patient's psychiatrist is essential because the underlying psychiatric condition must be taken into consideration and medications may not always be easily altered. When lithium is discontinued, symptoms typically subside within the first week after drug cessation.[5] In this patient, lithium was discontinued after 3 months, and she noticed significant improvement of the tremor with its discontinuation.

CASE 2: ASYMMETRIC TREMOR IN A MAN WITH COMPLAINTS OF IMPAIRED ACTIVITIES OF DAILY LIVING
Case Presentation

A 72-year-old right-handed man presented to the office with complaints of tremor for 1.5 years along with difficulty eating and writing. He was diagnosed with ET, and propranolol was prescribed by another physician. He did not have any clinical benefit from this medication. He decided to seek a second opinion.

Upon questioning, he said the tremor predominantly occurs at rest in the right hand. It extinguishes with most actions, but re-emerges when the patient is writing or eating. There is an intermittent resting tremor in the left hand as well. The patient reports loss of dexterity with the right hand, unrelated to tremor. He feels unsteady when walking, although he has not had any falls. On review of systems, the patient reports constipation for several years that improves with a stool softener. He denies any other autonomic symptoms, including urinary symptoms, excessive diaphoresis, or light-headedness. There is no exposure to dopamine-blocking medications and no history of head trauma. His mother had PD in her 60s.

What Features of the History Will Help to Achieve a Diagnosis?

Despite the prior diagnosis of ET, the patient endorses symptoms consistent with PD, including changes in dexterity and gait. Rest tremor can interfere with activities, especially when the tremor re-emerges when patients are holding an object in position such as a cup or a pen. Assessing ADLs is part of the Parkinson rating scale, and clinicians should be careful not to assume that ADL impairment is exclusive to the presence of action tremor.

Rest tremor is most commonly due to parkinsonism, and related questions should be queried. Specifically, patients should be asked about changes in their facial expression, voice (decreased volume, hoarseness, stuttering), hand dexterity, and gait and balance changes. Nonmotor symptoms should be specifically queried, including changes in smell, sleep behaviors (ie, restless leg, rapid eye movement sleep behavior, and apnea symptoms), constipation, mood, and anxiety.

When obtaining a medication history, it is important to specifically query about medications that block dopamine, such as antipsychotics and some of the antiemetics. A social history is important to screen for toxic habits or occupational exposures that could contribute to symptoms. Family history may also be helpful, and the patient should be specifically asked about a history of tremor or other movement disorder. When a history is present, it is ideal to obtain the age of onset of these conditions.

What Features of the Examination Will Help to Achieve a Diagnosis?

As in case 1, a thorough movement disorders examination and assessment of tremor in all modalities are crucial for an accurate diagnosis. Signs of dementia, cortical brain dysfunction (ie, apraxia, agraphesthesia), orthostatic dysfunction, and oculomotor impairment are suggestive of a diagnosis other than idiopathic PD.

Resting tremor is not always immediately present on examination, especially as the patient can have some volitional control. It is essential that the hand is truly at rest and supported against gravity. The clinician should position the patient's hand in the lap or on the armrest on the chair with the hand placed on its side or prone. Patients should remove socks before examination so that the feet may be examined as well. Several seconds may pass before the tremor emerges. The clinician may try to distract the patient by requesting the patient count backwards from 20 with eyes closed; this will diminish volitional control of the tremor and allow the tremor to emerge. This trick was used in Video 2. Tremor may emerge during other components of the examination, such as when the patient is walking.

A classic Parkinson rest tremor is 4 to 6 Hz in frequency and often has a "pill-rolling" quality that characterizes the movement of the thumb and/or forefinger. Alternatively, a pronation-supination of the forearm or flexion-extension of the wrist may be seen. The upper limb is the most common location at presentation, but tremor in the leg, jaw, lips, and tongue may be seen. The presentation is typically asymmetric in idiopathic PD. Secondary causes of parkinsonism or atypical parkinsonian conditions more frequently have symmetric presentations. However, asymmetric tremor can be present in these rare disease states and may even be characteristic of certain conditions such as corticobasal degeneration.

The Movement Disorder Society–United Parkinson's Disease Rating Scale is used by specialists for patient assessment. The accompanying instructions for testing bradykinesia, rigidity, and postural instability may be useful to the general practitioner. Bradykinesia is tested in the upper extremities by having the patient demonstrate 10 repetitions each of tapping the thumb and forefinger together, opening and closing the hand, and turning the wrist from pronation to supination as if turning a doorknob. In the lower extremities, patients are asked in the sitting position to lift the leg, hip flexed, up and down in order to stomp the heel on the ground as well as toe tapping. Each task is performed 10 times, and the examiner looks for slowness in movements, decreasing amplitude, and breaks in movement. Tone should be tested in the neck as well as the distal and proximal limb joints. If tone appears normal, patients should be asked to perform a task in another limb while tone is rechecked as rigidity may emerge with distraction. A pull test will assess postural stability. The patient is instructed to step backwards when the examiner forcefully pulls backwards on the shoulders. The strength of the pull must be strong enough for the patient to step back at least once for the test to be valid. An abnormal test occurs when the patient takes more than 2 steps to stop.

In this patient, aside from the movement examination, the neurologic examination was normal. The patient had trace hypomimia and hypophonia. Tone was mildly increased at the neck and the left leg. At rest, the patient had intermittent 4- to 5-Hz tremor in the fingers of the right hand; there was also rare tremor in the left hand. Tremor re-emerged with posture, encompassing the hands bilaterally, right more than left, and persisted on finger-to-nose bilaterally, although the amplitude during action was significantly reduced. On finger taps, handgrips, and heal taps, the patient had bradykinesia with decrementing amplitude bilaterally and freezing on the left hand. On writing examination, the patient's script was micrographic with minimal tremor. The patient was able to arise from a chair with his arms crossed over his chest without difficulty. He was slightly stooped. Stride was slow, but stride length and base were normal. There was diminished arm swing on the right with re-emergence of tremor. Pull test was negative.

Is Additional Testing Necessary?

In this case, the patient has a rest tremor (right > left), bradykinesia (left > right), and increased tone on the left. Posture was stooped and gait was slow, but balance was preserved. There were no history and examination findings consistent with atypical disease. Thus, the clinical picture is most consistent with PD. In clinical cases suggestive of PD, very few tests are needed.

In 2013, European guidelines reported there was good evidence for the use of MRI to differentiate PD from multiple system atrophy and evidence it will probably differentiate PD from progressive supranuclear palsy and symptomatic parkinsonism.[6] MRI brain scan can screen for normal pressure hydrocephalus and vascular disease. Unless there is a suggestive history for infection or cancer, gadolinium enhancement is not needed. There are no serum tests that diagnose PD. Low vitamin B12 and thyroid dysfunction are associated with tremor and parkinsonian symptoms; thus, a B12 level and TSH are useful serum screens. An initial screen for Wilson disease should be considered for patients younger than 50. The dopamine transporter (DaT) single-photon emission computed tomography scan was approved by the US Food and Drug Administration for use in PD diagnosis in 2011. A positive scan is one whereby there is reduced striatal uptake of the tracer. The routine use of DaTscan in the diagnosis of early PD has been questioned because of variability in reader interpretation, discrepancies between first and second readings, as well as sensitivity and specificity that are reported to be no better than a clinical diagnosis.[7,8]

What Is the Treatment and How Do I Counsel the Patient?

PD is the second most common neurodegenerative disease in the United States with an estimated prevalence of one million cases.[9] Although patients with PD commonly receive their diagnosis by a neurologist, the rates of misdiagnosis may be as high as 1:4.[10]

American Academy of Neurology (AAN) guidelines state that evidence suggests tremor as a presenting symptom is predictive of a more benign course and longer therapeutic benefit to levodopa (level C).[11] The treatment of PD is complex and depends on various factors, such as the patient's desire to treat, drug side-effect profiles, other medical conditions and medications taken, nonmotor complaints, and financial issues. Of all of the available drugs, carbidopa/levodopa is usually the most effective in tremor reduction. Patients may require higher than the starting dose of 25/100 mg 3 times daily in order to receive significant tremor relief. In this patient, there was significant tremor reduction and overall improvement of all symptoms with rasagiline 1 mg daily, carbidopa/levodopa 25/100 mg 3 times daily, and regular exercise.

CASE 3: A WOMAN WITH 1 YEAR OF NECK TREMOR
Case Presentation

A 35-year-old woman presents with neck tremor. She reports that over the past year she has developed head bobbing, which began after a motor vehicle accident. The neck movements do not occur all of the time. She cannot find a particular pattern to the tremor but is aware it occurs when reading. Her hairdresser noticed tremor with neck flexion. The tremor worsens with stress. She is unsure if the tremor improves with alcohol. She was assessed by a neurosurgeon and, after viewing her imaging, he diagnosed her with Arnold Chiari I; surgical intervention was proposed to help what was assessed to be titubation. She went to a neurologist for a second opinion regarding the surgery and was diagnosed instead with ET. She was not prescribed any medication because the neck symptoms were not continuous and appeared to be mild. However, in the year since the initial neurologist's assessment, the neck tremor has increased in amplitude and frequency and is now associated with neck pain, which she feels initiates migraines.

What Are the Key Features of the History Which Will Help Achieve the Diagnosis?

This patient has received 2 different diagnoses for her head tremor: titubation and ET. Patients with cerebellar disease can develop rhythmic oscillations of the trunk and head known as titubation. Other symptoms of cerebellar disease should be specifically queried, including changes of speech, ability to coordinate movements, balance, and gait

The patient then received a diagnosis of ET. Helpful questions to assess ET include the following:

1. *Do you have a hand tremor?* By definition, patients with ET must have hand tremor. ET was defined in a 1988 consensus statement as a "bilateral, largely symmetric postural or kinetic tremor involving hands and forearms that is visible and persistent."[12] Thus, it is important to ask the patient about hand tremor during activities.
   a. If so, when did neck tremor start in relation to hand tremor? Neck tremor is observed in up to 50% of patients with ET and is more often present in patients with long disease duration.[13] The neck tremor of ET is described as either a "yes-yes" vertical movement or a "no-no" horizontal tremor. Head tremor is more common in women, who are 6 times more likely to develop head tremor than men.[14]
   b. If so, did a voice tremor develop and did it emerge after the appearance of hand tremor?
2. *Do you have a family history of ET?* A history of ET is present in up to 50% of patients.
3. *Does the tremor improve with alcohol?* Alcohol sometimes alleviates tremor in ET. Alcohol-responsive patients may also experience a "rebound" period, typically 3 to 4 hours after consumption, during which time there is worsening of the tremor.

A third possibility in the differential diagnosis of neck tremor is a dystonic tremor, a clinical manifestation of cervical dystonia. Patients should be asked the following:

1. *Do you have a maneuver that you can do which improves symptoms?* Sensory tricks, also termed "geste antagoniste," are maneuvers that can be voluntarily performed by the patient to minimize the symptoms of dystonia. For example, a patient may note that wearing a scarf or touching the back of the head reduces tremor. Even the thought of the relieving the trick may diminish dystonic tremor.[15] Patients may have several tricks, and tricks may vary among individuals.[16]
2. *Do you have neck pain?* Pain is significantly more common in dystonia than it is in ET. Patients with cervical dystonia may have hand tremors. Hand tremor typically precedes neck tremor. Patients with hand tremors should be asked about the quality of their handwriting and the presence of writer's cramp.
3. *Is there a family history of dystonia or tremor?*

In this patient, there were no medication exposures and no family history of tremor. She had no complaints of a hand or voice tremor. The presence of worsening tremor looking downward suggests a possible positional component. Although she denied a sensory trick, she did endorse neck pain. The history is thus most suggestive of dystonia.

What Features of the Examination Will Help to Achieve Diagnosis?

During the examination, it is helpful to perform a close inspection of cervical muscle bulk because cervical dystonia is often associated with hypertrophy of the neck muscles; this is not true for other neck tremor conditions. The patient should be asked to move the neck in all directions and maintain the position at the furthest rotation possible in each direction (eg, "Turn the head all the way to the right."). The examiner should look for a null point where tremor stops. It is also helpful to watch as the patient returns to the center position as she or he may have to make small movements or perform tricks such as tucking the chin downward when returning to midline. Neck tremor may also be induced on bedside examination by asking the patient to sustain "ahh" or "eee" for 10 to 15 seconds. The sustained phonation can induce or amplify neck tremor and may be seen during the task or immediately after completing it.[17]

The differential diagnosis of a patient presenting with a chief complaint of neck tremor is limited and mainly includes ET and tremulous cervical dystonia. Although the presence of a null point, tremor directionality, neck pain, or a sensory trick all suggest cervical dystonia, it is the presence of associated hand tremor that can be most useful when trying to distinguish between these conditions. Video 3 shows a "yes-yes" tremor in a woman with long-standing ET. Video 4 shows a jerky horizontal tremor in a woman with cervical dystonia. **Table 2** highlights key differences, based on diagnosis, in the examination of a patient with neck tremor.

On this patient's examination, hypertrophic muscles were noted in the horizontal and vertical trapezius muscles. During neck flexion, a neck tremor emerged, and there was a jerky retrocollis movement. The tremor immediately resolved when the head was restored to neutral position. The tremor was not activated when speaking or during activity of the limbs. There was no arm tremor at rest, posture, or action. Coordination testing was normal. The SARA (Scale for the Assessment and Rating of Ataxia) score, an ataxia rating scale, was zero, signifying no signs of ataxia. Gait testing was normal. The remainder of the neurologic examination, including reflexes, was normal.

Is Additional Testing Necessary?

An isolated tremor in the neck is highly suggestive of dystonia.[18] The patient's history and examination support this diagnosis. Additional testing should be limited. An MRI of her brain was normal, and an MRI cervical spine could be performed to assess for cord abnormality given the history of trauma. Because of her young age, a screen for Wilson disease, including a serum ceruloplasmin and a slit-lamp examination, could be performed.

What Is the Treatment and How Do I Counsel the Patient?

The patient has a persistent focal isolated cervical dystonia. AAN guidelines report that botulinum toxin is safe and effective for patients with cervical dystonia. There is evidence that it is more efficacious and better tolerated in patients with cervical dystonia than treatment with trihexyphenidyl.[19] Of the 2 available strains for clinical use, strain A is used more often and is associated with less antibody development, somewhat longer period of efficacy, and a lower side-effect profile. Injections are frequently performed under electromyography (EMG) guidance because muscle involvement may include deep muscles, and EMG allows identification of affected muscles not easily visualized. Injections should be initiated at the lowest recommended doses

		Null Point/Tremor Amplitude Based	
	Hand Tremor	on Neck Position	Neck Muscle Hypertrophy
ET	Always present—bilateral, fairly symmetric; amplitude similar in all directions	No	No
Cervical dystonia	Sometimes present—often unilateral or asymmetric with amplitude based on position	Yes	Yes

Table 2
Examination findings for a patient with neck tremor based on diagnosis

and are usually repeated every 3 months as the effects of the previous injections abate. Various resources provide dose recommendations.[20] Potential side effects include dysphagia, dysarthria, and weakness in the injected muscle groups.

CASE 4: A MAN WITH AN ACUTE ONSET OF SEVERE TREMOR DURING REST AND ACTION
Case Presentation

A 58-year-old man presented with an acute onset of bilateral hand tremors. Before onset, he had persistent left arm pain for several months. This pain was evaluated by multiple doctors, including a cardiologist, orthopedist, and multiple neurologists. All testing was normal, including MRI of the brain and cervical spine. He had multiple interventional procedures and tried multiple medications, without relief. The tremors began 2 weeks after receiving an EMG/nerve conduction study. The tremors occur at both rest and action but appear more prominent with action. They occur all day. Nothing specifically aggravates or ameliorates the tremor. He reports that the tremors interfere with his ADL, but he is still able to perform them independently. At the same time he developed tremors, he developed balance difficulties. He has not had any falls but will consciously lower himself to the ground when his legs begin buckling. He endorses symptoms of poor memory, decreased concentration, depression, and disrupted sleep. He is a war veteran and reports vivid dreams associated with posttraumatic stress disorder.

He has no history of exposure to dopamine-blocking medication and no history of trauma or infection. Past medical history is positive only for hyperlipidemia for which he is taking a statin medication. Family history is significant for an autistic sibling who has hand tremors. He has a remote smoking history. He does not drink alcohol or use recreational drugs. He used to work as a cashier but is now receiving disability.

What Are the Key Features of the History Which Will Help Achieve the Diagnosis?

When a patient presents with resting and action tremor, there is a limited differential diagnosis. This diagnosis includes secondary causes such as medications (ie, valproic acid), underlying medical conditions (ie, Wilson disease), and structural lesions (ie, tumors, multiple sclerosis plaques, and cerebral infarctions in the midbrain or thalamus produce rubral tumors). A psychogenic or functional tremor should be considered as well, especially when the onset is acute and progression to maximum severity is rapid as in this case.

There are several historical clues that can suggest functional tremor. These clues include (a) the presence of a physical injury before tremor onset; (b) acute onset and a rapid generalization to maximum deficit, with tremor in multiple modalities (rest, action, posture); and (c) periods of remission that can occur rapidly and spontaneously.[21,22] The review of systems may include multiple somatic complaints. A history of work in the medical profession is a common historical feature in patients with functional disorders. When appropriate, the clinician should assess for secondary gain, such as pending litigation or potential monetary compensation for the present condition.

This patient has an acute onset with rapid progression of tremor occurring in all modalities. There was no recent change in medication, and testing to date is normal. A functional tremor is high in the differential diagnosis.

What Features of the Examination Will Help to Achieve the Diagnosis?

In patients wherein there is a high suspicion for functional tremor, there are several tests that can be performed in the examination room. Key strategies are highlighted here. The examiner should look for variability of the tremor in the speed, direction, or amplitude. If this is not obvious on testing, the examiner may try to *entrain* the tremor by asking the patient to perform a task with his hand at a different speed or direction than that of the tremor. Slower speeds may be more effective to entrain. The entrained tremor will match the speed or the direction of the new task. The tremor may also become disrupted during these tasks.

A functional tremor may be *distractible*. The examiner should observe the patient's tremor activity during the history taking, a time when the patient may not be focusing on the tremor. When the tremor is overtly tested, the tremor may significantly enhance. However, when the examiner appears to focus on another limb or engages the patient in a specific task, the tremor in the affected limb may diminish. The examiner can create a distracting task such as asking the patient to perform serial sevens.

Patients may show *selective disability*, such as when a patient demonstrates severe tremor on finger-to-nose testing but then is able to hold a cell phone to his ear to have a conversation. The tremor may be *suggestible*, changing in severity based on cue; for example, the tremor may increase with hyperventilation or decrease with vibration of a tuning fork, when the examiner suggests these responses before using these techniques.[21] A functional tremor may *worsen when the patient is provided a weighted object to hold*; an unusual finding for most central organic tremor, this may be seen in as many as 70% of patients with functional tremor.[23]

In addition to the tremor, the examiner should look for signs of multiple types of movement disorders, such as myoclonic-like jerks, parkinsonism, or dystonia. Patterns of movements are frequently sufficiently unique that they cannot be categorized as a recognizable movement disorder. On examination, these other movements may also have functional qualities. The examiner may want to note the patient's movements in the waiting room.

On examination, muscle tone was variable and improved with distraction. Tremor was variable in frequency and directionality and distractible. His gait was not typical of a parkinsonian gait and had several unusual components. There was a narrow-based stance, yet there were truncal movements forwards and backwards. There was frequent flexion of the knees that was slower than myoclonus. The remainder of the examination was normal.

Is Additional Testing Necessary?

In patients with functional tremor, the diagnosis is a clinical diagnosis and should be made by a neurologist, preferably a movement disorder specialist. A psychiatrist cannot make the diagnosis. In this case, the basic laboratory evaluation and MRI of the brain were normal. Further testing is unnecessary and can further reinforce the symptoms.

What Is the Treatment and How Do I Counsel the Patient?

It is critical that the clinician is honest and direct about the diagnosis. The patient's complaints should be validated, and counseling should occur in a nonjudgmental manner. A multidisciplinary treatment plan, including a psychologist or psychiatrist, is the most effective approach to management.

CASE 5: TREMOR IN A WOMAN WITH COGNITIVE AND MOTOR DECLINE
Case Presentation

A 70-year-old woman presents for evaluation of tremor, memory, and gait. Four years before presentation, she noted changes in her handwriting, which was shaky and sloppy. A tremor developed and is now most prominent during action, but is seen during rest as well. The tremor occurs intermittently during the day and is present in the legs at night. She was prescribed carbidopa/levodopa, up to 800 mg daily, in the past, and the tremor reportedly had no response to this dose. At the same time the tremor developed, she became more forgetful. However, she did not feel this interfered with ADL. In the year of presentation, she developed gait difficulties and multiple mechanical falls. She began to use a walker for poor balance and fear of falling. The family also noticed periods of confusion.

Her medical history is pertinent for diabetes mellitus type 2 and hypothyroidism. Medications include metformin, insulin glargine injections, and ezetimibe. She is unaware of her parents' medical history. She is a retired administrative assistant. She does not use alcohol, tobacco, or recreational drugs.

CLINICAL QUESTIONS
What Are the Key Features of the History Which Will Help Achieve the Diagnosis?

This patient presents with an unusual action > rest tremor. Despite the presence of resting tremor and gait difficulties, she has had minimal response to moderate to high doses of levodopa; this response is atypical for idiopathic PD. The cognitive complaints are not characteristic for early PD. A historical screen for oculomotor impairment (ie, difficulty reading or going down staircases) or autonomic dysfunction (ie, urinary incontinence, orthostatic hypotension) is important.

In this case, further exploration of family history was important. When queried further, it was revealed she had 2 sons with fragile X syndrome. Fragile X is the most common inherited cause of learning disability worldwide.[24] It is caused when there is more than 200 CGG repeat expansions in the fragile X mental retardation 1 (FMR1) gene. Patients who have a premutation range of 55 to 200 CGG repeat expansion may develop a tremor-ataxia syndrome (fragile X–associated tremor/ataxia syndrome or FXTAS) in later life.[25] Approximately 40% of male carriers become symptomatic, whereas only 16% of age-matched women manifest symptoms.[26]

Patients with FXTAS may have cognitive, balance, coordination, and tremor complaints. Endocrine dysfunction is common and may emerge in the past medical history. Thyroid disease occurs in approximately half of women with FXTAS, and primary ovarian deficiency is seen in 20% of women carrying premutation repeats.[27] Manifesting carriers may develop menopause before turning 40 years old.[28] Depression and anxiety occur at higher rates in FXTAS women than in the general population.

What Features of the Examination Will Help to Achieve the Diagnosis?

The abnormal findings on this patient's examination were as follows:

1. Cognitive impairment: She was bradyphrenic. Montreal Cognitive Assessment score was impaired.
2. Cerebellar dysfunction: There was saccadic intrusion into smooth pursuit on oculomotor testing. However, there was no dysmetria or ataxia on coordination testing.
3. Intention tremor: There was an irregular low-amplitude tremor at rest, posture, and action. The action tremor had an intention component. Writing sample showed invasion of the tremor, but there was no micrographia.
4. Parkinsonism: Tone was increased in the neck and all 4 limbs. Posture was mildly stooped. She required use of the walker for ambulation. She had frequent freezing with gait initiation.
5. Neuropathy: Vibration and proprioception were impaired bilaterally to the ankles. (Routine serum laboratory tests for neuropathy were normal.)

There are no clinical findings that are specific to the diagnosis of FXTAS. However, it is important to know the clinical criteria necessary for diagnosis. A definite diagnosis cannot be made without radiologic or pathologic support. However, a probable clinical diagnosis can be made if the patient has an intention tremor and cerebellar ataxia. Intention tremor is common and presents in as many as 70% of studied cases. Whereas intention tremor is frequently the presenting symptom in elderly men with FXTAS, tremor is not a prominent feature in manifesting women.[29,30] Although most tremors are similar to an ET or a coarse, slow cerebellar tremor, a parkinsonian tremor can be seen.[31] Patients with FXTAS may also have parkinsonism, cognitive problems (executive dysfunction, short-term memory deficits), and neuropathy. These findings can be used in combination with radiological changes to achieve the diagnosis.

Is Additional Testing Necessary?

An MRI brain scan should be ordered in patients wherein there is a suspicion of FXTAS. The middle cerebellar peduncles sign, the presence of T2 signal hyperintensities in the middle cerebellar peduncles, is a common finding in FXTAS, more often seen in men than women.[30] Approximately 60% of patients have white matter lesions in the splenium of the corpus callosum. White matter lesions are seen in 60% of patients with FXTAS and are seen equally among the sexes. The presence of either of these 2 radiologic findings warrants a genetic screen for FXTAS.[32] Moderate to severe general atrophy and T2 white matter signal changes in the periventricular region may also be seen.[25,31]

Nerve conduction studies can show a reduction of compound muscle action potential amplitude, slower conduction velocity, prolonged F-wave latency in the tibial nerve, and reduced sural sensory nerve action.[33] Studies are consistent with an axonal sensorimotor polyneuropathy.

Genetic testing for the premutation is not recommended as a screen for all patients with action tremor or parkinsonism. Considerations for screening include (a) a family history of fragile X or FXTAS, (b) women with a suggestive clinical presentation and a history of ovarian insufficiency, (c) the presence of intellectual disability or autistic features in the patient or family members, and (d) patients who present with tremor and ataxia of unknown cause.

In this patient, a vitamin B12 and folate serum test was sent because of the polyneuropathy on examination. An MRI brain scan showed periventricular white matter changes and diffuse moderate atrophy. On genetic testing, one FMR1 allele had 100 CGG repeats, and the other was in the normal range.

What Is the Treatment and How Do I Counsel the Patient?

There is no specific treatment for FXTAS, and thus, bothersome symptoms are generally targeted for treatment. When patients present with action tremor, medications such as propranolol, primidone, and topiramate are tried with variable success.[31] Parkinsonism may improve with dopaminergic medications and anticholinergics.[29] Although a controlled trial of memantine in patients with FXTAS did not show improvement in tremor, ataxia, or executive function, a subgroup of patients improved in verbal fluency and noncongruent word memory.[34,35] The role of deep brain stimulation in FXTAS is currently under study.[36]

SUPPLEMENTARY DATA

Supplementary data related to this article can be found at http://dx.doi.org/10.1016/j.ncl.2016.04.012.

REFERENCES

1. Jankovic J, Schwartz KS, Ondo W. Re-emergent tremor of Parkinson's disease. J Neurol Neurosurg Psychiatry 1999;67(5):646–50.
2. Gelenberg AJ, Jefferson JW. Lithium tremor. J Clin Psychiatry 1995;56(7):283–7.
3. Carroll JA, Jefferson JW, Greist JH. Treating tremor induced by lithium. Hosp Community Psychiatry 1987;38(12):1280–8.
4. Arbaizar B, Gomez-Acebo I, Llorca J. Postural induced-tremor in psychiatry. Psychiatry Clin Neurosci 2008;62(6):638–45.
5. Baek JH, Kinrys G, Nierenberg AA. Lithium tremor revisited: pathophysiology and treatment. Acta Psychiatr Scand 2014;129(1):17–23.
6. Berardelli A, Wenning GK, Antonini A, et al. EFNS/MDS-ES/ENS [corrected] recommendations for the diagnosis of Parkinson's disease. Eur J Neurol 2013; 20(1):16–34.
7. de la Fuente-Fernandez R. Role of DaTSCAN and clinical diagnosis in Parkinson disease. Neurology 2012;78(10):696–701.
8. Tolosa E, Borght TV, Moreno E, DaTSCAN Clinically Uncertain Parkinsonian Syndromes Study Group. Accuracy of DaTSCAN (123I-Ioflupane) SPECT in diagnosis of patients with clinically uncertain parkinsonism: 2-year follow-up of an open-label study. Mov Disord 2007;22(16):2346–51.
9. Smaga S. Tremor. Am Fam Physician 2003;68(8):1545–52.
10. Hughes AJ, Daniel SE, Kilford L, et al. Accuracy of clinical diagnosis of idiopathic Parkinson's disease: a clinico-pathological study of 100 cases. J Neurol Neurosurg Psychiatry 1992;55(3):181–4.
11. Suchowersky O, Reich S, Perlmutter J, et al. Practice parameter: diagnosis and prognosis of new onset Parkinson disease (an evidence-based review): report of the Quality Standards Subcommittee of the American Academy of Neurology. Neurology 2006;66(7):968–75.
12. Deuschl G, Bain P, Brin M. Consensus statement of the movement disorder society on tremor. Ad Hoc Scientific Committee. Mov Disord 1998;13(Suppl 3):2–23.
13. Whaley NR, Putzke JD, Baba Y, et al. Essential tremor: phenotypic expression in a clinical cohort. Parkinsonism Relat Disord 2007;13(6):333–9.
14. Hardesty DE, Maraganore DM, Matsumoto JY, et al. Increased risk of head tremor in women with essential tremor: longitudinal data from the Rochester Epidemiology Project. Mov Disord 2004;19(5):529–33.
15. Greene PE, Bressman S. Exteroceptive and interoceptive stimuli in dystonia. Mov Disord 1998;13(3):549–51.
16. Deuschl G. Dystonic tremor. Rev Neurol (Paris) 2003;159(10 Pt 1):900–5.
17. Wright BA, Michalec M, Louis ED. Triggering essential head tremor with sustained phonation: a clinical phenomenon with potential diagnostic value. Parkinsonism Relat Disord 2014;20(2):230–2.
18. Quinn NP, Schneider SA, Schwingenschuh P, et al. Tremor–some controversial aspects. Mov Disord 2011;26(1):18–23.
19. Simpson DM, Blitzer A, Brashear A, et al. Assessment: botulinum neurotoxin for the treatment of movement disorders (an evidence-based review): report of the Therapeutics and Technology Assessment Subcommittee of the American Academy of Neurology. Neurology 2008;70(19):1699–706.
20. Hallett M, Albanese A, Dressler D, et al. Evidence-based review and assessment of botulinum neurotoxin for the treatment of movement disorders. Toxicon 2013; 67:94–114.

21. Kenney C, Diamond A, Mejia N, et al. Distinguishing psychogenic and essential tremor. J Neurol Sci 2007;263(1–2):94–9.
22. Kim YJ, Pakiam AS, Lang AE. Historical and clinical features of psychogenic tremor: a review of 70 cases. Can J Neurol Sci 1999;26(3):190–5.
23. Deuschl G, Koster B, Lucking CH, et al. Diagnostic and pathophysiological aspects of psychogenic tremors. Mov Disord 1998;13(2):294–302.
24. Gallagher A, Hallahan B. Fragile X-associated disorders: a clinical overview. J Neurol 2012;259(3):401–13.
25. Hagerman RJ, Leehey M, Heinrichs W, et al. Intention tremor, parkinsonism, and generalized brain atrophy in male carriers of fragile X. Neurology 2001;57(1): 127–30.
26. Tassone F, Hagerman R. The fragile X-associated tremor ataxia syndrome. Results Probl Cell Differ 2012;54:337–57.
27. Al-Hinti JT, Nagan N, Harik SI. Fragile X premutation in a woman with cognitive impairment, tremor, and history of premature ovarian failure. Alzheimer Dis Assoc Disord 2007;21(3):262–4.
28. Reid JR, Wheeler SF. Hyperthyroidism: diagnosis and treatment. Am Fam Physician 2005;72(4):623–30.
29. Leehey MA. Fragile X-associated tremor/ataxia syndrome: clinical phenotype, diagnosis, and treatment. J Investig Med 2009;57(8):830–6.
30. Adams JS, Adams PE, Nguyen D, et al. Volumetric brain changes in females with fragile X-associated tremor/ataxia syndrome (FXTAS). Neurology 2007;69(9): 851–9.
31. Apartis E, Blancher A, Meissner WG, et al. FXTAS: new insights and the need for revised diagnostic criteria. Neurology 2012;79(18):1898–907.
32. Hagerman PJ, Hagerman RJ. Fragile X-associated tremor/ataxia syndrome. Ann N Y Acad Sci 2015;1338(1):58–70.
33. Soontarapornchai K, Maselli R, Fenton-Farrell G, et al. Abnormal nerve conduction features in fragile X premutation carriers. Arch Neurol 2008;65(4):495–8.
34. Seritan AL, Nguyen DV, Mu Y, et al. Memantine for fragile X-associated tremor/ataxia syndrome: a randomized, double-blind, placebo-controlled trial. J Clin Psychiatry 2014;75(3):264–71.
35. Yang JC, Niu YQ, Simon C, et al. Memantine effects on verbal memory in fragile X-associated tremor/ataxia syndrome (FXTAS): a double-blind brain potential study. Neuropsychopharmacology 2014;39(12):2760–8.
36. Weiss D, Mielke C, Wachter T, et al. Long-term outcome of deep brain stimulation in fragile X-associated tremor/ataxia syndrome. Parkinsonism Relat Disord 2015; 21(3):310–3.

Functional Disorders in Neurology: Case Studies

Jon Stone, MB ChB, PhD, FRCP[a],*, Ingrid Hoeritzauer, MB ChB, BSc, MRCP[a], Jeannette Gelauff, MD[b], Alex Lehn, MD, FRACP[c,d], Paula Gardiner, MSc, Dip CBT[a], Anne van Gils, MD[e], Alan Carson, MB ChB, MD, FRCP, FRCPsych[a,f]

KEYWORDS

- Functional • Psychogenic • Conversion disorder • Nonepileptic seizures
- Movement disorder • Dizziness • Physiotherapy • Psychotherapy

KEY POINTS

- Functional disorders in neurology should be diagnosed based on positive clinical features, not the absence of disease or normal investigations.
- Functional dizziness has now been conceptualized around the term persistent postural-perceptual dizziness and can be recognized based on typical features in the history.
- Axial jerking, sometimes labeled propriospinal myoclonus, is a functional movement disorder in most patients.
- Dissociative (nonepileptic) seizures are commonly preceded by prodromal autonomic and fear symptoms, which are a good target for evidence-based treatment.
- Functional movement disorders may respond well to physiotherapy designed to reverse states of abnormally focused attention and abnormal movement habits.

 Video content accompanies this article at http://www.neurologic.theclinics.com.

INTRODUCTION

Functional disorders, which within neurologic practice can also be described as psychogenic, nonorganic, or conversion disorders, are one of the most common reasons for referral to a clinical neurologist. Their frequency, around 1 in 6 to 1 in 3 new

[a] Department of Clinical Neurosciences, University of Edinburgh, Western General Hospital, Crewe Road, Edinburgh EH4 2XU, UK; [b] Department of Neurology, University of Groningen, University Medical Center Groningen, Hanzeplein 1, Groningen 9713 GZ, Netherlands; [c] Mater Centre for Neurosciences, 551 Stanley Street, South Brisbane, Queensland 4101, Australia; [d] School of Medicine, University of Queensland, St Lucia, Queensland 4072 Australia; [e] University of Groningen, University Medical Center Groningen, Interdisciplinary Center Psychopathology and Emotion regulation, Hanzeplein 1, Groningen 9713 GZ, Netherlands; [f] Department of Psychological Medicine, University of Edinburgh, Western General Hospital, Crewe Road, Edinburgh EH4 2XU, UK
* Corresponding author.
E-mail address: Jon.Stone@ed.ac.uk

Neurol Clin 34 (2016) 667–681
http://dx.doi.org/10.1016/j.ncl.2016.04.013   **neurologic.theclinics.com**

neurology patients in ambulatory care, is not matched by their representations in text-books and training for neurologists. In the last 15 years, research in the field has slowly emerged that allows a neurologist to approach the diagnosis and management of patients with functional disorders in a structured and logical way. The unique format of *Neurologic Clinics Case Studies* gives an opportunity to discuss some of the many challenges but also rewarding treatment opportunities that can be found in working constructively with patients who have functional symptoms and disorders.

This selection of case studies of functional disorders was written to complement those already found in a previous edition of *Neurologic Clinics: Case Studies* published in 2006.[1] Although the field has seen many advances since that time,[2,3] the fundamental principles of diagnosis and treatment of functional limb weakness, dissociative (nonepileptic) seizures, and movement disorders remain the same.

Therefore, in this article the authors take the opportunity to highlight advances with respect to the field in different symptoms of functional disorders (eg, dizziness, impaired cognition, and myoclonus). For a more comprehensive review of the field the reader is directed elsewhere.[2–4]

We use the term functional disorder throughout this article not because we insist others do the same, there are valid arguments for other terms,[5,6] but because we find it a more useful mechanistic term to use with our patients, which does not presuppose cause and fits best with a biopsychosocial approach to these often complex presentations.

CASE 1. JERKY BODY MOVEMENTS AFTER AN UNPLEASANT ANESTHETIC

A man in his middle 50s presents with frequent episodes of axial jerking that started after an inguinal hernia repair characterized by unusually long recovery time after anesthetic with some symptoms of dissociation. His jerks occur as frequently during sitting as when he is supine. Recently he has started having vocalizations during his jerks. Examination shows arrhythmic flexor axial jerking. He has associated bilateral jerking of his arms and legs and facial spasm. His partner notices that social situations or talking about his symptoms worsens them. When there is discussion about his vocalizations, he develops a brief grunt each time he jerks. On further questioning, the patient describes a feeling of "fizzing" in his legs, which builds up and is released when he jerks. He can postpone the jerks for a few seconds but is left with a very unpleasant feeling. Despite the frequency of jerks when seated, he has never had one when riding his motorbike. His partner says they are not present during sleep. A normal MRI of his whole spine has already been carried out when he attends the clinic. The patient is distressed by his symptoms and fearful of leaving the house or having visitors.

What Is the Diagnosis and How is It Confirmed?

The history and examination is in keeping with what has traditionally been termed idiopathic propriospinal myoclonus (PSM). PSM describes arrhythmical flexor jerking of the trunk, hips, and knees that increases when supine. PSM can be secondary to a structural spinal lesion or be idiopathic. Until recently, idiopathic PSM was thought to usually be an organic movement disorder. However, a large combined retrospective case series from London and the Netherlands (n = 176, n = 76, respectively) suggests that around two-thirds of idiopathic PSM is a functional movement disorder based on multiple clinical features and especially the demonstration of a Bereitschaftspotential (BP) in many cases (**Table 1**).[7–9] Functional PSM, also called psychogenic axial myoclonus, occurs as frequently in men as it does in women. Onset is later than other functional movement disorders, occurring usually in the 40s. A common trigger is a

Table 1
Clinical clues to help differentiate functional axial myoclonus from secondary and other organic causes

Functional Axial Myoclonus	Secondary, Structural, or Organic Axial Myoclonus
Bereitschaftspotential present	Bereitschaftspotential absent
Incongruous and variable neurophysiology	Slow conduction velocity (5–15 m/s), EMG burst <1000 ms
	Constant pattern of activation
Distractible and variable	Structural cause seen on spinal MRI
Premonitory sensation	Present during sleep
Facial involvement or vocalisation	Other clinical evidence of spinal lesion
Prolonged muscle contraction with jerks	Neck involvement
Temporary suppressibility	Rhythmic
Jerks internally inconsistent	—
Immediate response to botulinum toxin	—

Data from Refs.[7–9]

surgical or medical illness, often with physiologic triggers for myoclonus, such as sepsis or hypoxia combined with a health anxiety-inducing situation.

Some of the usual criteria for a functional movement disorder, such as acute onset and rapid progression, are unhelpful in differentiating secondary PSM due to a spinal cause from functional PSM. From the history, the main differentiating characteristics are variability over time and presence of alleviating or exacerbating factors.[8,9] Multi-focal onset of jerks, predominant lower limb or unilateral limb involvement, and pro-longed muscle contraction following jerks suggest a diagnosis of functional PSM.[8,9] Signs of a disorder outside of the spinal cord, such as coexisting facial involvement, vocalizations, or evidence of other functional movement disorders, reinforce a likely functional cause. Most patients with secondary PSM will have evidence of a myelop-athy on careful history and clinical examination.

Investigation

An MRI of whole spine is usually required to exclude a spinal lesion. The diagnosis of functional PSM should ideally be made with the assistance of electrophysiological testing. Polymyography in structural PSM will show slow conduction velocity (>15 m/s), electromyography (EMG) burst duration of less than 1000 millisecond, a constant pattern of muscle activation without involvement of facial muscles.[10] An elec-troencephalogram–EMG multichannel recording with jerk-locked back-averaging will often show a BP, a premovement potential seen in voluntary movement. The absence of a BP does not exclude functional PSM because BP can be affected by the level of attention, motivation, and task complexity, as well as technical difficulties during testing. Clinical suspicion of functional PSM is best verified by an incongruent EMG pattern for PSM (see previous discussion) and/or a BP.

Treatment

Treatment of functional PSM is uncertain. Medication such clonazepam or botulinum toxin can be tried but in many cases a symptomatic response may be related to pla-cebo. For example, in one study, 17 subjects achieved complete resolution of their symptoms after a single botulinum toxin injection (n = 17/39).[8]

CASE 2. PERSISTENT AND DISABLING DIZZINESS IN A YOUNG WOMAN

A 19-year-old woman presents with a history of persistent dizziness for the previous 2 years. She had an initial illness consistent with a viral labyrinthitis with intense rotatory vertigo and nausea, rendering her bedbound for a week. She was found to have rotatory nystagmus at the time but this settled. As she recovered her complaint of dizziness changed to a more nonspecific feeling of disequilibrium, light headedness with swaying, and a feeling of motion present mainly on standing and walking but also noticeable when lying in bed at night. She described feeling intermittently "spaced out," as if she was floating, and people seemed far away, which she found frightening. She also complained of sensitivity to objects moving in her environment when she was still, difficulty using a computer, or being in busy environments such as shops, as well as a fear of falling. Symptoms of fatigue, poor concentration, and anxiety about going outside were prominent and, consequently, she had stopped working. She had occasional migraine. Detailed vestibular testing and neuroimaging, although very uncomfortable for the patient, were all normal.

What Is the Diagnosis?

This is a typical history for a patient with dizziness presenting as part of a functional disorder. Commonly used terminology for this symptom cluster includes chronic subjective dizziness; phobic postural vertigo; visual vertigo; space and motion discomfort; and, most recently, persistent postural-perceptual dizziness (PPPD; or triple-P-D).

Neurologists and otologists working in balance clinics have long been aware that a significant proportion of patients referred with dizziness do not have one of the common vestibular disorders (eg, vestibular migraine, benign paroxysmal positional vertigo [BPPV], or canal dehiscence syndromes). For example, in a study of 547 subjects from the balance clinic in Munich, 19% had a nonorganic final diagnosis.[11]

In the 1980s, Thomas Brandt and Marianne Dieterich[12] proposed the concept of phobic postural vertigo, subsequently revised by Jeff Staab[13] who proposed the term chronic subjective dizziness to describe a symptom complex of dizziness that, importantly, the investigators recognized was not a diagnosis of exclusion and was clinically recognisable in their patient group. PPPD is the latest term agreed to bring together these diagnostic entities and to encourage more positive diagnosis. This is now described in the beta draft of the International Classification of Diseases (ICD)-11 (of the World Health Organization) as: "Persistent non-vertiginous dizziness, unsteadiness, or both lasting three months or more. Symptoms are present most days, often increasing throughout the day, but may wax and wane. Momentary flares may occur spontaneously or with sudden movement. Affected individuals feel worst when upright, exposed to moving or complex visual stimuli, and during active or passive head motion. These situations may not be equally provocative. Typically, the disorder follows occurrences of acute or episodic vestibular or balance-related problems."

The dizziness seen in PPPD or functional dizziness is not really vertigo. Although patients, as in this case, may complain of swaying, they typically also describe the feeling as lightheadedness or heaviness of the head. Dissociative symptoms of derealization and depersonalization may also occur, as in this case. Clinically, a useful clue is paradoxical improvement during more complex balance tasks, such as cycling or after alcohol. Fear of falling, worsening dizziness, or attacks of dizziness in crowded places or places with a lot of sensory stimulation (movement, visual, or auditory) can lead to a picture similar or overlapping with panic with agoraphobia. Onset after an identifiable vestibular trigger, such as migraine, labyrinthitis, BPPV, or minor head injury, is typical; whereas the rates of life events and stress before onset are not substantially different between functional and organic groups.[14] Obsessional personality traits or psychiatric disorder may or may not be present. Anxiety disorders, especially phobic disorders, occur in up to half of patients with organic vestibular disorders.[11] They are, therefore, not diagnostic in themselves, although they tend to worsen disability and distress associated with them.

Investigations

Vestibular studies and neuroimaging (MRI brain) should be normal in PPPD, although coexistence with other neurologic, vestibular, or psychiatric disorders may occur. Posturographic studies may demonstrate improved performance during distraction. Clinically, asking a patient to guess numbers written on their back or play a mobile telephone game while standing can be helpful when there is visible sway.[15]

Treatment

This new conception of functional dizziness or PPPD allows the clinical neurologist to make a positive diagnosis in the same way as for functional movement disorder or dissociative nonepileptic attacks, based on the characteristic nature of the symptoms themselves and not the presence or absence of psychopathology. This in itself is a major step forward for patients, their families, and for anyone attempting therapy.

PPPD can be explained to patients as a problem with the "software" of the nervous system that has arisen usually as a result of an earlier vestibular problem or dizzy experience. Normally, feelings of dizziness and imbalance settle after such episodes; however, in PPPD the "sensitivity settings" have become reset in an abnormal way such that the patient experiences sensation of movement and imbalance that are normally filtered out by the brain. The longer it goes on the more firmly this sensitivity gets stuck at these abnormal levels. If the person takes steps to avoid activities and situations that provoke dizziness, this only serves to make them more sensitive when they are exposed.

This kind of discussion can lead to discussion about superimposed anxiety and panic when present, as well as dissociation, a frightening symptom that patients are often relieved to discover is a common experience and not a sign of 'going crazy'.[16]

It is not hard to see the role here for physiotherapy using exercise[17] to help expose and desensitize patients to feared or avoided stimuli, as well as cognitive behavioral therapy (CBT) to help overcome unhelpful thoughts and fears.[18] There may also be a role for medication such as an SSRI in some patients.[13]

CASE 3. NEW ONSET STUTTERING IN AN ADULT

A 43-year-old man presents with new onset stuttering for 3 weeks. He had previously been well but earlier in the month was clipped by a car while riding his bike. He was wearing a helmet, there was no loss of consciousness or post-traumatic amnesia. On the way to hospital he recovered quickly (but was left with a severe headache) with no focal neurologic deficit, including normal speech. Computed tomography (CT) head scan was normal and he was kept overnight for observation because he felt unwell. The next morning nursing staff initially noticed some word finding difficulties, which rapidly deteriorated to a severe stutter. Apart from the speech disorder, no other neurologic deficit was found on re-examination and an MRI scan of the patient's head was entirely normal. Over the previous 3 weeks the stutter worsened, although the patient's partner reported significant variability in its severity.

What Is the Diagnosis?

The history is in keeping with a functional speech disorder (FSD) and there are several typical features of functional stutter. FSDs commonly occur in the setting of other functional disorders, particularly functional movement disorders,[18] but can also occur in isolation. After functional dysphonia, stuttering is the second most common functional speech abnormality, followed by articulation deficits and prosodic abnormalities (including foreign accent syndrome). The combination of different abnormalities is also seen frequently.[20] The diagnosis of FSD can be difficult as the clinical features of functional and organic speech deficits are sometimes similar and they can occur together.

Several features in history and on examination can be helpful in diagnosis (**Table 2**). The development of significant speech deficits after a minor ictus such as mild traumatic brain injury (mTBI), especially with delayed onset, makes an organic cause unlikely.[21] Sudden onset and rapid progression of a deficit in the absence of other associated deficits makes a functional disorder more likely. The severity of functional speech symptoms typically varies across different examination activities and some patients with FSD show significant distractibility and/or suggestibility in their deficit (whereas organic speech disorders are usually consistent during examination and do not fluctuate). Also, some patients with functional stutter show marked effortful physical struggle of face and head, as well as torso and limbs, which can be a helpful clue.[22] Speech may be more effortful and problematic when there is discussion of the speech symptoms. Stutter is a rare consequence of brain disease and in itself should be a red flag for a functional disorder. Finally, the presence of reversibility is a strong marker towards FSDs. Although organic speech disorders can improve with speech therapy, the improvement is rarely dramatic. With FSDs, on the other hand, some patients show rapid improvements even after just 1 or 2 therapy sessions.[22]

Investigations and Workup

MRI brain scans are normal in patients with pure FSDs but, as previously mentioned, the co-occurrence of organic and functional disturbances are not rare. An experienced

Table 2	
Clues to the presence of a functional speech disorder	
History	Development of severe speech deficit after uncomplicated mild traumatic brain injury
	Severe speech disorder in absence of other associated deficits
	Other functional neurologic symptoms may be present
	Other features of functional speech disturbance (eg, baby speech, telegraphic speech)
	Variability of deficit with significant fluctuations of speech disorder
Examination	Speech characteristics do not fit known patterns of organic speech disorders
	Inconsistencies between speech and cranial nerve or oral mechanism examination
	Variability of deficit during examination (eg, during conversation vs formal examination)
	Susceptibility to suggestion and/or distraction
	Paradoxic fatigability with deterioration of speech during examination due to increased muscle activity (eg, strained voice)
	Rapid improvement in speech with symptomatic therapy

Data from Duffy JR. Motor speech disorders: substrates, differential diagnosis, and management. 3rd edition. St Louis (MO): Elsevier Health Sciences; 2013.

speech therapist will often be able to define the organic and functional components through clinical assessment.

Treatment

Treatment of FSDs follows the same principles applicable to other functional disorders. The patient needs a clear positive diagnosis, preferably with transparency about the clinical features of inconsistency that allow the diagnosis to be made and indication that it is being taken as seriously as any other speech disorder. Speech therapy works on the principle of reducing abnormally focused attention and relearning normal movements or speech production.[20] In practice this may mean: identifying abnormal speech characteristics, which are often due to excessive and/or abnormal muscle activation patterns; asking the patient to imitate sounds that will approximate a normal response (eg, grunts, single syllables, simple words); and then normalizing the speech back to more natural speech sounds. Explain to the patient that these abnormal speech features are a barrier to speaking normally, "You are working so hard to talk that you are unable to speak naturally." No randomized, controlled trial data is available but experience suggests that symptomatic speech therapy can be helpful in a large proportion of cases.[20]

CASE 4. FATIGUE, HEADACHE, AND COGNITIVE SYMPTOMS AFTER A MILD TRAUMATIC BRAIN INJURY

A 22-year-old student presented with fatigue, headache, and cognitive symptoms. The symptoms had started 3 months earlier after he had been hit on the head by a hit on the head by a baseball. He had been unconscious for 5 minutes and described feeling as if he were "in a bubble" and having a severe headache afterwards. He was taken to the emergency department where physical examination and a CT scan were normal. In the weeks following the accident, he experienced extreme tiredness, general weakness, dizziness, and headaches. He spent most of his time in bed, at home with his parents. He was unable to read or watch TV because he had difficulty concentrating. His parents noticed that at times he was struggling to find the right words and that he had become rather irritable. The patient was worried that the accident might have caused permanent damage to his brain and he feared he would not be able to finish his studies.

What Is the Diagnosis?

This diffuse collection of physical, emotional, behavioral, and cognitive symptoms in the aftermath of a mild traumatic brain injury (mTBI), when it lasts longer than you would expect from the nature of the injury, is often referred to as postconcussion syndrome (PCS). More recent guidance[23] has cautioned against this term because the available evidence does not support a unique association with concussion and similar symptoms follow nonneurologic trauma. Typical symptoms after an mTBI include headache, dizziness, fatigue, irritability, poor concentration, hypersomnia, photosensitivity, and hyperacusis. They routinely settle down within weeks to 3 months.[24] However, in a minority of patients the reverse happens and the symptoms progressively increase in intensity, the reverse pattern from more severe brain injury in which improvement occurs. In the United Kingdom this affects approximately 15% of patients[25] but the rates vary considerably internationally. There is disagreement on the etiologic mechanisms underlying PCS. Some investigators believe PCS results from diffuse axonal injury with microtrauma to axons, although most consider PCS to be the result of an interaction between biological, psychological, and social factors.[25]

This might explain why similar symptoms are described after other types of injuries.[24] Risk factors for developing PCS are negative illness perceptions (believing symptoms will last a long time and will have a negative impact on your life), all-or-nothing behavior, and litigation and/or compensation issues.[24-28]

Treatment

The first step in the treatment is to explain to the patient what is wrong. The patient's primary concern is, almost always, the not unreasonable belief that these symptoms indicate brain damage and that she or he will not recover. The authors start treatment with a review of the injury severity, checking that the Glasgow coma scale was 13 or more at time of admission to hospital, the duration of total loss of consciousness was less than 15 minutes, and the duration of post-traumatic amnesia was less than 24 hours. When necessary, this is supplemented with reference to national clinical guidelines, such as the Scottish Intercollegiate Guidelines Network (SIGN) 130,[23] for additional reassurance. We will then explain that, although head injury commonly triggers such symptoms, they are just as common after severe injuries to legs or arms and their presence does not indicate brain damage. We will explain that recovery is the norm but the complicated course experienced is far from unusual and can also fully recover. We review analgesic use with a view to stopping opiate drugs and avoiding medication-overuse headaches and, if analgesia is required for headache or photosensitivity, using a tricyclic antidepressant. We use the principles of cognitive therapy and, sometimes, formal CBT[27] to structure a program of graded exposure to tackle avoidance and return to normal activity, stressing the need to avoid boom and bust cycles of excessive activity followed by collapse. We find a definite program, albeit arbitrary (eg, read for 15 minutes on days 1 to 3, then 30 minutes days 4 to 6), works better than vague advice. We challenge fearful cognitions. A common example is, "My memory is not working, I have damaged my brain," which usually relates to anxiety interfering with normal retrieval mechanisms. Memory symptoms can often be identified as functional in nature, for example, using that they can recount the memory problem in some detail, that memory performance is highly variable.[28] **Table 3** includes other features. We can also work on recognizing how often memory does actually

Table 3
Clues to the presence of functional cognitive symptoms either with or without preceding minor head injury

Functional	Neurologic Diseases
Young	Older
Attends alone	Attends with someone
Patient more aware of the problem than others	Others more aware of the problem than patient
Able to detail list of drugs, previous interactions with doctors	Less able
Watches television drama	Stops following drama
Marked variability	Less variability
Types of memory symptom are usually within most people's normal experience	Types of memory symptom are often not normal experiences
"I used to have a brilliant memory"	Does not highlight previous "brilliant memory"

Data from Stone J, Pal S, Blackburn D, et al. Functional (psychogenic) cognitive disorders: a perspective from the neurology clinic. J Alzheimers Dis 2015;48:S5–17.

work and have the patient challenge their anxious thoughts by talking these ideas through to themselves when they arise. In more intractable cases, particularly when there is considerable premorbid psychopathology, formal therapy can be required. However, for most cases, such as the previous example, these principles can be used within the confines of a neurology clinic appointment and resolution is usually reached within a couple of months. The authors have developed these principles in to a free-to-access patient self-help website: www.headinjurysymptoms.org.

CASE 5. TREATMENT OF DISSOCIATIVE (NONEPILEPTIC) ATTACKS OR SEIZURES

A 28-year-old woman presents with a 2-year history of blackouts occurring up to 5 times a day but sometimes with periods of 2 weeks with no episodes. The description given was of sudden motionless unresponsiveness lasting 5 to 10 minutes during which her eyes are usually closed. The patient initially said she had no warning symptoms when asked. However, when pressed she admitted she did often get brief symptoms lasting 10 to 20 seconds of light-headedness and a horrible feeling of "not really being there and floating," which she was reluctant to describe. She also described sweating and altered breathing pattern with a rising sense of fear. The patient admitted that, although she felt "wiped out" and upset after the seizure, she was relieved that the unbearable feelings preceding it had gone. Many of the seizures had happened outside, which caused embarrassment and a reluctance to go out.

What Is the Diagnosis?

The diagnosis is clearly that of a (nonepileptic) dissociative seizure (DS) or attack. In fact this kind of episode, which represents around 20% of all DS presentations, looks like syncope, not a seizure. Therefore, the term dissociative seizure or attack, as used in ICD-10, is potentially more inclusive. Recent studies of these patients indicate that they are more common than previously thought and often present to cardiology services more than neurology.[29] Sudden motionless, long duration episodes (more than 2 minutes) like this, especially with eyes closed, are usually diagnostic of DS. Further testing may be required to establish whether the patient also has cardiac or autonomic comorbidities.

Increasing evidence supports a hypothesis that in many patients DS is a dissociative response to a state of arousal similar to panic. Several studies have highlighted how common symptoms of panic and dissociation are in the prodromal state before a seizure.[30–32] As in this case, patients will typically be reluctant to admit they have warning symptoms,[33] partly because they do not like to think about them in case it brings an attack on, and partly because they are hard to describe and sound, in the case of dissociation, a bit 'crazy'. Not all patients do have prodromal symptoms, sometimes because they have lost them and sometimes because the patient is amnestic for the prodromal stage, which others may report as "looking glazed" or "they were staring through me." Patients may sometimes report mixed feelings of relief (that the prodromal symptoms have gone) combined with anxiety and distress at the blackout itself.[34] This helps clinicians to understand how the process becomes conditioned and keeps repeating.

What Can Be Learned from Treatment?

The patient was given a clear diagnosis backed up with written material (eg, as found on www.codestrial.org). They were referred to a cognitive behavioral therapist with expertise in seeing patients with DS. Over a period of 12 sessions the events stopped completely. Additional problems with past trauma arose and were approached with further therapy.

Increasing awareness of the arousal or dissociation mechanism in many patients with DS has led to advances in evidence-based treatment. This has developed from CBT approaches to panic disorder and other functional disorders. Two pilot randomized controlled trials of CBT for DS[35,36] produced promising data and a large multi-center trial is ongoing.[37]

CBT involves formulating an understanding of seizure development and agreeing on the reasons why the seizures may be happening. This understanding is often enough to reduce or stop seizures in some patients, probably through reducing fear. However, most patients need help overcoming learned cognitions and avoidant behaviors that perpetuate their seizures.

Understanding mechanism is only part of the picture. A multifactorial etiologic model can be used to understand that no single contributing factor has been identified sufficient to explain DS in all patients; in each individual, different factors will be relevant (**Fig. 1**).

In this patient, predisposing factors included post-traumatic stress disorder after being raped at gunpoint and only telling a close friend about it. There was also a history of bullying at school and perfectionistic traits. Precipitating factors identified included relationship breakdown, reports in media about rape, and a friend being attacked. Perpetuating factors included flashbacks that induced feelings of anxiety and the need to avoid the thoughts or memories. She had also been upset by feeling that health professionals did not know what was wrong and had avoidance of socializing, going outside, and travelling alone because of seizures. All these contributed to form a vicious circle that could be addressed with treatment.

The first step of treatment was to help the patient understand the diagnosis, its mechanism, and cause. Second, we worked to reduce seizure frequency by recognizing the prodromal sensations and used distraction techniques and exposure techniques to reduce anxiety over time to prodromal symptoms. Techniques to deal with the anxiety sensations, such as breathing techniques, imagery, and mindfulness,

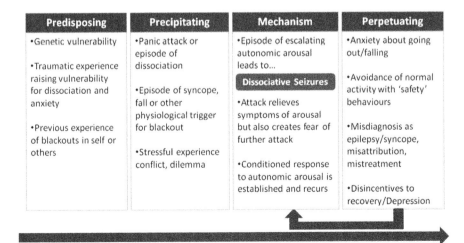

Predisposing	Precipitating	Mechanism	Perpetuating
•Genetic vulnerability •Traumatic experience raising vulnerability for dissociation and anxiety •Previous experience of blackouts in self or others	•Panic attack or episode of dissociation •Episode of syncope, fall or other physiological trigger for blackout •Stressful experience conflict, dilemma	•Episode of escalating autonomic arousal leads to... **Dissociative Seizures** •Attack relieves symptoms of arousal but also creates fear of further attack •Conditioned response to autonomic arousal is established and recurs	•Anxiety about going out/falling •Avoidance of normal activity with 'safety' behaviours •Misdiagnosis as epilepsy/syncope, misattribution, mistreatment •Disincentives to recovery/Depression

Fig. 1. A range of potential factors involved in the mechanism and cause of DSs. (*Data from* Reuber M. The etiology of psychogenic non-epileptic seizures: toward a biopsychosocial model. Neurol Clin 2009;27:909–24.)

allowed her to start going outside and face some of her fears. In this patient, dealing with the past trauma was also necessary and, therefore, exposure to imagery of the rape and being able to talk about it was helpful. Therapy also used thought and behavior diaries to find alternate thoughts for her abnormal cognitions around self-esteem and gradually challenge avoidant behavior. This patient's seizures ceased with treatment.

CASE 6. TREATMENT OF FIXED DYSTONIA

A 20-year-old woman with a history of chronic abdominal pain presented with pain and a fixed posture of her left leg and foot. Symptoms had started after she sprained her left ankle on a trampoline 3 years before. Persistent ankle pain and swelling in the presence of an inconclusive ankle MRI was treated with a cast for several weeks. When the cast came off, the foot looked different. It was swollen, more purple, and felt colder to the touch than the other side. In the following days to weeks, the ankle progressively inverted, to the point that the posture was mostly fixed and the pain persisted. Many specialists were consulted and she received various diagnoses of complex regional pain syndrome (CRPS), muscle dystrophy, dystonia, and a functional disorder, depending on the specialty of the physician.

Neurologic investigation showed a fixed inversion of the left ankle, with only small active movements of the toes and some passive movement of the ankle. The patient said, "My whole foot feels as if it's not there."

What Is the Diagnosis?

For a patient who presents with fixed abnormal posture of a limb with pain and sensory abnormalities, the diagnostic label depends partly on the preference and specialty of the physician. Functional dystonia, often called fixed dystonia, is characterized by the onset in an adult of an inverted ankle or clenched fist (**Fig. 2**, Video 1), although other types of functional dystonia, including at the shoulder, are also recognized.[38] It may occur in the absence of pain but it is recognized that onset after injury and chronic pain are common and there is a large overlap with CRPS. CRPS is now most commonly diagnosed using the Budapest Criteria[39] (**Box 1**).

Studies of movement and sensory disorders associated with CRPS have shown that they are common and have the same clinical characteristics as functional disorders.[40–42] Vasomotor, sudomotor, and trophic changes, such as hair growth, typically associated with the condition may also occur in healthy control subjects after 28 days

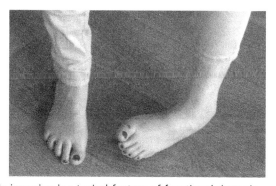

Fig. 2. Fixed ankle inversion is a typical feature of functional dystonia.

Box 1
Budapest Criteria for complex regional pain syndrome

1. Continuing pain disproportionate to an inciting event
2. Three symptoms from
   a. Sensory (eg, hyperesthesia, allodynia)
   b. Vasomotor (temperature or skin-color changes or asymmetry)
   c. Sweating or edema
   d. Motor (including weakness tremor dystonia) and/or trophic changes to hair, nail, or skin
3. Two signs from 2
4. No better diagnosis

---

of casting an upper limb hyperalgesia.[43] Arguments about the overlap between CRPS and functional disorders have unhelpfully polarized around arguments that psychogenic features of CRPS may suggest malingering and CRPS proponents pointing out the severe and genuine nature of the condition along with evidence along with lack of prior psychological factors in many patients. There is now common ground in that research on functional disorders also shows the severe and genuine nature of the condition and the lack of overt psychological factors in many patients.

What Can Be Learned from the Physiotherapy Approach in This Case?

The patient was given a positive diagnosis, with written material, of functional dystonia explaining the overlap with CRPS, and that it was a potentially reversible condition. She was prescribed physiotherapy to relearn normal movements. The physiotherapist found out normal posture could be evoked by exercises the patient used to do at her gymnastics practice. This was used to gain function and improve walking and posture.

Physiotherapy has been shown recently in a systematic review,[44] case series,[45,46] and a randomized controlled trial[47] to be potentially highly effective in functional motor disorders. Consensus recommendations exist that highlight that physiotherapy for these disorders departs in many significant ways from that used in other neurologic disorders.[48] For example, distraction techniques are used to enhance diagnostic confidence and regain automatic movement, preferably collaboratively and creatively with the patient as in this case. This may involve asking the patient to walk backwards or go on a treadmill even if they can barely walk. Treatment is more about movement retraining and can be explained as a way of altering abnormal movement habits that have developed as a consequence of pain, injury, or dissociation.

Nielsen and colleagues[45] studied 47 subjects with a mean duration of symptoms of 5.5 years who completed an intensive 5-day physiotherapy program. A good outcome (defined as very much improved or much improved on the 7 point Clinical Global Impression scale) was seen in 64% of subjects at the end of treatment and in 55% of subjects after a mean follow-up of 95 days. The physiotherapy approach was based on a combination of education, retraining of normal movement, and self-management. Such treatment is also commonly advocated in CRPS.[49] Arguably it is better to approach this clinical syndrome as fixed abnormal posturing that is most commonly functional in origin.[40] Helping the patient to understand that the potential for reversibility and the origin of the problem in the nervous system rather than the affected limb seem to be key components of treatment that this approach fosters.

SUPPLEMENTARY DATA

Supplementary data related to this article can be found at http://dx.doi.org/10.1016/j.ncl.2016.04.013.

REFERENCES

1. Stone J, Sharpe M. Functional symptoms in neurology: case studies. Neurol Clin 2006;24:385–403.
2. Carson AJ, Brown R, David AS, et al. Functional (conversion) neurological symptoms: research since the millennium. J Neurol Neurosurg Psychiatry 2012;83: 842–50.
3. Lehn A, Gelauff J, Hoeritzauer I, et al. Functional neurological disorders: mechanisms and treatment. J Neurol 2016;263(3):611–20.
4. Stone J, Carson A. Functional neurologic disorders. Continuum (Minneap Minn) 2015;21:818–37.
5. Edwards MJ, Stone J, Lang AE. From psychogenic movement disorder to functional movement disorder: it's time to change the name. Mov Disord 2014;29: 849–52.
6. Fahn S, Olanow CW. 'Psychogenic movement disorders': they are what they are. Mov Disord 2014;29:853–6.
7. van der Salm SMA, Koelman JHTM, Henneke S, et al. Axial jerks: a clinical spectrum ranging from propriospinal to psychogenic myoclonus. J Neurol 2010;257: 1349–55.
8. Erro R, Edwards MJ, Bhatia KP, et al. Psychogenic axial myoclonus: Clinical features and long-term outcome. Parkinsonism Relat Disord 2014;20:596–9.
9. van der Salm SM, Erro R, Cordivari C, et al. Propriospinal myoclonus: clinical reappraisal and review of literature. Neurology 2014;83:1862–70.
10. Erro R, Bhatia KP, Edwards MJ, et al. Clinical diagnosis of propriospinal myoclonus is unreliable: an electrophysiologic study. Mov Disord 2013;28:1868–73.
11. Lahmann C, Henningsen P, Brandt T, et al. Psychiatric comorbidity and psychosocial impairment among patients with vertigo and dizziness. J Neurol Neurosurg Psychiatry 2015;86:302–8.
12. Brandt T, Dieterich M. Phobischer Attacken Schwankschwindel, ein neues Syndrom? Munch Med Wochenschr 1986;28:247–50.
13. Staab JP. Chronic subjective dizziness. Continuum (Minneap Minn) 2012;18: 1118–41.
14. Radziej K, Schmid G, Dinkel A, et al. Psychological traumatisation and adverse life events in patients with organic and functional vestibular symptoms. J Psychosom Res 2015;79:123–9.
15. Wolfsegger T, Pischinger B, Topakian R. Objectification of psychogenic postural instability by trunk sway analysis. J Neurol Sci 2013;334:14–7.
16. Tschan R, Wiltink J, Adler J, et al. Depersonalization experiences are strongly associated with dizziness and vertigo symptoms leading to increased health care consumption in the German general population. J Nerv Ment Dis 2013; 201:629–35.
17. Thompson KJ, Goetting JC, Staab JP, et al. Retrospective review and telephone follow-up to evaluate a physical therapy protocol for treating persistent postural-perceptual dizziness: A pilot study. J Vestib Res 2015;25:97–104.
18. Schmid G, Henningsen P, Dieterich M, et al. Psychotherapy in dizziness: a systematic review. J Neurol Neurosurg Psychiatry 2011;82:601–6.

19. Balzabal-Carvallo JF, Jankovic J. Speech and voice disorders in patients with psychogenic movement disorders. J Neurol 2015;262(11):2420–4.

20. Duffy JR. Motor speech disorders: substrates, differential diagnosis, and management. 3rd edition. St Louis (MO): Elsevier Health Sciences; 2013.

21. Binder LM, Spector J, Youngjohn JR. Psychogenic stuttering and other acquired nonorganic speech and language abnormalities. Arch Clin Neuropsychol 2012; 27:557–68.

22. Duffy JR, Baumgartner J. Psychogenic stuttering in adults with and without neurologic disease. J Med Speech Lang Pathol 1997;5:75–95.

23. Scottish Intercollegiate Guidelines Network (SIGN). Brain injury rehabilitation in adults. Edinburgh (United Kingdom): SIGN; 2013.

24. Carroll L, Cassidy JD, Peloso P, et al. Prognosis for mild traumatic brain injury: results of the who collaborating centre task force on mild traumatic brain injury. J Rehabil Med 2004;36:84–105.

25. Reuben A, Sampson P, Harris AR, et al. Postconcussion syndrome (PCS) in the emergency department: predicting and pre-empting persistent symptoms following a mild traumatic brain injury. Emerg Med J 2014;31:72–7.

26. Hou R, Moss-Morris R, Peveler R, et al. When a minor head injury results in enduring symptoms: a prospective investigation of risk factors for postconcussional syndrome after mild traumatic brain injury. J Neurol Neurosurg Psychiatry 2012;83:217–23.

27. Al Sayegh A, Sandford D, Carson AJ. Psychological approaches to treatment of postconcussion syndrome: a systematic review. J Neurol Neurosurg Psychiatry 2010;81:1128–34.

28. Stone J, Pal S, Blackburn D, et al. Functional (psychogenic) cognitive disorders: a perspective from the neurology clinic. J Alzheimers Dis 2015;48:S5–17.

29. Blad H, Lamberts RJ, Gert van Dijk J, et al. Tilt-induced vasovagal syncope and psychogenic pseudosyncope: Overlapping clinical entities. Neurology 2015;85: 2006–10.

30. Hendrickson R, Popescu A, Dixit R, et al. Panic attack symptoms differentiate patients with epilepsy from those with psychogenic nonepileptic spells (PNES). Epilepsy Behav 2014;37:210–4.

31. Goldstein LH, Mellers JDC. Ictal symptoms of anxiety, avoidance behaviour, and dissociation in patients with dissociative seizures. J Neurol Neurosurg Psychiatry 2006;77:616–21.

32. Reuber M, Jamnadas-Khoda J, Broadhurst M, et al. Psychogenic nonepileptic seizure manifestations reported by patients and witnesses. Epilepsia 2011;52: 2028–35.

33. Reuber M, Monzoni C, Sharrack B, et al. Using interactional and linguistic analysis to distinguish between epileptic and psychogenic nonepileptic seizures: a prospective, blinded multirater study. Epilepsy Behav 2009;16:139–44.

34. Stone J, Carson AJ. The unbearable lightheadedness of seizing: wilful submission to dissociative (non-epileptic) seizures. J Neurol Neurosurg Psychiatry 2013;84:822–4.

35. Goldstein LH, Chalder T, Chigwedere C, et al. Cognitive-behavioral therapy for psychogenic nonepileptic seizures: a pilot RCT. Neurology 2010;74:1986–94.

36. LaFrance WC, Baird GL, Barry JJ, et al. Multicenter pilot treatment trial for psychogenic nonepileptic seizures: a randomized clinical trial. JAMA Psychiatry 2014;71:997–1005.

37. Goldstein LH, Mellers JDC, Landau S, et al. COgnitive behavioural therapy vs standardised medical care for adults with Dissociative non-Epileptic Seizures

(CODES): a multicentre randomised controlled trial protocol. BMC Neurol 2015; 15:98.

38. Sa DS, Mailis-Gagnon A, Nicholson K, et al. Posttraumatic painful torticollis. Mov Disord 2003;18:1482–91.

39. Harden RN, Bruehl S, Stanton-Hicks M, et al. Proposed new diagnostic criteria for complex regional pain syndrome. Pain Med 2009;8:326–31.

40. Hawley JS, Weiner WJ. Psychogenic dystonia and peripheral trauma. Neurology 2011;77:496–502.

41. Schrag A, Trimble M, Quinn N, et al. The syndrome of fixed dystonia: an evaluation of 103 patients. Brain 2004;127:2360–72.

42. Verdugo R, Ochoa J. Abnormal movements in complex regional pain syndrome: assessment of their nature. Muscle Nerve 2000;23:198–205.

43. Terkelsen AJ, Bach FW, Jensen TS. Experimental forearm immobilization in humans induces cold and mechanical hyperalgesia. Anesthesiology 2008;109: 297–307.

44. Nielsen G, Stone J, Edwards MJ. Physiotherapy for functional (psychogenic) motor symptoms: A systematic review. J Psychosom Res 2013;75:93–102.

45. Nielsen G, Ricciardi L, Demartini B, et al. Outcomes of a 5-day physiotherapy programme for functional (psychogenic) motor disorders. J Neurol 2015;262: 674–81.

46. Czarnecki K, Thompson JM, Seime R, et al. Functional movement disorders: successful treatment with a physical therapy rehabilitation protocol. Parkinsonism Relat Disord 2012;18:247–51.

47. Jordbru AA, Smedstad LM, Klungsøyr O, et al. Psychogenic gait disorder: a randomized controlled trial of physical rehabilitation with one-year follow-up. J Rehabil Med 2014;46:181–7.

48. Nielsen G, Stone J, Matthews A, et al. Physiotherapy for functional motor disorders: a consensus recommendation. J Neurol Neurosurg Psychiatry 2015;86: 1113–9.

49. Harden RN, Oaklander AL, Burton AW, et al. Complex regional pain syndrome: practical diagnostic and treatment guidelines, 4th edition. Pain Med 2013;14: 180–229.

Case Studies in Neurocritical Care

Amra Sakusic, MD[a,b,c], Alejandro A. Rabinstein, MD[d],*

KEYWORDS

- Acute stroke • Subdural hemorrhage • Seizures • Cardiac arrest
- Subarachnoid hemorrhage

KEY POINTS

- Timely recognition and adequate management of medical complications are essential to maximize the chances of recovery after a severe acute ischemic stroke.
- Autoimmune encephalitis can present with severe agitation and may be confused with a psychiatric disease. Search for seizures in these cases is necessary.
- Seizures are a common complication of subdural hemorrhage and they can be refractory.
- Aneurysmal subarachnoid hemorrhage can produce various neurologic and systemic complications, including hydrocephalus, delayed cerebral ischemia, central fever, and polyuria. Optimal management requires clinicians to be knowledgeable of these complications and remain highly vigilant to recognize them early.
- Seizures after cardiac arrest can be treatable, but they often portend poor prognosis. Yet, prognostication should be deferred until the seizures are controlled.

Neurocritical care is a specialty straddling fields of expertise. Its practitioners need to know neurology, internal medicine, and critical care. Critically ill neurologic and neurosurgical patients present unique challenges that demand special training and experience. The neurologic management of these patients requires in-depth knowledge of acute neurology while diagnosis and treatment of systemic complications necessitate critical care training. It is in the interface of these specialties, however, where the niche of the neurointensivist lies. As exemplified by the cases discussed later, the patients treated by a neurointensivist offer challenges that are not encountered in other fields.

This article discusses a few illustrative examples of patients the authors have seen over a single week in a neuroscience ICU. They are only a small sample of the variety of

Disclosures: The authors report no relevant disclosures.
[a] Department of Critical Care, Mayo Clinic, Rochester, MN, USA; [b] Department of Internal Medicine, Tuzla University Medical Center, Tuzla, Bosnia and Herzegovina; [c] Department of Pulmonary Medicine, Tuzla University Medical Center, Tuzla, Bosnia and Herzegovina; [d] Department of Neurology, Mayo Clinic, 200 First Street Southwest, Rochester, MN 55905, USA
* Corresponding author.
E-mail address: rabinstein.alejandro@mayo.edu

Neurol Clin 34 (2016) 683–697
http://dx.doi.org/10.1016/j.ncl.2016.04.007
0733-8619/16/$ – see front matter Published by Elsevier Inc.

conditions treated. They are selected because they serve well to highlight some useful practical messages.

CASE 1: COMPLICATIONS AFTER A STROKE

A 76-year-old woman suddenly developed left-sided weakness leading to a fall while at home with her husband. She had history of hypertension, impaired fasting blood glucose, and obesity. She had also been complaining of irregular palpitations and progressive exertional dyspnea for the past month but had never been diagnosed with atrial fibrillation. She arrived to the emergency department 60 minutes after symptom onset. On examination she had a systolic blood pressure ranging from 180 mm Hg to 200 mm Hg. ECG showed atrial fibrillation with accelerated ventricular rate (120–140 beats per minute). Neurologic examination demonstrated right gaze deviation; left visual field deficit; severe dysarthria; left hemiplegia involving face, arm, and leg; and left-sided neglect. Initial National Institutes of Health Stroke Scale (NIHSS) score was 20. Head CT scan showed some early ischemic changes (Alberta Stroke Program Early CT Score 7) (**Fig. 1**A) and CT angiogram confirmed the suspected occlusion of the right middle cerebral artery. Patient was treated with a total of 40 mg of intravenous (IV) labetalol and a nicardipine infusion (5 mg/h) for management of hypertension and atrial fibrillation. After control of the hypertension to a systolic blood pressure below 180 mm Hg, the patient was treated IV thrombolysis (bolus administered 115 minutes after symptom onset) and the patient was taken to an angiographic suite for endovascular therapy. The procedure was performed under conscious sedation and mechanical thrombectomy using a retrievable stent achieved successful recanalization and reperfusion (thrombolysis in cerebral infarction grade 3) 3 hours after symptom onset (see **Fig. 1**B, C). NIHSS score after the intervention was 15. She was then transferred to the neuroscience ICU. The sheath used for arterial access was kept in place and it was removed without complications the following morning.

By the following day, the patient had continued to improve (NIHSS score 11) although the repeat head CT scan at 24 hours showed a large infarction with hemorrhagic transformation within the right lateral basal ganglia (see **Fig. 1**D). That evening, the patient started to complain of right flank pain and examination revealed a rapidly expanding hematoma on the right groin (ie, the site of previous catheter access). She rapidly progressed to hemorrhagic shock, requiring 2 units of packed red blood cells and 2 L of crystalloids for emergent resuscitation. Systolic blood pressure reached a nadir of 68 mm Hg but recovered promptly. Prolonged direct pressure to the region was applied and an emergent ultrasound revealed a large femoral artery pseudoaneurysm, which was treated with thrombin injection. CT scan of the abdomen/pelvis did not show any retroperitoneal bleeding. After this hypotensive episode her neurologic deficits worsened (NIHSS score 16), and she developed transient oliguric acute kidney injury.

A repeat CT scan the following day revealed no significant expansion of the hemorrhage or major progression of mass effect. Her neurologic condition began to improve again until the fourth day of her hospitalization, when she developed fever after an episode of aspiration during formal swallowing testing by a dysphagia specialist. Shortly after, she became hypotensive and required fluid resuscitation. She was empirically started on broad-spectrum antibiotic therapy. Repeat groin ultrasound revealed continued persistent occlusion of the pseudoaneurysm. Tracheal secretions grew *Staphylococcus aureus* and chest radiograph disclosed a new left lower lobe consolidation. During her ICU hospitalization she also required infusions of diltiazem and esmolol for control of the rapid ventricular response to her atrial fibrillation and intermittent doses of furosemide for signs of pulmonary edema.

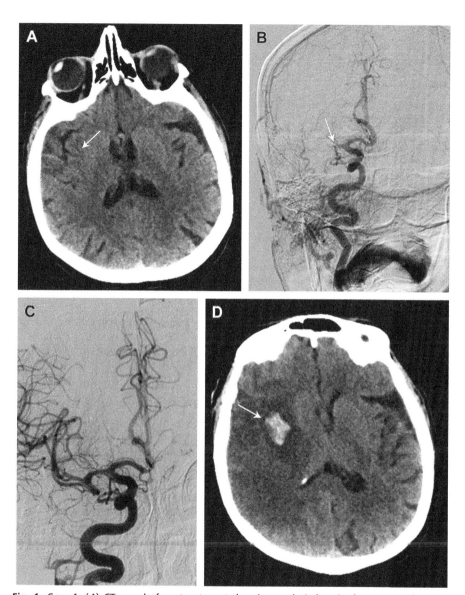

Fig. 1. Case 1. (*A*) CT scan before treatment showing early ischemic changes on the right middle cerebral artery territory, showing loss of insular ribbon and boundaries of the lenticular nucleus (*arrow*). Notice extreme right gaze deviation. (*B*) Catheter angiogram showing the proximal occlusion of the right middle cerebral artery (*arrow*) with poor collateral circulation. (*C*) Catheter angiogram demonstrating full recanalization and reperfusion after mechanical thrombectomy. (*D*) Follow-up CT scan showing a large infarction on the right middle cerebral artery territory with a hemorrhagic conversion in the region of the right basal ganglia (*arrow*).

Despite all these complications, she had begun to recover well by the time of her discharge to a skilled nursing facility. On outpatient follow-up 15 days later, she was walking 50 feet unassisted and was nearly ready to return home.

Clinical Messages

- Large infarctions can develop despite successful recanalization and reperfusion. In these cases, reperfusion injury, including edema and hemorrhage, can cause complications related to mass effect that should be anticipated.[1,2]
- The arterial site of catheter access should be closely monitored after any endovascular intervention, but this is particularly important in patients with acute stroke who have received IV thrombolysis. The most common occurrence is an inconsequential groin hematoma that can be limited with local pressure. As illustrated by this case, however, pseudoaneurysm formation may be accompanied by arterial rupture with massive bleeding that may present with hypovolemic shock. Unless the bleeding is promptly recognized and controlled, this complication can be fatal.
- Aspiration pneumonia is a common complication after a severe stroke and can occur despite appropriate assessment for dysphagia and in patients who are not allowed oral diet. The risk of aspiration may be higher when the infarction involves the insular cortex and frontal operculum.[3]
- Hypotension, even if brief, often causes worsening of neurologic deficits after an acute stroke.[4] This is possible even days after stroke onset.
- Patients with severe ischemic stroke may develop multiple treatable complications and still recover well if such complications are optimally addressed.

CASE 2: EXTREME AGITATION IN AUTOIMMUNE ENCEPHALITIS

A 23-year-old woman started to exhibit progressive behavioral changes accompanied by speech stuttering and spells of vertigo with nausea. She then developed visual illusions and hallucinations and episodes of left head turning and left hand gripping followed by transient confusion. Thought to have a psychiatric disorder, she was prescribed sertraline after having an electroencephalogram and a head CT scan that were interpreted as normal. Her condition worsened, however, over the following days. She became increasingly agitated and had paranoid ideation. Episodes of left facial twitching became more common but they were never associated with generalized convulsions or unresponsiveness. Finally she presented to another hospital where focal seizures arising from the right frontal region were detected and she was started on antiseizure medications. Cerebrospinal fluid analysis revealed 7 white blood cells/µL, protein of 20 mg/dL, and normal glucose content. Sedimentation rate was 96 mm but other markers of acute systemic inflammation were absent. Brain MRI was read as negative, although it actually revealed subtle changes on the limbic region bilaterally. Abdominal MRI demonstrated an ovarian teratoma that was subsequently removed by laparoscopic surgery. Autoimmune panel in serum and cerebrospinal fluid disclosed the presence of anti–N-methyl-D-aspartate (NMDA) receptor antibodies.

Her seizures were deemed refractory and she was treated with high doses of levetiracetam, lacosamide, phenytoin, and phenobarbital. Because of the seizures and the persistent intractable agitation, she was intubated and placed on a midazolam infusion (up to 30 mg/h) and then propofol and fentanyl were added in increasing doses. For the autoimmune encephalitis she received IV methylprednisolone (1 g/d) for multiple days and a 5-day course of IV immunoglobulin (IVIG). An infusion of rituximab was discontinued because of hypertension. She was then transferred to the authors' hospital for further care on request of the family. Her electroencephalogram revealed delta waves on the right frontal region that were semirhythmic at times but no seizures. The authors switched her to oral prednisone (60 mg/d), stopped phenytoin and phenobarbital, and gradually weaned off midazolam, fentanyl, and propofol. She progressively woke up with intermittent restlessness but no severe agitation. Spells of paroxysmal sympathetic hyperactivity (tachycardia, hypertension, tachypnea, diaphoresis, and fever) were successfully aborted with IV morphine (4 mg) and then made more infrequent with gabapentin (600 mg 3 times daily). Eight days after admission to the ICU she was stable to be safely transferred to the floor.

Clinical Messages

- Agitation mimicking psychosis from a primary psychiatric disease is a frequent manifestation of autoimmune encephalitis in its early phases. Conversely, catatonia can also be caused by autoimmune encephalitis. Thus, autoimmune encephalitis should be included in the differential diagnosis of new major behavioral changes, especially in young patients.[5,6]
- Autoimmune encephalitis is possible in patients with unremarkable or minimally abnormal cerebrospinal fluid and MRI of the brain.[7] When the clinical suspicion is high, autoantibodies should be tested regardless of the results of these investigations.
- Underlying seizures may be present in patients with severe agitation from autoimmune encephalitis. They can only be recognized by electroencephalography, which often needs to be prolonged to optimize detection.[8]
- The management of autoimmune encephalitis in the ICU can be challenging.[9] Multiple neurologic and systemic complications can occur during the hospitalization (**Table 1**). Aggressive sedation (and sometimes neuromuscular paralysis) may be necessary to control agitation, and multiple antiseizure medications may need to be used to abolish the seizures. Paroxysmal sympathetic hyperactivity is another common complication and it typically responds well to morphine as acute abortive treatment and to gabapentin as preventive agent.
- The response to immune therapy is commonly delayed. It is important to remember this to avoid overtreatment. Refractory cases demand increasingly

Table 1
Clinical manifestations and complications in patients with severe autoimmune encephalitis

Neurologic	Systemic
Severe agitation	Fever
Focal deficits	Respiratory failure
Seizures (focal or generalized)/status epilepticus	Sepsis
	Venous thromboembolism
Cognitive impairment	Gastrointestinal hemorrhage
Depressed level of consciousness	Ileus
Catatonia	Anemia
Headache	Hyperglycemia
Severe agitation	Atelectasis
Focal deficits	Rhabdomyolysis (related to seizures or extreme agitation)
Seizures (focal or generalized)	
Cognitive impairment	Others related to underlying tumor
Depressed level of consciousness	
Paroxysmal sympathetic hyperactivity	
Raised intracranial pressure	

aggressive treatment regimens (rituximab and cyclophosphamide). These second-line therapies, however, may be associated with greater risk of side effects and, therefore, it is prudent to delay the use of these medications in patients who remain stable with corticosteroids and IVIG or plasma exchange because a good proportion of these patients start improving over time.

- Searching for an underlying tumor, especially for an ovarian teratoma in young women with anti-NMDA receptor antibody encephalitis, should always be part of the evaluation of autoimmune encephalitis.[7]

CASE 3: SEIZURES AFTER SUBDURAL HEMORRHAGE

A 64-year-old woman on warfarin for atrial fibrillation had been having worsening headaches for 1 week after hitting her head with the door of a car. The day of the admission the headaches had worsened and then she became progressively drowsier. A head CT scan obtained in the emergency department showed an acute subdural hematoma over the right frontal cerebral convexity measuring 1 cm in maximal diameter and causing 5 mm of midline shift. The international normalized ratio was 2.7 and prompt reversal was achieved with prothrombin complex concentrate and IV vitamin K. The patient was then taken to surgery for craniotomy and evacuation of the subdural blood.

The surgery was uncomplicated and postoperative CT scan revealed resolution of the mass effect without parenchymal damage. The patient initially did well, but on the second postoperative day she developed worsening dysarthria and left arm weakness. No clinical seizure-like activity was reported by nurses. Subsequently, she became rapidly drowsier and required intubation for airway protection. Repeat brain imaging revealed no interval changes. An electroencephalogram disclosed frequent right frontal seizures. The patient was already on levetiracetam (750 mg twice daily) for seizure prophylaxis. Additional levetiracetam and loading with valproic acid and phenobarbital (after lack of improvement with phenytoin) eventually controlled the seizures. The patient remained stuporous after seizure control for several more days. The antiepileptic regimen was gradually narrowed back to monotherapy with levetiracetam with persistent seizure control proved by continuous electroencephalography. Eventually, her level of alertness began to improve. As she awakened, examination showed left arm apraxia, which improved over days. Twelve days after intubation she was successfully extubated and transferred to the floor the following day. Her subsequent recovery has been very favorable.

Clinical Messages

- Seizures are prevalent after acute subdural hemorrhage.[10] They can be focal or generalized and clinical or subclinical. Electroencephalography should be obtained in any patient with acute subdural hemorrhage who has unexplained depressed level of consciousness, altered content of consciousness, or new focal deficits. Continuous electroencephalography is advisable in patients with epileptiform discharges during the first 30 minutes of recording and necessary in patients with documented subclinical seizures.
- Seizures related to acute subdural hemorrhage are more common after hematoma evacuation, especially if craniotomy is needed.[10] Epileptiform discharges in the midline head regions predominate and the incidence of seizures correlates with the degree of preoperative midline shift.[11] Seizures can also occur, however, before surgery and in patients who do not require an operation.
- After subdural hemorrhage, seizures can be refractory to treatment and may require multiple antiseizure medications or even anesthetic agents before they

can be controlled. During this time, patients may present a concerning neurologic status (prolonged coma or persistent focal deficits without radiologic evidence of parenchymal injury). Yet, after resolution of the seizures and the sedative effects of the drugs used to control them, patients can make a favorable recovery.[10] Keeping this in mind is crucial to avoid premature withdrawal of intensive care measures.

CASE 4: COMPLICATIONS AFTER ANEURYSMAL SUBARACHNOID HEMORRHAGE

A 53-year-old woman developed a thunderclap headache while at work and was taken to the emergency department. She first became agitated and then became progressively less responsive to the point that she required intubation for airway protection (World Federation of Neurosurgical Surgeons [WFNS] grade V). Head CT scan demonstrated a severe subarachnoid hemorrhage (**Fig. 2**A, B). Her hypertension was reduced to a systolic blood pressure below 160 mm Hg with a combination of hydralazine and nicardipine. She received 1 gram of tranexamic acid in the emergency department. Because of the severity of the hemorrhage, the authors decided to take the patient directly to the angiographic suite for endovascular coiling of the suspected aneurysm. While on the table ready to undergo the procedure, she developed sudden severe hypertension (up to 230/120 mm Hg despite a nicardipine infusion at 7.5 mg/h), a brief episode of ventricular tachycardia, and bilateral extensor posturing. Examination also showed anisocoria with preserved light reactivity. After emergent hemodynamic stabilization, the angiogram was performed and a 7-mm basilar tip aneurysm was successfully coiled. The patient also underwent placement of a ventriculostomy. Repeat CT scan confirmed that she had rebled and developed worsened IV hemorrhage with hydrocephalus (see **Fig. 2**C, D).

After the intervention, she was treated with mannitol because of increased intracranial pressures. Ventricular drain was kept open at 5 mm Hg. She gradually improved and the authors were able to extubate her on day 4. Fevers that had begun on day 3 became more persistent over subsequent days. Infectious work-up was negative. On day 6 she became more agitated and, at times, drowsy. Transcranial Doppler revealed borderline increased blood flow velocities in the left anterior cerebral artery (112 cm/s) but was otherwise unremarkable. CT angiogram was suspicious for distal bilateral anterior cerebral artery vasospasm and there was slight prolongation of mean transient times on the watershed distribution (between anterior and middle cerebral arteries) on the upper frontal lobes. She was spontaneously hypertensive (systolic blood pressures up to 220 mm Hg and mean arterial pressures up to 140 mm Hg). Despite the fairly unimpressive results of the investigations, the authors attributed the neurologic change to delayed cerebral ischemia and allowed her to remain hypertensive (permissive hypertension). On day 8, her mean arterial pressure briefly dropped below 100 mm Hg and she became stuporous. Her condition improved immediately after a fluid bolus and initiation of a phenylephrine infusion restored the previous level of hypertension. For the following 4 days she remained intermittently on hemodynamic augmentation. Between days 7 and 11 she developed severe polyuria (up to 18 L of urinary output per day), which the authors treated with fluid and sodium replacement but allowing her to be up to 2 L to 3 L negative as long as the blood pressure remained within target. The patient was also receiving fludrocortisone and she did not develop any substantial hyponatremia.

By day 12, her condition was more stable. The level of ventricular drainage was progressively raised and the drain could be removed on day 14. Repeat CT scan showed

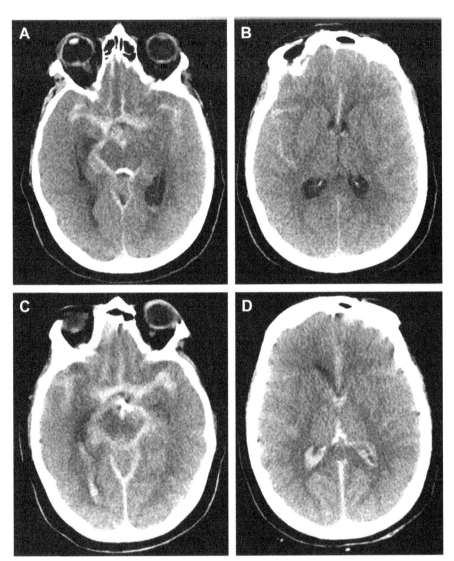

Fig. 2. Case 4. CT scans (*A, B*) at presentation with aneurysmal subarachnoid hemorrhage and (*C, D*) after aneurysmal rebleeding.

no evidence of infarctions. The patient is now undergoing a short course of rehabilitation. The authors expect her to make a full recovery.

Clinical Messages

- Aneurysmal subarachnoid hemorrhage is characteristically associated with an increased risk of multiple neurologic and systemic complications, both early after aneurysm rupture and over the following days (**Table 2**).[12,13] Many of these complications are predictable and being prepared for their occurrence is indispensable to optimize the chances of good functional recovery.[14,15]
- During the first few hours, the 2 main cerebral complications are aneurysm rebleeding and hydrocephalus (obstructive or communicating).[13] Rebleeding

Table 2
Neurologic and systemic complications in patients with aneurysmal subarachnoid hemorrhage

Complication	Therapeutic Measures
Before aneurysm treatment	
Hydrocephalus	Place external ventricular or lumbar drain
Aneurysmal rebleeding	Early aneurysm repair Tranexamic acid 1 g IV every 6 h not exceeding 48–72 h
Increased intracranial pressure	Elevate head of bed to 30° Control fever and agitation Short-term hyperventilation Osmotherapy (20% mannitol, hypertonic saline) Surgical evacuation/decompression for lesions with mass effect and clinical deterioration
Stress-induced cardiomyopathy (neurogenic stunned myocardium, apical ballooning syndrome, takotsubo cardiomyopathy)	Consider β-blockers if no cardiogenic shock If cardiogenic shock, adrenergic agents are not contraindicated, but placement of an intra-aortic balloon pump may be advisable in the most severe cases Diuretics if pulmonary edema
Neurogenic pulmonary edema	Increase level of positive end-expiratory pressure Add diuretics if necessary
After aneurysm treatment	
Delayed cerebral ischemia (most commonly caused by symptomatic vasospasm)	Nimodipine, 60 mg every 4 h for up to 21 d (for prevention) Maintain euvolemia with crystalloids or colloids If symptomatic, induce hypertension with phenylephrine, norepinephrine, or dopamine If refractory, proceed to endovascular treatment (transluminal angioplasty or intra-arterial vasodilators)
Hyponatremia (most often combined with polyuria)	Strict avoidance of free water Hydration with saline solutions (1.5% or 3%) Fludrocortisone acetate up to 0.2 mg twice daily
Hyperglycemia	Use insulin to maintain normoglycemia (100–180 mg/dL)
Fever	Rule out infection Maintain normothermia with acetaminophen, cooling blankets, or surface cooling devices

carries high morbidity and mortality; its risk can be reduced by the early administration of an antifibrinolytic agent, such as tranexamic acid.[16] It is typically manifested with sudden hypertension, tachycardia (sometimes followed by bradycardia), and posturing (often confused with a seizure) and can be confirmed by the presence of new blood on the CT scan. Hydrocephalus has a less dramatic presentation. Patients become less responsive, bradycardic, and mildly hypertensive; downgaze deviation may be noticed. Ventriculomegaly on brain imaging may be more subtle than expected in patients with global brain swelling.[17]

- During the acute phase (first 12–24 hours), cardiopulmonary complications may also be observed, more commonly in patients with poor-grade hemorrhages (WFNS score IV–V). ECG changes are frequent and include repolarization changes (widespread giant T-wave inversions known as cerebral T waves are most characteristic but certainly not the most common), supraventricular and ventricular arrhythmias, and prolongation of the QTc interval.[18] The ECG changes caused by aneurysmal subarachnoid hemorrhage can also mimic an acute ST-elevation myocardial infarction.[19] Neurogenic cardiopulmonary injury can produce pulmonary edema (neurogenic, cardiogenic, or mixed) and other signs of congestive heart failure in patients with preexistent cardiac disease and in those who develop stress-induced cardiomyopathy.[20,21] Stress-induced cardiomyopathy is more common in postmenopausal women and its most typical echocardiographic pattern is apical hypokinesis or akinesis (apical ballooning syndrome or takotsubo cardiomyopathy).[21,22]

- Delayed cerebral ischemia is the most severe neurologic complication occurring days after aneurysm rupture (maximal risk between days 4 and 10).[13,23] It is primarily caused by vasospasm.[23,24] Vasospasm is mainly caused, however, by endothelial dysfunction that starts affecting the microcirculation.[25] Consequently, symptoms of delayed cerebral ischemia may develop in the absence of visible luminal narrowing in the larger intracranial arteries.[26] For this reason, delayed cerebral ischemia remains a clinical diagnosis.[27] CT perfusion (combined with CT angiogram) may be useful in some instances to confirm the diagnosis,[28] but the sensitivity of this modality is not perfect.

- The medical treatment of delayed cerebral ischemia consists of hemodynamic augmentation.[12–15] Spontaneous hypertension should not be treated and vasopressors should be added when delayed cerebral ischemia is diagnosed or suspected. Endovascular therapy (balloon angioplasty for vasospasm involving larger arterial segments and selective intra-arterial infusion of calcium channel blockers for more distal vasospasm) should be used as a rescue treatment in patients who remain symptomatic despite hemodynamic augmentation or cannot tolerate vasopressors.[12–15]

- Polyuria is common in patients with aneurysmal subarachnoid hemorrhage. Its most common pathophysiology is cerebral salt wasting syndrome (ie, excessive secretion of natriuretic peptides leading to increased urinary sodium losses with concomitant dragging of water resulting in intravascular volume depletion).[29] Inappropriate secretion of antidiuretic hormone may contribute. These 2 mechanisms lead to hyponatremia.[30] Treatment consists of fluid and sodium replacement.[29] Fludrocortisone can also be beneficial to ameliorate the negative sodium balance.[29] Diabetes insipidus is uncommon in aneurysmal subarachnoid hemorrhage. When it occurs, it tends to appear early and in patients with the most severe forms of hemorrhage. Finally, polyuria may be perpetuated by excessive administration of fluids as it may have occurred in this case. Although often difficult to avoid because of concerns that the patient may develop ischemia if volume contraction is not avoided, excessive fluid administration can be problematic. In the authors' experience, positive fluid balance is independently associated with worse outcomes.[31] Thus, the authors always prefer to "chase the fluid losses" from behind if at all possible and do not try to induce hypervolemia at any point.

- Aneurysmal subarachnoid hemorrhage is the most common cause of central fever in neuroscience ICU.[32,33] Early onset of fever (within the first 72 hours) and absence of infiltrates on chest radiograph increase the chances that the fever is central.[32] Central fever tends to be prolonged and refractory to antipyretics. It has also been associated with greater risk of vasospasm.[33] Although fever is often central in subarachnoid hemorrhage, infections (including ventriculitis in patients with a ventriculostomy or lumbar drain) should be excluded. Controlling fever is advisable because fever (regardless of its cause) has been associated

with worse outcomes in aneurysmal subarachnoid hemorrhage.[34] The benefit of aggressive fever control in these patients, however, has not been formally studied.
- Patients with poor-grade aneurysmal subarachnoid hemorrhage can achieve an excellent outcome even after developing multiple complications, as long as irreversible brain tissue damage is avoided during the acute phase.[35]

CASE 5: STATUS EPILEPTICUS AFTER CARDIAC ARREST

A 53-year-old man with previously documented coronary artery disease suffered a witnessed out-of-hospital arrest. The first rhythm was ventricular fibrillation. Time to recovery of spontaneous circulation was 20 minutes. The patient remained comatose after resuscitation. On arrival to the hospital, he was diagnosed with an ST-elevation myocardial infarction. Emergency coronary angiography revealed critical left main coronary artery disease extending into the circumflex and left anterior descending arteries and he received implantation of an intra-aortic balloon pump to support his blood pressure and improve his coronary perfusion. He was treated with targeted temperature management to keep the body temperature at 36°C for the first 24 hours. During this time he was treated with midazolam and fentanyl for sedoanalgesia and required atracurium infusion to control the shivering. There was no report of myoclonus before initiation of the pharmacologic neuromuscular paralysis.

Electroencephalography during cooling demonstrated continuous epileptiform discharges, predominantly involving the posterior head regions that were consistent with status epilepticus (**Fig. 3**A). After loading with levetiracetam, valproic acid, and lacosamide, the status epilepticus was aborted, although he continued to exhibit frequent multifocal spikes in the posterior head regions and occasional generalized epileptiform discharges. The patient remained comatose after seizure control and discontinuation of all sedative drugs. Physical examination demonstrated preserved brain stem reflexes with absent motor responses to pain. At times the patient would

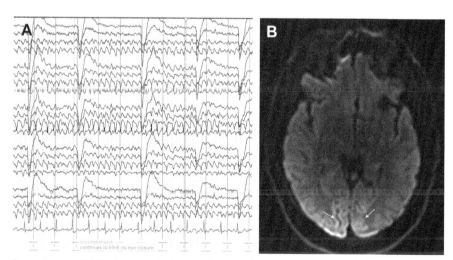

Fig. 3. Case 5. (*A*) Electroencephalogram (longitudinal bipolar montage) showing posterior predominant continuous epileptiform discharges consistent with status epilepticus. Eye opening was semirhythmic and spontaneous. (*B*) MRI scan (diffusion-weighted sequence) shows diffusion restriction affecting the medial occipital cortex bilaterally (*arrows*).

have spontaneous eye opening, with some deviation upwards, and no visual fixation or tracking. Serial neuron specific enolase levels ranged from 29 ng/mL to 43 ng/mL over the first 3 days. A brain MRI on day 4 disclosed restricted diffusion involving the medial occipital cortex bilaterally (**Fig. 3B**). Repeat electroencephalography on day 7 showed persistent generalized epileptiform discharges but no organized seizures.

Because of the lack of neurologic improvement, his family requested withdrawal of life-sustaining measures on day 12. He expired shortly after.

Clinical Messages

- Myoclonic status epilepticus has been traditionally considered an ominous prognostic sign after cardiac arrest.[36] It is manifested by multisegmental or generalized myoclonic jerks with an electroencephalogram typically demonstrating polyspike and wake discharges or, more often, a burst-suppression pattern. The prognostic impact of isolated segmental myoclonus with a continuous, non-epileptiform background or electrographic status epilepticus without myoclonus is less certain. In the authors' experience, the latter has also been associated with poor outcome, as illustrated by this case.

- Knowledge of seizures after cardiac arrest has been considerably expanded because of the frequent use of continuous electroencephalography for neurologic monitoring while patients are sedated (and often paralyzed) during targeted temperature management.[37] Targeted temperature management has undergone a recent shift from a target temperature of 33°C to 36°C.[38] Seizures occurring despite therapeutic hypothermia at 33°C were consistently predictive of poor outcome (which was not necessarily the case for seizures that occurred before induction of hypothermia or during or after rewarming).[39,40] Although 33°C has antiepileptic properties,[41] it is unlikely that 36°C affects significantly the seizure threshold. Hence, aggressive treatment of seizures occurring during targeted temperature management at 36°C should be pursued, particularly when the underlying background is continuous.

- In patients having seizures after cardiac resuscitation, prognostication must be delayed until the seizures are controlled and the sedative effect of the medications used to treat the seizures is resolved.

- The electroencephalographic features that portend poor chances of recovery of awareness after cardiac arrest are discontinuous background (ie, burst-suppression pattern), epileptiform discharges, and lack of reactivity to various forms of stimulation.[39,42] Neither electroencephalography nor any other parameter, however, should be considered in isolation when prognosticating in these patients. Prognosis should be estimated after considering multiple parameters, including the characteristics of the arrest (shockable vs nonshockable initial rhythm, witnessed or unwitnessed, time to return of spontaneous circulation), serial findings on physical examination (brainstem reflexes and motor responses to pain) after excluding confounders (residual effects of sedatives, metabolic failure, or hypothermia itself), somatosensory evoked potentials (N20 cortical responses), electroencephalography, biochemical markers (serum neuron-specific enolase), and brain imaging scans (CT scan or MRI).[43]

SUMMARY

These cases exemplify some of the problems seen in neurocritical care units every day and evince the need for subspecialty expertise to ensure their appropriate management. Not discussed are myriad other diagnosis and complications, including infectious meningoencephalitis, traumatic brain injury, spinal cord injury, intracerebral hemorrhage, coma of unclear cause, other forms of super-refractory status epilepticus, and neuromuscular respiratory failure, to mention a few. Neurointensivists should also be trained to recognize and treat postneurosurgical emergencies and neurologic complications of general medical and surgical diseases. The spectrum of disorders treated and the chance of changing the lives of patients with decisions make the specialty uniquely exacting but also singularly stimulating.

REFERENCES

1. Lansberg MG, Straka M, Kemp S, et al. MRI profile and response to endovascular reperfusion after stroke (DEFUSE 2): a prospective cohort study. Lancet Neurol 2012;11:860–7.
2. Wijdicks EF, Sheth KN, Carter BS, et al. Recommendations for the management of cerebral and cerebellar infarction with swelling: a statement for healthcare professionals from the American Heart Association/American Stroke Association. Stroke 2014;45:1222–38.
3. Galovic M, Leisi N, Muller M, et al. Lesion location predicts transient and extended risk of aspiration after supratentorial ischemic stroke. Stroke 2013;44: 2760–7.
4. Castillo J, Leira R, Garcia MM, et al. Blood pressure decrease during the acute phase of ischemic stroke is associated with brain injury and poor stroke outcome. Stroke 2004;35:520–6.
5. Kayser MS, Titulaer MJ, Gresa-Arribas N, et al. Frequency and characteristics of isolated psychiatric episodes in anti-N-methyl-d-aspartate receptor encephalitis. JAMA Neurol 2013;70:1133–9.
6. Kruse JL, Jeffrey JK, Davis MC, et al. Anti-N-methyl-D-aspartate receptor encephalitis: a targeted review of clinical presentation, diagnosis, and approaches to psychopharmacologic management. Ann Clin Psychiatry 2014;26:111–9.
7. Dalmau J, Lancaster E, Martinez-Hernandez E, et al. Clinical experience and laboratory investigations in patients with anti-NMDAR encephalitis. Lancet Neurol 2011;10:63–74.
8. Toledano M, Pittock SJ. Autoimmune epilepsy. Semin Neurol 2015;35:245–58.
9. Mittal MK, Rabinstein AA, Hocker SE, et al. Autoimmune encephalitis in the ICU: analysis of phenotypes, serologic findings, and outcomes. Neurocrit Care 2015; 24(2):240–50.
10. Rabinstein AA, Chung SY, Rudzinski LA, et al. Seizures after evacuation of subdural hematomas: incidence, risk factors, and functional impact. J Neurosurg 2010;112:455–60.
11. Rudzinski LA, Rabinstein AA, Chung SY, et al. Electroencephalographic findings in acute subdural hematoma. J Clin Neurophysiol 2011;28:633–41.
12. Rabinstein AA, Lanzino G, Wijdicks EF. Multidisciplinary management and emerging therapeutic strategies in aneurysmal subarachnoid haemorrhage. Lancet Neurol 2010;9:504–19.
13. Rabinstein AA. Critical care of aneurysmal subarachnoid hemorrhage: state of the art. Acta Neurochir Suppl 2015;120:239–42.
14. Connolly ES Jr, Rabinstein AA, Carhuapoma JR, et al. Guidelines for the management of aneurysmal subarachnoid hemorrhage: a guideline for healthcare professionals from the American Heart Association/American Stroke Association. Stroke 2012;43:1711–37.

15. Diringer MN, Block TP, Claude Hemphill J 3rd, et al. Critical care management of patients following aneurysmal subarachnoid hemorrhage: recommendations from the Neurocritical Care Society's Multidisciplinary Consensus Conference. Neurocrit Care 2011;15:211–40.

16. Hillman J, Fridriksson S, Nilsson O, et al. Immediate administration of tranexamic acid and reduced incidence of early rebleeding after aneurysmal subarachnoid hemorrhage: a prospective randomized study. J Neurosurg 2002;97:771–8.

17. Dupont S, Rabinstein AA. Extent of acute hydrocephalus after subarachnoid hemorrhage as a risk factor for poor functional outcome. Neurol Res 2013;35:107–10.

18. Liu Q, Ding YH, Zhang JH, et al. ECG change of acute subarachnoid hemorrhagic patients. Acta Neurochir Suppl 2011;111:357–9.

19. Delelis F, Calais G, Ennezat PV, et al. Subarachnoid haemorrhage mimicking acute myocardial infarction. BMJ Case Rep 2012;2012 [pii:bcr1120115134].

20. Busl KM, Bleck TP. Neurogenic pulmonary edema. Crit Care Med 2015;43:1710–5.

21. Boland TA, Lee VH, Bleck TP. Stress-induced cardiomyopathy. Crit Care Med 2015;43:686–93.

22. Lee VH, Connolly HM, Fulgham JR, et al. Tako-tsubo cardiomyopathy in aneurysmal subarachnoid hemorrhage: an underappreciated ventricular dysfunction. J Neurosurg 2006;105:264–70.

23. Macdonald RL. Delayed neurological deterioration after subarachnoid haemorrhage. Nat Rev Neurol 2014;10:44–58.

24. Rabinstein AA, Wijdicks EF. Cerebral vasospasm in subarachnoid hemorrhage. Curr Treat Options Neurol 2005;7:99–107.

25. Rabinstein AA. Secondary brain injury after aneurysmal subarachnoid haemorrhage: more than vasospasm. Lancet Neurol 2011;10:593–5.

26. Rabinstein AA, Friedman JA, Weigand SD, et al. Predictors of cerebral infarction in aneurysmal subarachnoid hemorrhage. Stroke 2004;35:1862–6.

27. Frontera JA, Fernandez A, Schmidt JM, et al. Defining vasospasm after subarachnoid hemorrhage: what is the most clinically relevant definition? Stroke 2009;40:1963–8.

28. Cremers CH, Vos PC, van der Schaaf IC, et al. CT perfusion during delayed cerebral ischemia after subarachnoid hemorrhage: distinction between reversible ischemia and ischemia progressing to infarction. Neuroradiology 2015;57:897–902.

29. Rabinstein AA, Bruder N. Management of hyponatremia and volume contraction. Neurocrit Care 2011;15:354–60.

30. Rabinstein AA, Wijdicks EF. Hyponatremia in critically ill neurological patients. Neurologist 2003;9:290–300.

31. Kissoon NR, Mandrekar JN, Fugate JE, et al. Positive fluid balance is associated with poor outcomes in subarachnoid hemorrhage. J Stroke Cerebrovasc Dis 2015;24:2245–51.

32. Hocker SE, Tian L, Li G, et al. Indicators of central fever in the neurologic intensive care unit. JAMA Neurol 2013;70:1499–504.

33. Rabinstein AA, Sandhu K. Non-infectious fever in the neurological intensive care unit: incidence, causes and predictors. J Neurol Neurosurg Psychiatry 2007;78:1278–80.

34. Scaravilli V, Tinchero G, Citerio G. Fever management in SAH. Neurocrit Care 2011;15:287–94.

35. Bing Z, Rabinstein AA, Murad MH, et al. Surgical and endovascular treatment of poor-grade aneurysmal subarachnoid hemorrhage: a systematic review and meta-analysis. J Neurosurg Sci 2015. [Epub ahead of print].

36. Wijdicks EF, Hijdra A, Young GB, et al. Practice parameter: prediction of outcome in comatose survivors after cardiopulmonary resuscitation (an evidence-based review): report of the Quality Standards Subcommittee of the American Academy of Neurology. Neurology 2006;67:203–10.

37. Crepeau AZ, Britton JW, Fugate JE, et al. Electroencephalography in survivors of cardiac arrest: comparing pre- and post-therapeutic hypothermia eras. Neurocrit Care 2015;22:165–72.

38. Nielsen N, Wetterslev J, Cronberg T, et al. Targeted temperature management at 33°C versus 36°C after cardiac arrest. N Engl J Med 2013;369:2197–206.

39. Crepeau AZ, Rabinstein AA, Fugate JE, et al. Continuous EEG in therapeutic hypothermia after cardiac arrest: prognostic and clinical value. Neurology 2013;80:339–44.

40. Rabinstein AA, Wijdicks EF. The value of EEG monitoring after cardiac arrest treated with hypothermia. Neurology 2012;78:774–5.

41. Corry JJ, Dhar R, Murphy T, et al. Hypothermia for refractory status epilepticus. Neurocrit Care 2008;9:189–97.

42. Juan E, Kaplan PW, Oddo M, et al. EEG as an Indicator of Cerebral Functioning in Postanoxic Coma. J Clin Neurophysiol 2015;32:465–71.

43. Ben-Hamouda N, Taccone FS, Rossetti AO, et al. Contemporary approach to neurologic prognostication of coma after cardiac arrest. Chest 2014;146:1375–86.

Case Studies Illustrating Focal Alzheimer's, Fluent Aphasia, Late-Onset Memory Loss, and Rapid Dementia

 CrossMark

Gamze Balci Camsari, MD[a], Melissa E. Murray, PhD[b],
Neill R. Graff-Radford, MBBCh, FRCP (UK)[a],*

KEYWORDS

• Atypical Alzheimer's • Fluent aphasia • Late-onset dementia • Rapid dementia

KEY POINTS

• The differential diagnosis of dementia can be challenging because the initial clinical presentation can be variable and different neuropathologies can coexist.
• Visual impairment can be the only symptom early in the course of focal Alzheimer's.
• The clinical picture of CBS may have Alzheimer's as the underlying pathology.
• Patients with logopenic aphasia frequently have Alzheimer's pathology, whereas TDP-43 is the most common pathology in semantic dementia.
• Different neuropathologic processes can result in similar clinical presentations. It is important to not to overlook treatable causes of rapidly progressive dementia.

INTRODUCTION

Many dementia subtypes have more shared signs and symptoms than defining ones. We review 8 cases with 4 overlapping syndromes and demonstrate how to distinguish the cases. These include focal cortical presentations of Alzheimer's disease (AD; posterior cortical atrophy and CBS), fluent aphasia (semantic dementia and logopenic aphasia), late-onset slowly progressive dementia (hippocampal sclerosis [HpScl] limbic and predominant AD), and rapidly progressive dementia (Creutzfeldt–Jakob disease and limbic encephalitis). We shall illustrate each syndrome with a case and then describe the characteristic clinical features, commonly associated pathophysiology, and main differential diagnoses.

Disclosures: Dr. Murray is partly supported by Donors Cure Foundation New Vision Award and Gerstner Family Career Development Award. The study is supported in part by Mayo Clinic Alzheimer's Disease Research Center (ADRC) grant P50AG 16574-14 (PI: Ronald Petersen, MD, PhD). The authors have nothing to disclose.
[a] Department of Neurology, Mayo Clinic, 4500 San Pablo Road, Jacksonville, FL 32224, USA;
[b] Department of Neuroscience, Mayo Clinic, 4500 San Pablo Road, Jacksonville, FL 32224, USA
* Corresponding author.
E-mail address: graffradford.neill@mayo.edu

Neurol Clin 34 (2016) 699–716
http://dx.doi.org/10.1016/j.ncl.2016.04.008
0733-8619/16/$ – see front matter © 2016 Elsevier Inc. All rights reserved.

neurologic.theclinics.com

FOCAL CORTICAL PRESENTATIONS OF ALZHEIMER'S DISEASE

Posterior Cortical Atrophy

Clinical case

A 74 year-old, right-handed woman with a PhD in English was evaluated for memory impairment with visuospatial difficulties. The first symptom she noticed 10 years previously was being unable to follow the correct line when reading a book and used a magnification device to follow the right line. She had difficulty finding objects in her refrigerator and failed to recognize objects. She had difficulty attending to stimuli on the left. Memory difficulties began 2 years previously. She had to stop driving owing to her visual impairment and was functioning well otherwise. She was referred to the behavioral neurology clinic by her ophthalmologist, who had ruled out primary ocular abnormality. Her Kokmen Short Test of Mental Status[1] score was 28 of 38. She registered 4 words over 1 trial but did not recall any with a delay. Her constructional abilities were severely impaired, and she had a tendency to neglect the left visual field. She was able to name primary colors, but had difficulty discriminating visually between like colors. She was unable to see numbers on the Ishihara plates and had prominent simultagnosia as well as ocular apraxia. No significant Parkinsonism, dyspraxia, dysphasia, cortical sensory loss, or surface dyslexia were noted. Her brain MRI showed bilateral occipitoparietal atrophy (**Fig. 1**). ^{18}F-fluorodeoxyglucose-PET scan (**Fig. 2**) revealed severe right more than left occipital hypometabolism.

Clinical features

- Early age of onset compared with typical AD.
- Relative preservation of orientation and episodic memory early in the disorder.
- Visual field deficits.
- Simultanagnosia.
- Acalculia.
- Alexia.
- Anomia.

Pathophysiology

The term posterior cortical atrophy (PCA) was first used by Benson and colleagues[2] to describe a syndrome characterized by progressive decline in higher order visual

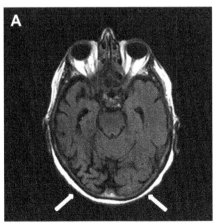 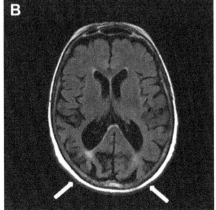

Fig. 1. MRI of the brain showing bilateral occipitoparietal atrophy in posterior cortical atrophy seen at two levels *A* and *B* (*arrows*).

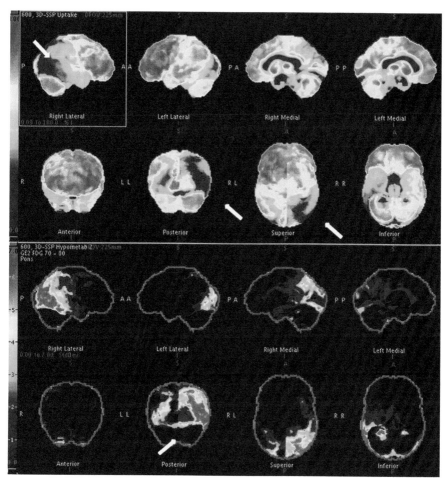

Fig. 2. Corresponding ^18F-fluorodeoxyglucose PET scan in posterior cortical atrophy revealing severe right more than left occipital hypometabolism (*arrows*).

processing with relatively intact memory and language in the early stages along with posterior brain atrophy. Hof and colleagues[3] were the first to report that the majority of these cases had Alzheimer pathology with a high tangle count in the posterior cortical areas. In a large series by Tang-Wai and colleagues[4] described the frequent associated symptoms and confirmed the neuritic pathology in the posterior cortical area and hippocampal sparing, which is related to the early preservation of anterograde memory. The typical presentation as in this case is that patient goes to the ophthalmologist who does not find an ocular cause for the visual impairment and then is referred to neurology. Because there is relative preservation of anterograde memory, doctors may not recognize that AD is the most frequent cause. Common clinical features are early age of onset (mean age of 60.5 years in the Tan-Wai series), simultanagnosia (inability to see all the details of a picture quickly and efficiently), visual field deficits, acalculia, alexia, and anomia. Because of the preserved anterograde memory, good insight is often preserved. Other diseases that should be included in the differential diagnosis include corticobasal degeneration (2 of the cases reported by Tang-Wai and colleagues had this), Lewy body disease (these patients often have visuospatial difficulty) and Creutzfeldt–Jakob disease (which can present with visual difficulty). Amyloid PET scan is abnormal in PCA patients with AD, although the distribution is difficult to distinguish from AD[6]; however, tau PET scan shows disproportionate tau deposits in the visual areas.[6] Recently, Carrasquillo and colleagues[7] found apolipoprotein E (ApoE) to be related to PCA and indicated that, CLU, BIN1, and ABCA7 may be related, but further study is needed.

Corticobasal Syndrome

Clinical case

A 55-year-old, right-handed woman was evaluated for a 1-year history of progressive memory impairment, limb apraxia, bradykinesia, and gait instability. Her husband noted that she also developed difficulty understanding spatial relations. She was still able to perform her job as a nurse and drive without accidents. Neurologic examination revealed ideomotor and limb–kinetic apraxia, focal dystonia of the right hand, asymmetric (right > left) Parkinsonism, and decreased graphesthesia bilaterally. No myoclonus, alien limb phenomena, or eye movement abnormalities were noted. Detailed neuropsychological assessment revealed marked impairment in memory, language, and visuospatial skills. MRI of the brain showed diffuse mild cortical atrophy, more prominent bifrontally. Comprehensive laboratory workup, cerebrospinal fluid (CSF) studies and electroencephalogram (EEG) were unremarkable. The working diagnosis was CBS. The medical disability process was initiated and she graciously stopped driving. She was seen yearly and progressive cognitive impairment continued. She was placed on donepezil and memantine eventually as atypical AD was a consideration. She died 7 years after the initial assessment. The autopsy revealed advanced[8] (Braak stage VI) AD with relatively less neuronal loss and neurofibrillary degeneration in hippocampus compared with the cortex (hippocampal-sparing AD; **Fig. 3**).

Clinical features

- Progressive cognitive impairment.
- Apraxia.
- Asymmetric Parkinsonism and dystonia.
- Decreased graphestesia bilaterally.
- Visuospatial Impairment.

Pathophysiology

The clinical picture of CBS may have many pathologic causes in addition to corticobasal degeneration, such as in this case which had AD.[9] Other causes include progressive supranuclear palsy, Picks disease, and Creutzfeldt–Jakob disease. Although hippocampal atrophy rates have been used to monitor progression of AD and to predict cognitive decline,[10–12] a subset of AD cases has less hippocampal atrophy relative to the predominance of cortical atrophy,[13,14] which challenges the Braak staging scheme of neurofibrillary changes[8] and results in symptomatic heterogeneity, as in our case. Murray and colleagues[14] looked into a large cohort (n = 889) of autopsy-proven AD cases and showed that AD has distinct clinicopathologic subtypes: typical, hippocampal sparing, and limbic predominant. They pointed out that, compared with the other subtypes, hippocampal-sparing cases were mostly presented as focal cortical clinical syndromes, such as CBS, behavioral variant frontotemporal dementia (FTD), progressive aphasia, or PCA. Hippocampal-sparing cases were mostly men and were younger at death, with early onset and rapid progression. They had higher neurofibrillary tangle densities in the association cortices and the motor cortex, with significantly lower H1H1 MAPT genotype. Murray and

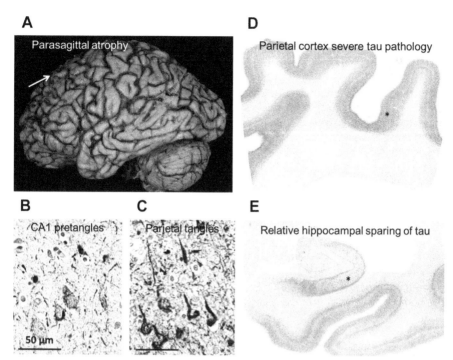

Fig. 3. Autopsy revealed neuropathologic changes consistent with Alzheimer's disease in a patient with corticobasal syndrome. (*A*) Parasagittal atrophy (*arrow*) was noted when examining the fixed tissue. Immunohistochemical evaluation with a tau antibody revealed (*B*) a paucity of neurofibrillary tangles, (*C*) relative to the abundance of mature and extracellular tangles noted in the parietal lobe. A 1× magnification of the (*D*) parietal cortex shows an appreciably higher tau burden compared with the (*E*) hippocampus. Scale bar at 50 μm for 20 × images and * in *D* and *E* refer to location in *C* and *B* respectively.

colleagues[14] added that atypical AD (hippocampal sparing and limbic predominant) might account for 25% of the cases, and so should be considered in diagnostic evaluation and treatment studies. In a recent study by Paterson and colleagues,[15] the typical and atypical AD groups were matched for age, sex, and rate and severity of cognitive decline and had similar biomarker profiles, both different from controls. The atypical AD group seemed to be an heterogeneous entity with evidence of subtle differences in amyloid processing and neurodegeneration between subsets. For example, they showed that PCA patients had the lowest CSF total tau (T-tau), phospho-tau (p-tau) T-tau/Ab1-42 ratio, and the slowest rate of cognitive decline as opposed to frontal variant group which had the highest T-tau, P-tau T-tau/Ab1-42 ratio, and fastest rate of cognitive decline. Overall, these findings may have practical implications for CSF biomarker interpretation.

FLUENT APHASIA
Semantic Dementia

Clinical case
A 72-year-old, right-handed woman with a master's degree in speech pathology presented with a 5-year history of progressive word finding problems followed by difficulty recognizing faces even of familiar people. She was functioning well otherwise,

was able to manage her finances and drive without getting lost. On examination, she scored 26 of 30 on the Folstein Mini Mental Status Examination (MMSE),[16] 8 of 10 on the orientation and 1 of 3 on the memory items. Her score was 0 of 20 on the first 20 words of the Boston Naming Test. On the famous faces test, she scored 0 of 20. On naming the last 3 presidents and their wives, first names, she scored 1 of 6. Her speech was fluent without any articulation difficulty. Her sentence repetition was intact. She had difficulty understanding sentences in the passive voice. Neuropsychological assessment revealed impaired semantic retrieval, including confrontation naming and speeded semantic fluency, with intact phonemic fluency, visual spatial skills, cognitive speed, executive function, and immediate attention. Brain MRI showed severe left more than right temporal lobe atrophy (**Fig. 4**). Autopsy was not available.

Clinical features

- Impaired confrontation naming.[17]
- Impaired single-word comprehension.
- Impaired object/person knowledge.
- Intact repetition.
- Intact motor speech.
- Surface dyslexia and/or dysgraphia.

Pathophysiology

Arnold Pick[18] was first to describe the clinical syndrome in late 19th century, long before Mesulam[19] reawakened the interest in 1982, and the term "semantic dementia" was coined by Snowden and colleagues.[20] The underlying pathology is usually TDP-43, characterized by dystrophic neurites,[21] categorized as FTLD-TDP type. Hodges and Patterson[22] reported an autopsy-proven case series of 20 patients: 14 with TDP-43, 4 with Pick's disease, and 2 with AD pathology. Neurodegeneration in semantic dementia seems to begin in the anterior temporal lobe, more left than

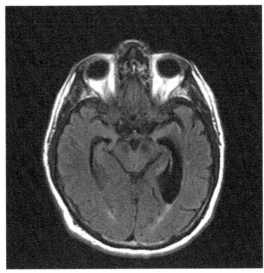

Fig. 4. MRI of the brain showing left temporal lobe atrophy in a patient with semantic dementia.

right, then spreads to entorhinal cortex, hippocampus, and the inferior, middle, and superior (anterior) parts of temporal gyrus. Hodges and Patterson[22] have suggested that sparing of the cingulate in semantic dementia might explain intact orientation and ability to learn new information despite severe degeneration of the hippocampal and entorhinal cortices, which leads to disorientation and poor anterograde memory in AD. Using lesion method and PET scanning, Damasio and colleagues[23] pointed out that different parts of the left temporal lobe take an intermediary role in naming and organization of conceptual knowledge of different categories—faces in the anterior temporal lobe, animals in the inferior temporal lobe and tools in the postero-lateral temporal lobe. Gefen and colleagues[24] demonstrated that impaired face naming was correlated with atrophy of the left anterior temporal lobe whereas impaired face recognition was correlated with bilateral anterior temporal lobe atrophy, as in this case.

Logopenic Aphasia

Clinical case
A 72-year-old, right-handed man with 18 years of formal education presented with a 3-year history of progressively worsening memory and naming difficulties that had not interfered with his daily functioning. He noted no difficulty carrying out his volunteer job and was able to drive without getting lost. Although he was able to manage his household finances, it was taking him longer to complete the task and his wife started double checking after several errors were noted. Family history was significant for his mother developing dementia in her early 70s. On examination his Folstein MMSE[16] was 22 of 30; he scored 8 of 10 on the orientation items, 0 of 3 on the memory items, and his sentence repetition was impaired. He named 12 out of first 15 items on Boston Naming Test. Although his speech was fluent his rate was slow. He made a few phonemic paraphasic errors. Grammar and articulation were preserved. Brain MRI showed diffuse cortical atrophy, more in the left temporoparietal region.

Clinical features

- Impaired word finding.[17]
- Impaired sentence repetition.
- Preserved single word comprehension.
- Phonetic paraphasic errors.
- No agrammatism.
- Normal motor speech.

Pathophysiology
Gorno-Tempini and colleagues[17] described that impaired single-word retrieval and sentence repetition are main features of logopenic aphasia. Phonological paraphasic errors may also be seen. Object knowledge, single-word comprehension, motor speech, and grammar are typically preserved. They have suggested phonological loop deficit as core mechanism.[25] Neuropathologic and biomarker studies[26] have linked logopenic aphasia with AD. Mesulam[27] described that memory is preserved early in the disease owing to relative sparing of the medial temporal lobe, which was shown in a pathologic comparison of a patient with logopenic aphasia and a patient with typical AD. In the patient with logopenic aphasia, there were more tangles in temporoparietal junction and fewer tangles in the entorhinal area; the reversal of the pattern was seen in the patient with typical AD. Neuroimaging studies revealed prominent atrophy in the left posterior temporal and inferior parietal regions in logopenic aphasia.

LATE-ONSET DEMENTIA
Hippocampal Sclerosis

Clinical case

An 85 year old, right handed man presented with a 6 month history of subtle memory difficulties. His wife noted that he had started to repeat his stories and was having difficulty remembering his fellow golfers' names. He was functioning very well otherwise. He was able to drive without problems, perform his activities of daily living and play golf 3 times a week. He scored 26 of 30 on the Folstein MMSE,[16] scoring 9 of 10 on the orientation and 0 of 3 on the memory items. Neuropsychological assessment was suggestive of amnestic mild cognitive impairment with high-average performance across all domains, except inefficient learning and poor retention of information over time. Brain MRI was unremarkable, showing diffuse mild cortical atrophy, compatible with his age. He was seen 3 years after the initial evaluation. Although he reported progressive memory difficulties, he had continued to function well, was still driving, managing his finances, and was playing golf once a week. His performance on Folstein MMSE was similar (25/30) to his initial evaluation. Neuropsychological assessment revealed relatively isolated memory dysfunction, remained to be consistent with amnestic mild cognitive impairment, although his performance had declined comparing to his baseline evaluation (Dementia Rating Scale scores of 109/144 and 129/144, respectively). He died at age 92, and the autopsy revealed moderate temporal lobe atrophy. The histology showed HpScl with TDP-43 pathology limited to medial temporal and limbic lobes with predominant neuronal cytoplasmic inclusions along with tangle dominant (Braak stage IV) AD-type pathology (**Fig. 5**).

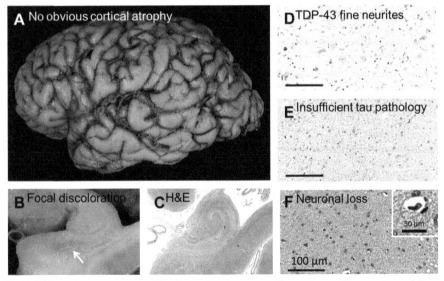

Fig. 5. This patient presented with a long-standing amnestic syndrome. Upon autopsy (A), no obvious cortical atrophy was noted when examining the fixed tissue. (B) When the hippocampus was observed, however, focal discoloration of the subiculum was noted in the fixed tissue at the *arrow* and (C) upon examination with hematoxylin and eosin (H&E) without observable senile plaques. Immunohistochemical evaluation with a TDP-43 antibody revealed (D) fine neurites consistent with hippocampal sclerosis of a neurodegenerative etiology. (E) By definition, there was insufficient tau pathology to account for the (F) extensive neuronal loss (*inset*: pyknotic neuron). Scale bar at 100 μm for 20× images and 50 μm for inset.

Clinical features compared with typical AD

- Older age of onset.[28]
- Slower rate of cognitive decline.
- Stronger family history of dementia.

Limbic-Predominant Alzheimer's Disease

Clinical case

A 74-year-old, left-handed woman presented with a 3-year history of progressive memory difficulties. She was able to perform her activities of daily living, run her house, and drive without problems. She scored 28 of 30 on the Folstein MMSE,[16] scoring 1 of 3 on the memory items. Comprehensive neuropsychological assessment was suggestive of amnestic mild cognitive impairment with isolated memory difficulty, particularly list learning and logical memory difficulties, despite above average performance in most areas. Brain MRI was unremarkable. She was seen 2 years after the initial presentation and was placed on donepezil by her primary care physician in the interim. She stopped driving and was functioning well otherwise. She scored 25 of 30 on the Folstein MMSE and her neuropsychological testing showed some deterioration in memory and language domains. She continued to follow-up yearly. Progressive cognitive deterioration was noted to the point that she was unable to perform her activities of daily living and eventually moved into a retirement home at age 83 with her husband. She died when she was 87. The autopsy revealed limbic-predominant AD with predominance of neurofibrillary degeneration in the medial temporal lobe structures without any significant atrophy (**Fig. 6**).

Clinical features

- Age of onset and cognitive decline are similar to typical AD.

Pathophysiology

Differentiating late-onset amnestic dementias can be difficult because the clinical presentations are similar and multiple pathologies can coexist.[29] Pathologic subtypes of AD are described based on the relative density of neurofibrillary tangles in the hippocampus and cortex: typical AD, hippocampal-sparing AD, and limbic-predominant AD.[14,30] Whereas typical AD follows the Braak staging,[8] limbic-predominant AD has disproportionately greater neurofibrillary tangles in the hippocampus than in the neocortex. HpScl is characterized by severe hippocampal volume loss and neuronal loss in CA1 and the subiculum, which is disproportionate to the number of neurofibrillary tangles.[01] Considering the medial temporal lobe involvement in both HpScl and limbic-predominant AD, neuroimaging and pathologic analysis can be limited in distinguishing.[32] Concomitant HpScl and AD can further blur the picture. Murray and colleagues[28] examined a large cohort of autopsy-confirmed cases of typical AD, limbic-predominant AD, HpScl, and HpScl-AD to identify distinct clinical, genetic, and pathologic characteristics. They showed that existence of AD pathology (typical AD, limbic-predominant AD, HpScl-AD) dominates the phenotype, whereas "pure HpScl" phenotype is distinct with significantly older age of onset (79 vs 71 years in typical AD) and slower cognitive decline. They pointed out that AD groups were more likely to be carriers of ApoE ε4, the strongest genetic risk factor for AD, whereas HpScl groups (HpScl and HpScl-AD) were more likely to exhibit genetic variants in GRN and TMEM106B that are associated with frontotemporal lobar degeneration[33–35] and ApoE status was independent of risk for HpScl,[34,36,37] which may have diagnostic value along with a novel polymorphism that was recently described in the adenosine triphosphate-binding cassette, subfamily C member 9 in HpScl.[38] Murray and

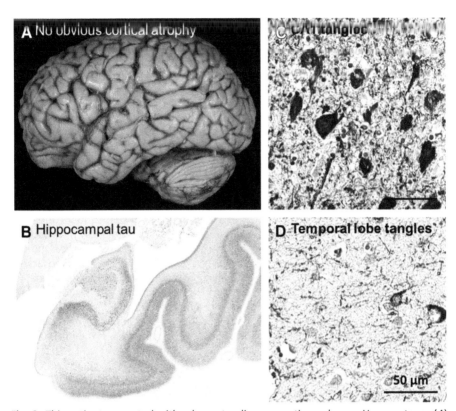

Fig. 6. This patient presented with a long-standing amnestic syndrome. Upon autopsy (*A*), no obvious cortical atrophy was noted when examining the fixed tissue. (*B*) The hippocampus, however, was greatly atrophied with extensive tau pathology. (*C*) Frequent neurofibrillary tangles were noted with extensive neuronal loss in CA1 and subiculum of the hippocampus. (*D*) Consistent with the limbic predominant form of Alzheimer's disease, sparse neurofibrillary tangles were noted in the neocortex as illustrated by the temporal lobe. Scale bar at 50 μm for 20× images.

colleagues also showed that HpScl groups had a high frequency of TDP-43 pathology that was most often type A morphology and distribution,[33] whereas AD groups had a significantly lower frequency of TDP-43 pathology that was most often type B.[14,30] Taken together, it is suggested that HpScl and AD are pathologically and genetically distinct and nonsynergistic neurodegenerative processes, despite similar clinical presentations.[28,39,40]

RAPIDLY PROGRESSIVE DEMENTIA
Creutzfeldt–Jakob Disease

Clinical case
An 82-year-old, right-handed otherwise healthy woman presented with a 1-year history of rapidly progressive cognitive impairment. Despite her short-term memory problems and word-finding difficulties, she was functioning well. She was able to live alone and drive without getting lost. She reported some difficulty standing from a sitting position. She was feeling increasingly unsteady and most recently started using a cane to ambulate. No falls or abnormal movements were reported. She scored

26 of 30 on the Folstein MMSE[16] examination, 2 of 10 on orientation and 1 of 3 on the memory items. She scored 14 of 20 on the first 20 items of Boston Naming Test. She had significant simultanagnosia. Examination did not reveal ataxia, myoclonus, or Parkinsonism. Serum and CSF paraneoplastic panels were unremarkable. CSF 14-3-3 protein was positive and T-tau level was high (3615 pg/mL). Diffusion-weighted MRI brain images showed cortical ribboning in the occipital and temporal lobes bilaterally, left more than right (**Fig. 7**). EEG was not performed. The patient died within 2 months of her evaluation. Autopsy was not performed.

Clinical features

- Progressive dementia.[41]
- Visual disturbances.
- Myoclonus.
- Cerebellar and pyramidal/extrapyramidal findings.
- Akinetic mutism.
- CSF 14-3-3 positivity.
- Periodic sharp wave complexes on the EEG.

Pathophysiology

Considering the diagnosis of Creutzfeldt–Jakob disease can be delayed irrespective of the age of onset,[42] older age can further complicate the picture. The World Health Organization criteria for Creutzfeldt–Jakob disease[41] require either a typical EEG (periodic sharp wave complexes) or a positive CSF 14-3-3 along with progressive dementia resulting in fatality within 2 years. Diagnostic accuracy of protein 14-3-3 has been questioned because an approximation of its sensitivity differs anywhere between 50% to 92% with an approximate specificity of 80%[43,44] compared with T-tau with sensitivity and specificity of greater than 90%.[45,46] Forner and colleagues[47] recently looked into diagnostic tools for sporadic Creutzfeldt–Jakob disease, and noted that diffusion-weighted MRI had a higher diagnostic accuracy (97%) than CSF biomarkers (14-3-3, neuron-specific enolase, night eating syndrome, T-tau) among which T-tau had the highest diagnostic accuracy (79.6%). The newer real-time quaking-induced conversion may also be helpful.[48] Despite its high

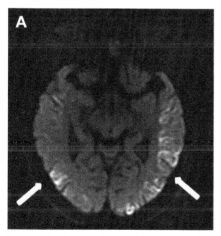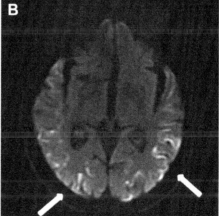

Fig. 7. (*A, B*) Diffusion-weighted imaging shows cortical ribboning in the occipital and temporal lobes bilaterally, left more than right (*arrows*).

diagnostic accuracy for Creutzfeldt–Jakob disease, similar diffusion-weighted MRI hyperintensity patterns can be seen in nonprion rapidly progressing dementia. Several other conditions, particularly autoimmune encephalitis and rapidly progressive neurodegenerative diseases, can mimic Creutzfeldt–Jakob disease.[49] In a case series of 15 subjects who had an initial diagnosis of Creutzfeldt–Jakob disease but eventually confirmed to have voltage-gated potassium channel (VGKC) autoantibody–associated encephalopathy, Geschwind and colleagues[50] noted that more than one-half (60%) of the subjects satisfied World Health Organization diagnostic criteria for Creutzfeldt–Jakob disease, with rapidly progressive dementia, elevated CSF 14-3-3 protein, or night eating syndrome. The T2-weighted and fluid-attenuated inversion recovery hyperintensities of the medial temporal regions were noted in 5 subjects, which is classic for autoimmune limbic encephalitis, but can also be seen in Creutzfeldt–Jakob disease. EEG showed no periodic sharp wave complexes despite diffuse slowing along with frontal intermittent rhythmic delta activity and focal epileptogenic activity. Hyponatremia was common (60%) and was thought to have an important diagnostic value favoring an autoimmune etiology. Neoplasia was confirmed histologically in 5 patients (33%) and was suspected in another 5. Most patients (92%) improved after immunomodulatory therapy. Rapidly progressive AD (rpAD) is another consideration, in a cohort (n = 89) of autopsy-confirmed rpAD, Schmidt and colleagues[51] showed that rpAD is a different clinical syndrome than typical AD, at least in the early stages, and is similar to Creutzfeldt–Jakob disease symptomatology. Fast decline seems to be associated with certain symptoms, such as motor signs. Although CSF AD biomarkers did not differ from that of typical AD pattern, protein 14-3-3 was detected frequently (42%) in rpAD.

Limbic Encephalitis

Clinical case

A 71-year-old, right-handed engineer presented with a 1-year history of seizures and cognitive impairment. After being evaluated by multiple providers, he was referred to behavioral neurology by an epileptologist. His initial symptom was a sudden onset of focal amnesia, followed by persistent memory impairment and paroxysmal episodes of olfactory hallucinations, diaphoresis, oral automatisms, and dysarthria lasting for several minutes. He was placed on memantine and donepezil without any significant benefit. Oxcarbazepine had diminished the frequency and severity of the seizures; however, the seizures persisted with intermittent generalization. Medical and family history indicated no autoimmunity. He scored 19 of 30 on the Folstein MMSE. Neurologic examination was otherwise unremarkable. Comprehensive neuropsychological assessment revealed profound memory impairment with mild frontal–subcortical involvement. Laboratory workup showed hyponatremia (125 mmol/L) and VGKC antibodies in the serum at a level of 0.59 nmol/L (normal, <0.02 nmol/L). CSF studies were unremarkable. EEG revealed subclinical electrographic seizure activity arising from bilateral temporal lobes in the sleep states. MRI of the brain was unremarkable with no evidence for encephalopathy (**Fig. 8**). Full-body ^{18}F-fluorodeoxyglucose PET scan revealed no abnormality. Diagnosis of limbic encephalitis with VGKC antibodies was considered and the patient was placed on intravenous (IV) methylprednisolone (1 g IV daily for 3 days then weekly for 6 weeks and then biweekly for 6 weeks). Blood count, and liver and kidney function were monitored closely. He was placed on vitamin D and calcium replacement along with trimethoprim/sulfamethoxazole (1 double-strength tablet 3 times a week) for *Pneumocystis carinii* pneumonia. He returned 12 weeks after the initiation of immunotherapy. He reported significant cognitive improvement, which was also noted by his wife with particular improvement in the days immediately after infusions, then slow gradual decline until the following infusion. His seizures were resolved. Detailed neuropsychological assessment confirmed notable improvement across domains relative to his initial evaluation, except persistent memory impairment. His blood sodium was normalized (135 mmol/L). He was switched to oral prednisolone (60 mg daily for 3 months) and azathioprine was started (50 mg twice a day) simultaneously with an aim to increase his mean corpuscular volume by 5 points. Thiopurine methyltransferase enzyme activity was checked and was normal before initiation of azathioprine.[52] He was seen 12 weeks after initiation of azathioprine. Neuropsychological assessment revealed stable cognitive function, although the patient and his wife reported cognitive improvement. Azathioprine was titrated (100 mg twice a day) and oral prednisolone was continued at the dose of 60 mg daily for 12 weeks, until his return visit. Neuropsychological assessment revealed stable cognitive function, with subjective report of continuous cognitive improvement. His mean corpuscular volume had increased by 10 (Na, 139 mmol/L), and liver and kidney function were normal. Steroid taper was initiated (10 mg per month until 10 mg daily followed by 1 mg/d per month decrements until completion). He was seen upon completion of steroid taper. He reported stable cognitive function, which was confirmed by the neuropsychological assessment. Azathioprine (100 mg twice a day) was continued.

Clinical features

- Rapidly progressive or fluctuating course.[53]
- One or more symptoms of memory impairment, behavioral disturbance, hallucinations, focal seizures.
- Inflammatory markers in the CSF.
- Coexisting organ-specific autoimmunity (particularly thyroid).
- Response to immunotherapy.

Pathophysiology

When evaluating a patient with rapidly progressing dementia, it is important to not to overlook potentially treatable conditions. Systematic approach is needed to ensure

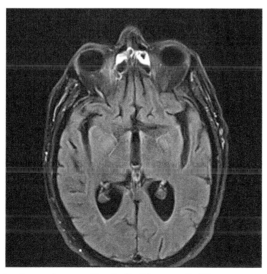

Fig. 8. MRI of the brain can be negative in limbic encephalitis.

that all possibilities are considered. The mnemonic VITAMIN C (vascular, Infectious, toxic–metabolic, autoimmune, metastatic, iatrogenic, neurodegenerative, congenital/systemic) can come in handy. Flanagan and colleagues[34] looked into 72 consecutive patients who received immunotherapy for suspected autoimmune dementia and showed that more than one-third (35%) of the immunotherapy responders were initially diagnosed with a neurodegenerative or prion disorder. If an autoimmune dementia is suspected, several points are worth noting[53]:

- The clinical manifestations are diverse and often multifocal;
- A personal or family history of autoimmunity/seropositivity is a risk factor;
- Neural-specific autoantibody positivity serves as a marker of neurologic autoimmunity;
- Identification of neural-specific autoantibodies may lead a targeted oncological evaluation in the context of a known cancer association (eg, N-methyl-D-aspartate receptor antibody and teratoma); and
- Immunotherapy trial may have a "diagnostic" value.

For evaluation and treatment of patients with suspected autoimmune dementia, McKeon and colleagues[53] outlined practical guidelines, starting with the exclusion of other causes of cognitive decline, followed by objective documentation of cognitive and neurologic abnormalities (comprehensive neuropsychological assessment, EEG, MRI, and functional imaging) to provide a pretreatment baseline by which response to immunotherapy can be measured. CSF analysis, comprehensive antibody testing (serum and CSF), and paraneoplastic investigation (eg, whole-body CT or PET scan) may lead to further clues about autoimmune etiology. Although the phenotype associated with any given autoantibody seems to be broader,[55] there are several direct associations that are identified, such as limbic encephalitis with VGKC antibodies, ANNA-1 (antineuronal nuclear antibody/anti-Hu), and α-amino-3- hydroxy-5-methyl-4-isoxazolepropionic acid receptor antibodies[56]; fluctuating hemiplegia with complete recovery and thyroid autoantibodies[57]; and diverse psychiatric presentations early in the course with N-methyl-D-aspartate receptor antibody.[58] The positive predictive values for cancer detection rates vary from 33% for VGKC antibodies (various cancer types)[59] to more than 80% for ANNA-1 (almost always small-cell lung carcinoma).[60] Once autoimmune dementia is suspected, immunotherapy should be initiated promptly because a lesser delay to treatment is shown[61] to be one of the predictors of treatment response along with subacute onset, fluctuating course, detection of a cation channel- specific autoantibody (calcium channel, VGKC, ganglionic acetylcholine receptor) and CSF findings of elevated protein (>100 mg/dL) or pleocytosis. Treatment of autoimmune dementias remains empirical. McKeon and colleagues[53] recommended starting a trial of IV corticosteroid "pulse therapy" with methylprednisolone 1 g IV daily for 3 to 5 days then weekly for 6 to 8 weeks (alternatively IVIG 0.4–1.0 g/kg IV daily for 3–5 days then weekly for 6–8 weeks). They pointed out that plasma exchange can be tried for critically ill or when corticosteroids/IV immunoglobulin (IVIG) is poorly tolerated. They recommended a return visit following 4 to 8 weeks of immunotherapy to investigate subjective and objective evidence of clinical improvement (reported functional/cognitive improvement, comprehensive neuropsychological assessment, neuroimaging, etc). In the absence of objective evidence of improvement, a trial of IVIG can be considered, followed by reevaluations. The investigators noted that a favorable response to immunotherapy supports the diagnosis and prompts long-term immunotherapy as relapse is common owing to withdrawal of acute therapies. Extending the interval between infusions of IV corticosteroids (or IVIG) from weekly to biweekly, then every 3 weeks and then monthly, over a period of 4 to 6 months while bridging with oral steroid-sparing immunosuppressants (azathioprine 1–2 mg/kg/d in a 2 daily divided doses or mycophenolate mofetil 500–2000 mg/d in a 2 daily divided doses) to ensure reduction in corticosteroid (or IVIG) dependence. Some overlap in corticosteroid (or IVIG) and oral immunosuppressant treatment is required, approximately 12 weeks for azathioprine and 6 to 8 weeks for mycophenolate mofetil.[62] If no cognitive improvement occurs after infusion, corticosteroid (or IVIG) can be discontinued. No data are available to determine the appropriate duration of immunosuppression treatment in autoimmune dementia. Although spontaneous remission is possible, some patients are dependent lifelong on immunosuppressants. McKeon and colleagues[53] recommend a trial of immunosuppressant medication withdrawal after 2 to 3 years. Appropriate calcium (1000–1500 mg/d) and vitamin D (800 IU/d) intake is recommended for patients taking corticosteroids long term.[63] Prophylaxis against *P carinii* pneumonia (trimethoprim/sulfamethoxazole, 1 double-strength tablet 3 times a week) is recommended for patients receiving long-term corticosteroids or a purine analog.[64] Withdrawal of chronic oral corticosteroids may lead to adrenocortical failure if not done cautiously; collaborating with an endocrinologist or internist would be beneficial. Close monitoring of blood count, and liver and renal function is required for patients on immunotherapy, weekly for the first month then biweekly for 2 months, and monthly thereafter.

DISCUSSION

The differential diagnosis of dementia can be challenging as initial clinical presentation can be variable and different neuropathologies can coexist, particularly in the elderly. It is important not to overlook focal cortical presentations of AD: visual impairment can be the only symptom early in the course leading to unfruitful ophthalmologic visits and the clinical picture of CBS may have AD as the underlying pathology. Patients with logopenic aphasia frequently have AD, whereas TDP-43 is the most common pathology in semantic dementia. Different neuropathologic processes can result in similar clinical presentations, as discussed in limbic-predominant AD and HpScl. Early diagnosis in rapidly progressing dementia is of paramount importance, because it can be reversible, such as autoimmune encephalitis. Recognizing the different syndromes described in this paper can help the clinician to improve their diagnostic skills leading to improved patient outcomes by early and accurate diagnosis, prompt treatment, appropriate counseling and guidance.

REFERENCES

1. Kokmen E, Naessens JM, Offord KP. A short test of mental status: description and preliminary results. Mayo Clin Proc 1987;62(4):281–8.
2. Benson DF, Davis RJ, Snyder BD. Posterior cortical atrophy. Arch Neurol 1988; 45(7):789–93.
3. Hof PR, Vogt BA, Bouras C, et al. Atypical form of Alzheimer's disease with prominent posterior cortical atrophy: a review of lesion distribution and circuit disconnection in cortical visual pathways. Vision Res 1997;37(24):3609–25.
4. Tang-Wai DF, Graff-Radford NR, Boeve BF, et al. Clinical, genetic, and neuropathologic characteristics of posterior cortical atrophy. Neurology 2004;63(7): 1168–74.
5. Rosenbloom MH, Alkalay A, Agarwal N, et al. Distinct clinical and metabolic deficits in PCA and AD are not related to amyloid distribution. Neurology 2011; 76(21):1789–96.

6. Osseukuppele H, Schwarthout DN, Baker CL, et al. Tau, amyloid, and hypometabolism in a patient with posterior cortical atrophy. Ann Neurol 2015;77(2):338–42.

7. Carrasquillo MM, Khan Qu, Murray ME, et al. Late-onset Alzheimer disease genetic variants in posterior cortical atrophy and posterior AD. Neurology 2014; 82(16):1455–62.

8. Braak H, Braak E. Neuropathological stageing of Alzheimer-related changes. Acta Neuropathol 1991;82(4):239–59.

9. Boeve BF, Maraganore DM, Parisi JE, et al. Pathologic heterogeneity in clinically diagnosed corticobasal degeneration. Neurology 1999;53(4):795–800.

10. Jack CR Jr, Petersen RC, Xu Y, et al. Rate of medial temporal lobe atrophy in typical aging and Alzheimer's disease. Neurology 1998;51(4):993–9.

11. Frisoni GB, Ganzola R, Canu E, et al. Mapping local hippocampal changes in Alzheimer's disease and normal ageing with MRI at 3 Tesla. Brain 2008; 131(Pt 12):3266–76.

12. Desikan RS, Sabuncu MR, Schmansky NJ, et al. Selective disruption of the cerebral neocortex in Alzheimer's disease. PLoS One 2010;5(9):e12853.

13. Giannakopoulos P, Gold G, Kövari E, et al. Assessing the cognitive impact of Alzheimer disease pathology and vascular burden in the aging brain: the Geneva experience. Acta Neuropathol 2007;113(1):1–12.

14. Murray ME, Graff-Radford NR, Ross OA, et al. Neuropathologically defined subtypes of Alzheimer's disease with distinct clinical characteristics: a retrospective study. Lancet Neurol 2011;10(9):785–96.

15. Paterson RW, Toombs J, Slattery CF, et al. Dissecting IWG-2 typical and atypical Alzheimer's disease: insights from cerebrospinal fluid analysis. J Neurol 2015; 262(12):2722–30.

16. Folstein MF, Folstein SE, McHugh PR. Mini-mental state. A practical method for grading the cognitive state of patients for the clinician. J Psychiatr Res 1975; 12(3):189–98.

17. Gorno-Tempini ML, Hillis AE, Weintraub S, et al. Classification of primary progressive aphasia and its variants. Neurology 2011;76(11):1006–14.

18. Pick A. Über die Beziehungen der senilen Hirnatrophie zur Aphasie. Prag Med Wochenschr 1892;17:165–7.

19. Mesulam MM. Slowly progressive aphasia without generalized dementia. Ann Neurol 1982;11(592):8.

20. Snowden JS, Goulding PJ, Neary D. Semantic dementia: a form of circumscribed cerebral atrophy. Behav Neurol 1989;2(167):82.

21. Mackenzie IR, Neumann M, Baborie A, et al. A harmonized classification system for FTLD-TDP pathology. Acta Neuropathol 2011;122(1):111–3.

22. Hodges JR, Patterson K. Semantic dementia: a unique clinicopathological syndrome. Lancet Neurol 2007;6(11):1004–14.

23. Damasio H, Grabowski TJ, Tranel D, et al. A neural basis for lexical retrieval. Nature 1996;380(6574):499–505.

24. Gefen T, Wieneke C, Martersteck A, et al. Naming vs knowing faces in primary progressive aphasia: a tale of 2 hemispheres. Neurology 2013;81(7):658–64.

25. Gorno-Tempini ML, Dronkers NF, Rankin KP, et al. Cognition and anatomy in three variants of primary progressive aphasia. Ann Neurol 2004;55(3):335–46.

26. Teichmann M, Kas A, Boutet C, et al. Deciphering logopenic primary progressive aphasia: a clinical, imaging and biomarker investigation. Brain 2013;136(Pt 11): 3474–88.

27. Mesulam MM. Primary progressive aphasia and the language network: the 2013 H. Houston Merritt Lecture. Neurology 2013;81(5):456–62.

28. Murray ME, Cannon A, Graff-Radford NR, et al. Differential clinicopathologic and genetic features of late-onset amnestic dementias. Acta Neuropathol 2014; 128(3):411–21.

29. Jellinger KA, Attems J. Challenges of multimorbidity of the aging brain: a critical update. J Neural Transm (Vienna) 2014;122(4):505–21.

30. Janocko NJ, Brodersen KA, Soto-Ortolaza AI, et al. Neuropathologically defined subtypes of Alzheimer's disease differ significantly from neurofibrillary tangle-predominant dementia. Acta Neuropathol 2012;124(5):681–92.

31. Dickson DW, Davies P, Bevona C, et al. Hippocampal sclerosis: a common pathological feature of dementia in very old (> or = 80 years of age) humans. Acta Neuropathol 1994;88(3):212–21.

32. Dutra JR, Cortes EP, Vonsattel JP. Update on hippocampal sclerosis. Curr Neurol Neurosci Rep 2015;15(10):67.

33. Amador-Ortiz C, Ahmed Z, Zehr C, et al. Hippocampal sclerosis dementia differs from hippocampal sclerosis in frontal lobe degeneration. Acta Neuropathol 2007; 113(3):245–52.

34. Nelson PT, Schmitt FA, Lin Y, et al. Hippocampal sclerosis in advanced age: clinical and pathological features. Brain 2011;134(Pt 5):1506–18.

35. Nelson PT, Smith CD, Abner EL, et al. Hippocampal sclerosis of aging, a prevalent and high-morbidity brain disease. Acta Neuropathol 2013;126(2):161–77.

36. Troncoso JC, Kawas CH, Chang CK, et al. Lack of association of the apoE4 allele with hippocampal sclerosis dementia. Neurosci Lett 1996;204(1–2):138–40.

37. Leverenz JB, Agustin CM, Tsuang D, et al. Clinical and neuropathological characteristics of hippocampal sclerosis: a community-based study. Arch Neurol 2002; 59(7):1099–106.

38. Nelson PT, Jicha GA, Wang WX, et al. ABCC9/SUR2 in the brain: implications for hippocampal sclerosis of aging and a potential therapeutic target. Ageing Res Rev 2015;24(Pt B):111–25.

39. Pao WC, Dickson DW, Crook JE, et al. Hippocampal sclerosis in the elderly: genetic and pathologic findings, some mimicking Alzheimer disease clinically. Alzheimer Dis Assoc Disord 2011;25(4):364–8.

40. Brenowitz WD, Monsell SE, Schmitt FA, et al. Hippocampal sclerosis of aging is a key Alzheimer's disease mimic: clinical-pathologic correlations and comparisons with both Alzheimer's disease and non-tauopathic frontotemporal lobar degeneration. J Alzheimers Dis 2014;39(3):691–702.

41. WHO Global surveillance, diagnosis and therapy of human transmissible spongiform encephalopathies: report of a WHO consultation. Geneva (Switzerland): WHO; 1998.

42. Paterson RW, Torres-Chae CC, Kuo AL, et al. Differential diagnosis of Jakob-Creutzfeldt disease. Arch Neurol 2012;69(12):1578–82.

43. Muayqil T, Gronseth G, Camicioli R. Evidence-based guideline: diagnostic accuracy of CSF 14-3-3 protein in sporadic Creutzfeldt-Jakob disease: report of the guideline development subcommittee of the American Academy of Neurology. Neurology 2012,79(14):1499–506.

44. Kim MO, Geschwind MD. Clinical update of Jakob-Creutzfeldt disease. Curr Opin Neurol 2015;28(3):302–10.

45. Coulthart MB, Jansen GH, Olsen E, et al. Diagnostic accuracy of cerebrospinal fluid protein markers for sporadic Creutzfeldt-Jakob disease in Canada: a 6-year prospective study. BMC Neurol 2011;11:133.

46. van Harten AC, Kester MI, Visser PJ, et al. Tau and p-tau as CSF biomarkers in dementia: a meta-analysis. Clin Chem Lab Med 2011;49(3):353–66.

47. Forner OA, Takada LT, Bottuhur BM, et al. Comparing CSF biomarkers and brain MRI in the diagnosis of sporadic Creutzfeldt-Jakob disease. Neurol Clin Pract 2015;5(2):116–25.

48. Atarashi R, Satoh K, Sano K, et al. Ultrasensitive human prion detection in cerebrospinal fluid by real-time quaking-induced conversion. Nat Med 2011;17(2):175–8.

49. Geschwind MD. Rapidly progressive dementia: prion diseases and other rapid dementias. Continuum (Minneap Minn) 2010;16(2 Dementia):31–56.

50. Geschwind MD, Tan KM, Lennon VA, et al. Voltage-gated potassium channel autoimmunity mimicking Creutzfeldt-Jakob disease. Arch Neurol 2008;65(10):1341–6.

51. Schmidt C, Haïk S, Satoh K, et al. Rapidly progressive Alzheimer's disease: a multicenter update. J Alzheimers Dis 2012;30(4):751–6.

52. Liu YP, Xu HQ, Li M, et al. Association between thiopurine S-methyltransferase polymorphisms and azathioprine-induced adverse drug reactions in patients with autoimmune diseases: a meta-analysis. PLoS One 2015;10(12):e0144234.

53. McKeon A, Lennon VA, Pittock SJ. Immunotherapy-responsive dementias and encephalopathies. Continuum (Minneap Minn) 2010;16(2 Dementia):80–101.

54. Flanagan EP, McKeon A, Lennon VA, et al. Autoimmune dementia: clinical course and predictors of immunotherapy response. Mayo Clin Proc 2010;85(10):881–97.

55. Mittal MK, Rabinstein AA, Hocker SE, et al. Autoimmune encephalitis in the ICU: analysis of phenotypes, serologic findings, and outcomes. Neurocrit Care 2015; 24(2):240–50.

56. Lai M, Hughes EG, Peng X, et al. AMPA receptor antibodies in limbic encephalitis alter synaptic receptor location. Ann Neurol 2009;65(4):424–34.

57. Shaw PJ, Walls TJ, Newman PK, et al. Hashimoto's encephalopathy: a steroid-responsive disorder associated with high anti-thyroid antibody titers–report of 5 cases. Neurology 1991;41(2 (Pt 1)):228–33.

58. Dalmau J, Gleichman AJ, Hughes EG, et al. Anti-NMDA-receptor encephalitis: case series and analysis of the effects of antibodies. Lancet Neurol 2008;7(12): 1091–8.

59. Tan KM, Lennon VA, Klein CJ, et al. Clinical spectrum of voltage-gated potassium channel autoimmunity. Neurology 2008;70(20):1883–90.

60. Lucchinetti CF, Kimmel DW, Lennon VA. Paraneoplastic and oncologic profiles of patients seropositive for type 1 antineuronal nuclear autoantibodies. Neurology 1998;50(3):652–7.

61. Flanagan E, McKeon A, Lennon V. Immunotherapy responsive dementia or encephalopathy: clinical course and predictors of improvements. Ann Neurol 2009;66:S41.

62. Meriggioli MN, Ciafaloni E, Al-Hayk KA, et al. Mycophenolate mofetil for myasthenia gravis: an analysis of efficacy, safety, and tolerability. Neurology 2003; 61(10):1438–40.

63. American College of Rheumatology Ad Hoc Committee on glucocorticoid-induced osteoporosis. Recommendations for the prevention and treatment of glucocorticoid-induced osteoporosis: 2001 update. Arthritis Rheum 2001;44(7): 1496–503.

64. Stern A, Green H, Paul M, et al. Prophylaxis for pneumocystis pneumonia (PCP) in non-HIV immunocompromised patients. Cochrane Database Syst Rev 2014;(10):CD005590.

Neurology of Pregnancy
A Case-Oriented Review

Mary Angela O'Neal, MD

KEYWORDS

- Pregnancy • Stroke • Eclampsia • Multiple sclerosis • Epilepsy

KEY POINTS

- The anatomic and physiologic changes of pregnancy, although advantageous, may in some instances predispose to pathology.
- Treatment of women with an ischemic stroke during pregnancy should be based on their stroke characteristics. Both intravenous t-PA and endovascular therapy should be offered for qualifying strokes.
- Eclampsia and reversible cerebral vasospasm syndrome have a shared pathology and occur along a clinical spectrum.
- Pregnancy has no effect on multiple sclerosis severity or disability.
- Women with epilepsy planning to become pregnant should have their seizures under optimal control, on the least teratogenic anticonvulsant that controls their epilepsy, and be maintained on folate. Serum levels of many antiepileptic medications need to be followed in pregnancy because of altered metabolism.
- Compression neuropathies in pregnancy and the postpartum period are common and usually resolve.

PREGNANCY PHYSIOLOGY

In pregnancy, the blood volume increases by about 1500 mL mainly because of the expansion of plasma volume. In fact, the blood volume may increase by 10% by 7 weeks of pregnancy.[1] The red cell mass also increases, but not in proportion to the change in plasma volume. This results in the physiologic anemia of pregnancy, which is maximal by 30 to 32 weeks. In pregnancy, blood pressure (BP) decreases to reach a nadir at 28 weeks of gestation. The decrease in BP is caused by lower systemic vascular resistance. The result is an increase in cardiac output and heart rate.[2] Thus the hemodynamic changes of pregnancy are characterized primarily by volume expansion and a decrease in vascular resistance.[3]

Conflicts of Interest. The author has no conflicts of interest or relevant financial disclosures.
Department of Neurology, Brigham and Women's Hospital, 75 Francis Street, Boston, MA 02115, USA
E-mail address: maoneal@partners.org

Neurol Clin 34 (2016) 717–731
http://dx.doi.org/10.1016/j.ncl.2016.04.009
0733-8619/16/$ – see front matter © 2016 Elsevier Inc. All rights reserved.

Drug metabolism is affected in several ways. First, systemic absorption is altered for many medications. In addition, glomerular filtration rate increases by 40% to 50% in pregnancy with increased renal clearance of medications. Both the increase in maternal total body water and the decrease in albumin changes drug distribution and the bioavailability or free drug. Finally, alterations in hepatic function may affect drug metabolism. Serum levels of medication may also be decreased by the induction of the cytochrome P-450 system and because of increased hepatic extraction related to increased blood flow.[4]

Pregnancy is a hypercoaguable state particularly in the last trimester and post-partum as a means to prepare for labor and delivery. Fibrin generation is increased. This occurs because of increased levels of the procoagulant factors II, VII, VIII, IX, X, XII, and XIII, and because of a decrease in the anticoagulant proteins antithrombin III, protein S, and acquired resistance to activated protein C. Uncomplicated pregnancy is accompanied by substantial increase in markers of thrombosis and fibrinolytic activation, the latter reflected by increased D-dimer levels.[5]

Lastly, pregnancy is a state of relative immune tolerance. This immune tolerance seems to be mediated by regulatory T cells, which suppress maternal recognition of the semiallogeneic tissue of the fetus.[6] Immune tolerance may affect those disorders that are T-cell mediated.

CASE 1: ACUTE ISCHEMIC STROKE DURING PREGNANCY

A 28-year-old woman G2P1 (G = gravidum, number of pregnancies; P = partum, number of births) at 30 weeks gestation was last seen well at 10 AM. She was found on the ground not speaking or moving her right side at 10:50 AM. On initial examination, she was mute with a left gaze deviation and a dense right hemiplegia.

Questions

What is the most appropriate initial imaging test?
Should she receive intravenous tissue plasminogen activator (IV t-PA)?
Is she a potential candidate for intra-arterial (IA) therapy?
What are the most likely mechanisms for stroke during pregnancy?

Imaging During Pregnancy

Imaging during pregnancy is often necessary. In general, MRI is the imaging modality of choice. There have been no fetal harmful effects related to MRI in field strengths up to 3 T. The mother's health is the most important factor in maintaining the health of the fetus. Therefore radiation and contrast concerns should not delay critical imaging. Computed tomography imaging raises concern about fetal exposure to ionizing radiation. The level of radiation exposure from most diagnostic imaging is far below that known to cause fetal anomalies. However, not all effects of radiation are dose dependent. Therefore a risk-benefit analysis should be done to weigh the importance of a computed tomography scan on deciding emergent therapy. In an emergency the most appropriate imaging to take care of the mother and give the necessary answer to enable treatment is appropriate. In this case, a head computed tomography without contrast was done and was unremarkable.

Safety of Intravenous Tissue Plasminogen Activator in Pregnancy

Acute stroke treatment within 3 hours from onset with IV t-PA is a Food and Drug Administration approved treatment of ischemic stroke, and the American Stroke Association/American Heart Association endorses the extension of the treatment window to 4.5 hours.[7,8] There are only a few case reports of using IV t-PA in pregnancy, but the benefit seems to outweigh the risk. The studies of using IV t-PA are summarized in **Table 1**. The patient did receive IV t-PA.

Safety of Intra-Arterial Therapy in Pregnancy

The number of pregnant women who have received IA therapy is small. A summary of the maternal and fetal outcomes following IA therapy is shown in **Table 2**. Given the recent validation of the benefit of IA therapy in ischemic stroke, pregnant women should be offered IA therapy if they are appropriate candidates.[20–23] This patient was considered for IA therapy, but during the preparation for the arteriogram, fetal monitoring showed prominent decelerations. The risks of further therapy were believed to outweigh the potential benefit and IA therapy was not done. Her brain MRI and brain magnetic resonance angiogram are shown in **Figs. 1** and **2**.

Mechanisms of Stroke During Pregnancy

The types of strokes reported in various studies depend on the population studied, the detail of evaluation, and the classification system used. In data acquired from a hospital-based study most ischemic strokes in pregnancy and the postpartum period were caused by cardiac embolus or are associated with preeclampsia/eclampsia (PEE).[24,25] In community populations the causes of pregnancy-related stroke differ with no reported strokes related to cardiac embolus and a large group of patients with stroke of undetermined cause.[26,27] Both hemorrhagic and ischemic strokes are most common in the last trimester and postpartum period reflecting the timing of PEE and the maximum time of hypercoagulability (**Boxes 1** and **2**).

In our patient there was a family history of hypercoagulability, but extensive evaluation did not reveal the cause of her stroke. She was discharged to a rehabilitation facility on low-molecular-weight heparin. Two months later, she was readmitted for an elective cesarean section (C-section) and delivered a healthy male infant weighing 3033 g. A year later, the patient had almost normal language with only mild dysfluency with excellent comprehension and expression. She walked with mild right leg weakness, but had persistent severe spastic weakness of the right arm.

Table 1 Use of IV t-PA in pregnancy		
Study, Year	**Maternal Outcome**	**Fetal Outcome**
Dapprich,[9] 2002	Improved	No complications
Weise,[10] 2006	No complications	No complications
Leonhardt,[11] 2006	No complications	No complications
Murugappan,[12] 2006; three cases	1. Minor intrauterine bleed 2. No complications 3. Died	1. Medically terminated 2. Medically terminated 3. Died
Yamaguchi,[13] 2010	Improved	No complications
Hori,[14] 2013	Improved	No complications
Tassi,[15] 2013	Improved	No complications
Ritter,[16] 2014	Improved	No complications

Table 2		
Use of IA t-PA in Pregnancy		
Study, Year	**Maternal Outcome**	**Fetal Outcome**
Elford,[17] 2002	Minor intracranial hemorrhage	No complications
Johnson,[18] 2005	Improved	No complications
Murugappan,[12] 2006	No complications	No complications
Li,[19] 2012	Improved	No complications

CASE 2: ECLAMPSIA

A 29-year-old woman G1P0 at 30 weeks gestation presented with headache, blurry vision, and vomiting. Her BP was 197/110. She received magnesium, labetalol, and hydralazine. She had a generalized seizure while in the emergency room, and underwent an emergent C-section. She had another generalized seizure while a spinal epidural was attempted. She continued to have recurrent seizures. Her BP was normal after the C- section. Laboratory studies were notable for white blood cell count (4.0–11.0), normal hematocrit and platelet count, and urinalysis with 3+ protein. She was transferred for further management of her seizures. Her brain MRI is shown in **Fig. 3**.

Questions

What is the definition of PEE?
What are the risks of PEE?
What is the pathophysiology of PEE?
How should this patient be managed?

Definition of Preeclampsia/Eclampsia

Preeclampsia is defined by a rise in systolic BP (>140 mm Hg or >30 points from the women's baseline systolic BP) and proteinuria greater than 3 g in 24 hours. Eclampsia

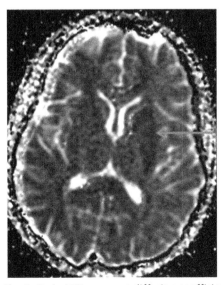
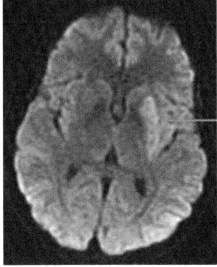

Fig. 1. Brain MRI apparent diffusion coefficient imaging on the left and diffusion-weighted imaging on the right showing an acute infarct in the lenticulostriate territory (*arrows*).

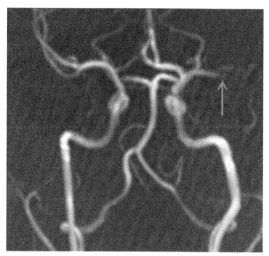

Fig. 2. Brain magnetic resonance angiography showing occlusion (*arrow*) of the left middle cerebral artery.

is defined by a change in mentation and seizures. A subset of patients with eclampsia can develop the syndrome of hemolytic anemia, liver abnormalities, and low platelets (HELLP). Case 2 is an example of eclampsia.

Risks of Preeclampsia/Eclampsia

PEE is a cause of significant morbidity and mortality for the mother and the fetus. Maternal risks include an increase in the risk of abruptio placenta, aspiration, acute renal failure, development of disseminated intravascular coagulopathy/HELLP, and death. Fetal complications may include growth restriction, hypoxic injury, preterm delivery, and death.[28] In addition, PEE is a major contributor of future maternal cardiovascular risk.[29]

Pathophysiology

PEE is caused by endothelial dysfunction. Placental ischemia is the cause of this condition, not the fetus. The genesis of PEE occurs early in pregnancy, likely at the time of placental implantation. It is believed that the cytotrophoblasts do not adequately penetrate the maternal myometrium, so a low capacitance placental vascular system

---

Box 1
Causes of ischemic stroke to consider in pregnancy and postpartum

Cardiac emboli

Dissection

Preeclampsia/eclampsia

Cerebral venous thrombosis

Reversible cerebral vasoconstriction syndrome

Other (amniotic fluid emboli, choriocarcinoma, air emboli, Sheehan syndrome, fat emboli)

Box 2
Causes of hemorrhagic stroke in pregnancy and postpartum

Vascular malformation

Preeclampsia/eclampsia

Cerebral venous thrombosis

Reversible cerebral vasoconstriction syndrome

Cerebral aneurysm

is not established. This sets up a milieu of ischemia causing an imbalance with high levels of antiangiogenic factors, and low levels of proangiogenic factors, such as vascular endothelial growth factor and placental growth factor. Inflammation also contributes to endothelial damage.[30] This leads to hypertension, additional ischemia, and endothelial damage in end organs: in the kidney causing proteinuria; in the liver causing abnormal liver function tests and a coagulopathy; and in the brain, changes occur in the posterior white matter. The posterior circulation vessels have less ability to autoregulate and are more prone to endothelial injury. Injury is manifested by edema in posterior white matter. This syndrome is called posterior reversible encephalopathy syndrome (PRES) (see **Fig. 3**). The neurologic sequelae of eclampsia include seizures, confusion, headache, and visual symptoms. In addition, ischemic stroke and hemorrhage can also occur.

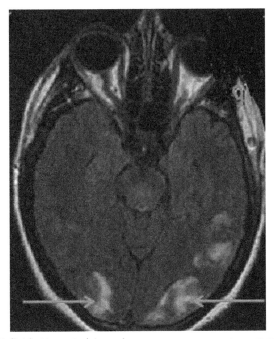

Fig. 3. Brain MRI fluid-attenuated inversion recovery sequence; *arrows* depict posterior white matter changes consistent with posterior reversible encephalopathy syndrome.

Management

The definitive treatment of PEE is delivery of the infant and placenta. The decision as to timing and mode of delivery is related to the severity of the PEE and gestational age of the fetus. BP management is critical; the usual agents used include labetolol, hydralazine, and calcium channel blockers. Steroids may be given to accelerate fetal lung development for infants with a gestational age of 24 to 34 weeks.[31] First-line seizure prophylaxis and treatment is with magnesium sulfate. Studies have shown that magnesium sulfate reduces the risk of seizure in women with severe preeclampsia and is more efficacious than phenytoin.[32]

CASE 3: REVERSIBLE VASOSPASM SYNDROME

A 39-year-old woman G3P3 on postpartum Day 4 following an urgent C-section for PEE with a severe manifestation of hemolytic anemia, elevated liver enzymes and low platelets, and HELLP syndrome complained of a severe bifrontal headache that was maximal at onset. She was markedly hypertensive with systolic BPs in the 230s. Temperature was 99.0°F; BP was 143/77; heart rate was 69; respiratory rate was 16. The neurologic examination was normal. Laboratory studies showed persistently abnormal liver function tests; white blood cell count, 10.7 K/µL (4.0–11.0); hematocrit, 31.2%; platelet count, 155 K/µL (150–450); and fibrinogen, 790 mg/dL (200–450). **Fig. 4** shows the imaging.

Questions

How does reversible cerebral vasoconstriction syndrome (RCVS) usually present?
What is the underlying pathophysiology?
What are the usual precipitants?
How should this patient be managed?

Presentation

A thunderclap headache, a headache that is severe and maximal intensity at onset, is the core and most common feature of this syndrome. Repetitive thunderclap

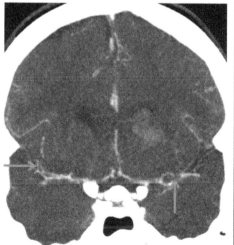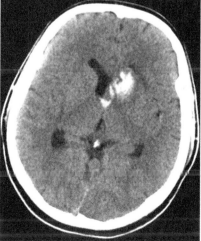

Fig. 4. On the left is the computed tomography angiogram; *arrows* show vascoconstriction involving both middle cerebral arteries. On the right is the noncontrast head computed tomography showing a hemorrhage in the left caudate with intraventricular extension.

headaches may also occur. The headache may be the only feature (as in our case) or associated with focal neurologic deficits. The deficits can be gradual in onset mimicking migraine or occur abruptly.[33] RCVS can cause major complications including seizure, ischemic stroke, and hemorrhage either intracranial or subarachnoid.[33]

Pathophysiology

The pathophysiology of RCVS strongly overlaps that associated with PRES. The endothelial changes that occur as part of PRES can also cause vessel constriction or rupture leading to RCVS. The vasoconstriction when severe can cause ischemic stroke often in border zone territories. Subarachnoid and intracranial hemorrhage is caused by vessel dilatation and rupture.[34,35]

Precipitants

In pregnancy women who develop PEE (as illustrated in the case) are at risk for RCVS because of the underlying shared pathophysiology. There are several medications known to cause RCVS either by increasing sympathetic tone or by directly altering endothelial function. In the postpartum period bromocriptine given to suppress lactation is a common culprit. Serotonergic medications including many used for migraine and antidepressants can also precipitate RCVS in vulnerable individuals.[36]

Management

The mainstay of management is similar to that for PEE with magnesium and antihypertensive agents. If there is a medication trigger, that should be removed and other agents in that class avoided. The headache can be treated symptomatically. There is some evidence to suggest that the thunderclap headaches of RCVS respond to calcium channel blockers.[33]

CASE 4: MANAGEMENT OF MULTIPLE SCLEROSIS

A 28-year-old woman with relapsing remitting multiple sclerosis (MS) who has stable disease wants to get pregnant. She has had no relapses in the last year. She is on interferon-β1b and an oral contraceptive. Her neurologic examination is normal.

Questions

  What is the risk her child will have MS?
  What should be done about her medications?
  How is pregnancy likely to affect her MS?
  Should she breastfeed?

Multiple Sclerosis Genetics

Available data suggest that MS is inherited as a complex disorder from the interaction of genetic and environmental factors. There is some genetic predisposition. The risk of developing MS for an offspring of a parent with MS is 2% to 3% higher than the general population and higher if both parents have MS.[37]

Medication Management

As a rule, none of the MS disease-modifying therapies (DMT) are continued during pregnancy. **Table 3** shows the Food and Drug Administration classification and breastfeeding recommendations for the common medications used to treat MS. The length of time after discontinuing the DMT to wait before attempting to conceive

Table 3 MS therapies		
Treatment	Pregnancy Class	Breastfeeding
Interferons	C	Caution
Glatiramer acetate	B	Compatible
Fingolimod	C	Unknown
Azathioprine	D	Contraindicated
Methotrexate	X	Contraindicated
Corticosteroids	C	Compatible
Teriflunomide	X	Contraindicated
Dimethyl fumarate	C	Caution
Natalizumab	C	Caution

depends on the drug half-life. For example, a 1- to 2-month washout is recommended for the interferons, whereas a 3-month washout period is recommended for natalizumab. This patient should be counseled to stop her oral contraceptive. Once her menstrual cycle resumes she should discontinue her disease-modifying drug and attempt to conceive after a 1-month period.

Effect of Pregnancy on Multiple Sclerosis

MS is believed to be mediated by an upregulation of the ratio of T helper cells to T suppressor cells. The rate of pregnancy relapse in a MS study published in 1998 demonstrated that the relapse rate in the third trimester decreased, postpartum there was an increase in the relapse rate, but by 1 year postpartum the relapse rate had returned to the prepregnancy baseline.[38] This means that it is important to plan for pregnancy after disease stability has been achieved. Those women with active disease before pregnancy should be restarted on their DMT promptly postpartum. A flare during pregnancy can be treated with IV methylprednisolone sodium succinate (Solumedrol).

Breastfeeding

Breastfeeding may be protective. In one study comparing patients with MS who did not breastfeed with those who breastfed exclusively, of those who did not breastfeed 87% had a postpartum relapse, compared with 36% of the women with MS who breastfed exclusively for at least 2 months postpartum.[39] However, this study did not control for MS severity, so the women who chose not to breastfeed may have had more severe disease. Women with mild or moderately severe MS like the patient presented should be encouraged to breastfeed given the well-known benefits. However, those women with severe or active disease need to restart their DMT postpartum and forego breastfeeding.

CASE 5: EPILEPSY

A 22-year-old woman presents to clinic for evaluation of epilepsy. She is after a right parietal oligoastrocytoma resection and radiation, 2 years previously with epilepsy well controlled on phenytoin. She is actively trying to become pregnant. She had initially presented after a generalized seizure. Her neurologic examination is normal.

Questions

What are the teratogenic risk profiles of various antiepileptic drugs (AEDs)?
What are the maternal and fetal risks from seizure during pregnancy?
How does the management of AEDs change during pregnancy?

Teratogenicity Profiles of Antiepileptic Drugs

The background teratogenic risk for a general population of healthy women is 1.6% to 2.1%. The North American registry reported the following percent risks for major congenital malformation with monotherapy exposure: valproate, 10.7% (confidence interval [CI], 6.3%–16.9%); phenobarbital, 6.5% (CI, 2.1%–14.5%); lamotrigine, 2.7% (CI, 1.5%–4.3%); and carbamazepine, 2.5% (CI, 1.6%–3.7%).[40] Multiple studies have corroborated the relatively higher risk for malformations with valproate exposure.[41–43] A comparison of major congenital malformations among the AEDs when used as to monotherapy showed a low rate of major congenital malformation with lamtotrigine, 2.0% (CI, 1.4%–2.8%); levetriacetam, 2.4% (CI, 1.2%–4.3%); an intermediate rate for phenytoin, 2.9% (CI, 1.5%–5.0%); and a high rate for valproate, 9.3% (CI, 6.4%–13%).[41] In our patient treating her epilepsy with either levetriacetam or lamotrigine would lower the teratogenic risk. A switch to levetriacetam can be accomplished over several days, which is an advantage over the longer switch over time for lamotrigine. Furthermore, the teratogenic effects of AEDs seem to be dose related. Therefore, monotherapy at the lowest effective dose is recommended. In addition, folate supplementation of 0.4 to 5 mg daily should be begun before conception to lower the incidence of neural tube defects.[43]

Maternal and Fetal Risks from Seizure During Pregnancy

The risks of generalized seizures during pregnancy include maternal and fetal hypoxia and acidosis, fetal heart rate decelerations, and possibly miscarriages and stillbirths. Seizures can also result in trauma to mother and baby leading to membrane rupture, premature labor, and even death.[44] The effect of pregnancy on seizure frequency is variable with 20% to 33% of women experiencing an increase in seizure frequency and up to 50% to 83% having no change in their seizure frequency.[45] It is generally recommended that a woman have good seizure control for 6 to 9 months before conception.

The following recommendations were given to the patient: to initiate levetriacetam, after several days begin a phenytoin taper, and folate at 1 mg daily was also prescribed. Finally, it was recommended that she refrain from trying to conceive for 6 months to ensure that her epilepsy was controlled on the new AED.

Changes in Management of Antiepileptic Drugs During Pregnancy

Maintaining epilepsy control depends on keeping the predetermined preconception level of the AED stable. Because of the physiologic changes during pregnancy including increased volume of distribution, increased renal and hepatic clearance, decreased gastric absorption, and decreased albumin, AEDs levels tend to fall during pregnancy. During pregnancy the levels of lamotrigine, phenytoin, levetriacetam, carbamazepine, and oxcarbazepine all decrease in variable amounts and require drug level monitoring.[46]

In our patient, before conception the levetriacetam level that controlled her epilepsy should be determined and levels followed monthly during the pregnancy. This allows one to change levetriacetam dosing to maintain the prepregnancy therapeutic level. Postpartum the dose should be adjusted to slightly higher than the preconception baseline over 2 weeks to 3 months, depending on the AED. It is also important to educate the mother about newborn care and safety concerns for mothers with epilepsy including the importance of sleep disruption as a seizure trigger.

CASE 6: FEMORAL NEUROPATHY

The neurology service was asked to evaluate a 32-year-old woman G1P1 for right leg weakness 2 days postpartum. She had an uneventful vaginal delivery of a 3266-g baby with epidural analgesia. Initially, she noted right leg numbness and perceived knee weakness with weight bearing. On the first postpartum day, her leg buckled and she fell when she stood. She had no back or leg pain.

On examination, she had 4/5 weakness in right hip flexion and knee extension, diminished right patellar deep tendon reflex, and a sensory loss in her medial thigh and calf. Her hip abductor and adductor strength were normal. Her back was not tender and back range of motion was normal. She had some tenderness over the right inguinal ligament.

Questions

How common are lower extremity postpartum compression neuropathies?
What is the cause of this neuropathy?
What is the prognosis?

Incidence of Postpartum Lower Extremity Neuropathy

An obstetric postpartum neuropathy occurs in about 1% of deliveries. Risk factors for developing a lower extremity peripheral neuropathy include prolonged second stage of labor, instrumental delivery, short stature, and nulliparity. The lateral femoral cutaneous nerve is the most commonly injured nerve in the lower extremity, followed by the femoral, peroneal, lumbosacral plexus, sciatic, and obturator nerves in decreasing incidence.[47] The incidence of a postpartum femoral neuropathy is estimated at 2.8 per 100,000 of which 25% are bilateral.[48] This contrasts with the rarity of major complications from neuroaxial anesthesia. In one review of complications related to obstetric neuraxial anesthesia, the risk of an epidural hematoma was 1 in 183,383 patients and epidural abscess 1 in 168,391 patients.[49]

Causes of Femoral Neuropathy in the Postpartum Period

The femoral nerve can be compressed by retroperitoneal processes or more commonly as it passes under the inguinal ligament. Compression of the femoral nerve as the nerve passes under the inguinal ligament can occur related to abdominal distention from excessive weight gain, a large fetus, instrumental vaginal delivery, and maintenance of lithotomy position associated with prolonged second stage of labor. Other more rare causes include retroperitoneal hemorrhage and intrapelvic pathology.[48]

Prognosis

The mechanism of injury of postpartum lower extremity peripheral neuropathies and most plexopathies is related to nerve compression or a stretch injury at a vulnerable site. This usually results in a segmental demyelinating nerve injury with the axon remaining intact and no change in the neuronal body. Overall, the prognosis for recovery of obstetric nerve palsies is thought to be excellent because axonal injury is usually limited in this setting. Treatment is mostly supportive and symptomatic, including medication for neuropathic pain, bracing when appropriate, and physical therapy for motor impairment. The time for recovery of the neuropathy can range from days to 6 to 8 weeks, but may be longer if there is a component of axonal injury.

CASE 7: CARPAL TUNNEL SYNDROME

A 32-year-old woman G1P0 at 35 weeks of gestation came in for evaluation of bilateral hand pain. The pain had been a problem for several weeks. It woke her from sleep and was associated with hand numbness.

On examination she had normal hand intrinsic strength. There was a positive Tinel sign over both median nerves at the wrist and her sensory examination showed diminished pinprick in bilateral median nerve distributions.

Questions

How common is carpal tunnel syndrome (CTS) in pregnancy?
What are the differences in CTS in pregnancy and CTS outside of pregnancy?
How is CTS in pregnancy best managed?

Incidence

Carpal tunnel is the most common compressive neuropathy during pregnancy. In nonpregnant women the prevalence of CTS ranges from 0.7% to 9.2%.[50] In pregnancy the prevalence is as high as 62%.[51] There is a great deal of variability in the reported incidence depending on how CTS is defined, clinically or by nerve conduction studies.

How Is Carpal Tunnel Syndrome in Pregnancy Different?

The cause of CTS in pregnancy is not entirely understood. The most probable cause is believed related to edema in the carpal tunnel causing compression of the median nerve. This mechanism is supported by studies showing an increased incidence of CTS in women with hand swelling, gestational hypertension, and PEE.[51] This also explains why CTS is worst in the last trimester and why in pregnancy CTS is usually bilateral.

This is in contrast to the nonpregnant state where the dominant hand is most often affected. The common mechanism of injury outside of pregnancy is believed related to repetitive wrist movement. This repetitive movement leads to friction between the tendons and their sheaths causing inflammation, swelling, and finally fibrous tissue formation. The result is squeezing the median nerve in the carpal tunnel.[52]

Management of Carpal Tunnel Syndrome in Pregnancy

CTS in pregnancy is generally mild, so usually only symptomatic therapy is required. This means limiting aggravating activities and using cock-up splints primarily at night. If pain cannot be controlled steroid injections are efficacious with 50% of patients showing sustained symptom improvement at 15 months.[53] CTS in pregnancy generally does not require surgery and resolves in the first several weeks postpartum. However, in only half of the affected women does CTS completely disappear 1 year after delivery.[51]

REFERENCES

1. Pritchard JA. Changes in the blood volume during pregnancy and delivery. Anesthesiology 1965;26:393–9.
2. Metcalfe J, Ueland K. Maternal cardiovascular adjustments to pregnancy. Prog Cardiovasc Dis 1974;16:363–74.

3. Cheung KL, Lafayette RA. Renal physiology of pregnancy. Adv Chronic Kidney Dis 2013;20(3):209–14.
4. Pennell P. Antiepileptic drug pharmacokinetics during pregnancy and lactation. Neurology 2003;61(6 Suppl 2):S35–42.
5. Francalanci I, Comeglio P, Alessandrello A, et al. D-dimer concentrations during normal pregnancy, as measured by ELISA. Thromb Res 1995;78:399–403.
6. Leber A, Teles A, Zenclussen AC. Regulatory T cells and their role in pregnancy. Am J Reprod Immunol 2010;63:445–59.
7. Tissue plasminogen activator for acute ischemic stroke. The National Institute of Neurological Disorders and stroke rt-PA Stroke Study Group. N Engl J Med 1995; 333(24):1581–7.
8. Hacke W, Markku K, Bluhmki E, et al. Thrombolysis with alteplase 3 to 4.5 hours after acute ischemic stroke. N Engl J Med 2008;359:1317–29.
9. Dapprich M, Boessenecker W. Fibrinolysis with alteplase in a pregnant woman with stroke. Cerebrovasc Dis 2002;13:290.
10. Wiese KM, Talkad A, Mathews M, et al. Intravenous recombinant tissue plasminogen activator in a pregnant woman with cardioembolic stroke. Stroke 2006;37: 2168–9.
11. Leonhardt G, Nietsch GC, Buerke M, et al. Thrombolytic therapy in pregnancy. J Thromb Thrombolysis 2006;21(3):271–6.
12. Murugappan A, Coplin WM, Al-Sadat AN, et al. Thrombolytic therapy of acute ischemic stroke during pregnancy. Neurology 2006;66(5):768–70.
13. Yamaguchi Y, Kondo T, Ihara M, et al. Intravenous recombinant tissue plasminogen activator in an 18-week pregnant woman with embolic stroke. Rinsho Shinkeigaku 2010;50:315–9.
14. Hori H, Yamamoto F, Yasoyuki I, et al. Intravenous recombinant tissue plasminogen activator in a 14-week pregnant woman with embolic stroke due to protein S deficiency. Rinsho Shinkeigaku 2013;53:212–6.
15. Tassi R, Acampa M, Maroth G, et al. Systemic thrombolysis for stroke in pregnancy. Am J Emerg Med 2013;31:448.e1–3.
16. Ritter ML, Schuler A, Gangopadhyay R, et al. Successful thrombolysis of stroke with intravenous alteplase in the third trimester of pregnancy. J Neurol 2014; 261:632–4.
17. Elford K, Leader A, Wee R, et al. Stroke in ovarian hyperstimulation syndrome in early pregnancy treated with intra-arterial rt-PA. Neurology 2002;59:1270–2.
18. Johnson DM, Kramer DC, Cohen E, et al. Thrombolytic therapy for acute stroke in late pregnancy with intra-arterial recombinant tissue plasminogen activator. Stroke 2005;36:e53–5.
19. Li Y, Margraf J, Kluck B, et al. Thrombolytic therapy for ischemic stroke secondary to paradoxical embolism in pregnancy: a case report and literature review. Neurologist 2012;18:44–8.
20. Goyal M, Demchuk AM, Menon BK, et al. Randomized assessment of rapid endovascular treatment of ischemic stroke. N Engl J Med 2015;372:1019–30.
21. Campbell BCV, Mitchell PJ, Kleinig TJ, et al. Endovascular therapy for ischemic stroke with perfusion-imaging selection. N Engl J Med 2015;372:1009–18.
22. Berkhemer OA, Fransen PS, Beumer D, et al. A randomized trial of intraarterial treatment for acute ischemic stroke. N Engl J Med 2014;372:11–20.
23. Saver JL, Goyal M, Bonafe A, et al. Stent-retriever thrombectomy after intravenous t-PA vs. t-PA alone in stroke. N Engl J Med 2015;372:2285–95.
24. Feske SK, Klein AM, Ferrante KL. Clinical risk factors predict pregnancy-associated strokes. Stroke 2009;40(4):e18.

25. Jaigobin O, Silver FL. Stroke and pregnancy. Stroke 2000;31(12):2948–51

26. Sharshar T, Lamy C, Mas JL. Incidence and causes of stroke associated with pregnancy and puerperium. A study in public hospitals of Ile de France. Stroke in Pregnancy Study Group. Stroke 1995;26(6):930–6.

27. Kittner SJ, Stern BJ, Feeser BR, et al. Pregnancy and the risk of stroke. N Engl J Med 1996;335(11):768–74.

28. Baha Sibai B, Dekker G, Kupferminc M. Pre-eclampsia. Lancet 2005;365:785–99.

29. Ahmed R, Dunford J, Mehran R, et al. Pre-eclampsia and future cardiovascular risk among women, a review. J Am Coll Cardiol 2014;63:1815–22.

30. Maynard SE, Karumanchi SA. Angiogenic factors and preeclampsia. Semin Nephrol 2011;31:33–46.

31. Turner J. Diagnosis and management of pre-eclampsia: an update. Int J Womens Health 2010;2:327–37.

32. Lucas MJ, Leveno KJ, Cunningham G. A comparison of magnesium sulfate with phenytoin for the prevention of eclampsia. N Engl J Med 1995;333:201–5.

33. Chen SP, Fuh JL, Lirng JF, et al. Recurrent primary thunderclap headache and benign CNS angiopathy: spectra of the same disorder? Neurology 2006;67:2164–9.

34. Ducros A, Bousser MG. Reversible cerebral vasoconstriction syndrome. Pract Neurol 2009;9:256–67.

35. Singhai AB, Hajj-Ali RA, Topcuoglu MA, et al. Reversible cerebral constriction syndromes: analysis of 130 cases. Arch Neurol 2011;68(8):1005–12.

36. Singhal AB, Caviness VS, Begleiter AF, et al. Cerebral vasoconstriction and stroke after use of serotonergic drugs. Neurology 2002;58:130–3.

37. Alonso A, Hernan MA. Temporal trends in the incidence of multiple sclerosis: a systematic review. Neurology 2008;71(2):129–35.

38. Confavreux C, Huthinson MD, Hours MM, et al. Rate of pregnancy-related relapse in multiple sclerosis. N Engl J Med 1998;339:285–91.

39. Langer-Gould A, Huang SM, Gupta R, et al. Exclusive breastfeeding and the risk of postpartum relapses in women with multiple sclerosis. Arch Neurol 2009;66(8):958–63.

40. Hernández-Díaz S, Smith CR, Shen A, et al, For the North American AED Pregnancy Registry. Comparative safety of antiepileptic drugs during pregnancy. Neurology 2012;78(21):1692–9.

41. Morrow JI, Russell A, Gutherie E, et al. Malformation risks of anti-epileptic drugs in pregnancy: a prospective study from the UK Epilepsy and Pregnancy Register. J Neurol Neurosurg Psychiatry 2006;77:193–8.

42. Vajda FJ, Eadie MJ. Maternal valproate dosage and foetal malformations. Acta Neurol Scand 2005;112:137–43.

43. Van Allen M, Fraser FC, Dallaire L, et al. Recommendations on the use of folic acid supplementation to prevent the recurrence of neural tube defects. Can Med Assoc J 1993;149:1239–43.

44. Chen YH, Chiou HY, Lin HC, et al. Effect of seizures during gestation on pregnancy outcomes in women with epilepsy. Epilepsy Curr 2010;10(2):40–1.

45. EURAP Study Group. Seizure control and treatment in pregnancy: observations from the EURAP epilepsy pregnancy registry. Neurology 2006;66(3):354–60.

46. Harden CL, Pennell PB, Koppel BS, et al. Practice parameter update: management issues for women with epilepsy—focus on pregnancy (an evidence-based review): vitamin K, folic acid, blood levels, and breastfeeding: report of the Quality Standards Subcommittee and Therapeutics and Technology

Assessment Subcommittee of the American Academy of Neurology and American Epilepsy Society. Neurology 2009;73(2):142–9.

47. Wong CA, Scavone BM, Dugan S, et al. Incidence of postpartum lumbosacral spine and lower extremity nerve injuries. Obstet Gynecol 2003;101:279–88.

48. Massey EW, Stolp KA. Peripheral neuropathy in pregnancy. Phys Med Rehabil Clin N Am 2008;19:149–62.

49. Ruppen W, Derry S, McQuay H, et al. Incidence of epidural hematoma, infection, and neurological injury in obstetric patients with epidural analgesia/anesthesia. Anesthesiology 2006;104:394–9.

50. Andersen JH, Thomsen JF, Overgaard E, et al. Computer use and carpal tunnel syndrome: a 1-year follow-up studhy. JAMA 2003;289(22):2963–9.

51. Pazzaglia C, Caliandro P, Aprile I, et al. Multicenter study on carpal tunnel syndrome and pregnancy incidence and natural course. Acta Neurochir Suppl 2005;92:35–9.

52. Burt S, Deddens JA, Crombie K, et al. A prospective study of carpal tunnel syndrome: workplace and individual risk factors. Occup Environ Med 2013;70(8):568–74.

53. Osterman M, Ilyas AM, Matzon JL. Carpal tunnel syndrome in pregnancy. Orthop Clin North Am 2012;43:515–20.

Sports Neurology in Clinical Practice: Case Studies

Tad Seifert, MD

KEYWORDS

- Sports • Concussion • Headache • Traumatic brain injury
- Chronic traumatic encephalopathy • Exercise

KEY POINTS

- With regard to persistent posttraumatic headache, there is legitimate concern that duration of symptoms may have an impact on the efficacy of future treatment attempts.
- Without neuropathologic confirmation, a clinical diagnosis of chronic traumatic encephalopathy (CTE) cannot be made with a high degree of confidence.
- Sport-related headaches are challenging in a return-to-play context, because it is often unclear whether an athlete has an exacerbation of a primary headache disorder, has new-onset headache unrelated to trauma, or is in the recovery phase after concussion.
- Regular physical exercise may prove beneficial to multiple neurologic disease states.

It is only recently that neurologists have become more active participants in the realm of sports medicine. The field of sports neurology specifically addresses the neurologic aspects of sports and sports-related injuries. Many major professional and amateur sports programs have found neurologists to be crucial in determining when an athlete can return to play after an injury. Whether a general neurologist, designated subspecialist, or dedicated sports neurologist, however, each clinical neurologist ultimately encounters patients whose neurologic disorders either are a consequence of or have an impact on participation in an athletic activity. The 4 cases discussed provide a framework for a general neurologist's participation with such patients.

CASE 1. SPORT-RELATED CONCUSSION AND ASSOCIATED HEADACHE

A 22-year-old Division I male football player presented 3 months after his second lifetime concussion. The injury occurred via head-to-head collision with no associated loss of consciousness; however, the subject experienced approximately 4 hours of anterograde amnesia immediately postinjury. His initial recovery course was fairly typical, with expected headache, light and sound sensitivity, positional dizziness, and cognitive slowing. All symptoms resolved over the ensuing 2 weeks with the exception of

Sports Concussion Program, Norton Healthcare, NCAA Headache Task Force, 3991 Dutchmans Lane, Suite 310, Louisville, KY 40207, USA
E-mail address: tad.seifert@nortonhealthcare.org

Neurol Clin 34 (2016) 733–746
http://dx.doi.org/10.1016/j.ncl.2016.04.010
0733-8619/16/$ – see front matter © 2016 Elsevier Inc. All rights reserved.

continued persistent headache. For this reason, he was held out of all physical activity and was unable to return to practice and/or game participation the remainder of the season. The headache was unresponsive to various over-the-counter medical regimens; however, no prescription medication was attempted. His neurologic examination as well as MRI of the brain were all noted to be within normal limits despite his prolonged recovery. Due to this ongoing singular complaint of persistent posttraumatic headache, his primary care sports medicine physician ultimately referred him to a regional sports neurologist for further input.

Discussion

After concussion occurs, a complex neurophysiologic cascade is initiated resulting in the disruption of axonal and membrane function, including ionic flux with widespread neurotransmitter release, cerebral blood flow alterations, and synaptic dysfunction.[1,2] These physiological changes results in an injury of transient neurologic dysfunction, as evidenced by the clinical syndrome of concussion. The metabolic mismatch of decreased cerebral blood flow and increased glucose requirement is thought to be a potential cause of central nervous system (CNS) vulnerability and the presence of associated symptoms.[3] Headache is consistently the most common symptom after concussion and occurs in approximately 86% of athletes with sports-related concussion.[4] Approximately 90% of adults experience clinical recovery from concussion within 7 to 21 days, whereas up to 10% progress to postconcussion syndrome, which often includes persistent headache.[5] Prolonged recovery courses are more common in the pediatric population, with 15% still reporting postconcussion symptoms 90 days after injury.[6]

Multiple studies suggest that posttraumatic headache (PTH) characteristics after concussion are associated with cognitive impairments and prolonged symptoms, highlighting the considerable overlap of typical postconcussive symptoms and those commonly described in migraine.[7,8] Most recently, Kontos and colleagues[8] reported that patients with posttraumatic migraine had 7.3-times and 2.6-times increased risks of a protracted recovery compared with those with no headache or headache without migrainous symptoms, respectively. Previous research raises the possibility of a common molecular pathophysiologic cause of migraines and posttraumatic headache.[9–11] Mild head trauma can activate trigeminal nociception, similar to that seen in migraine. This, in turn, results in the sequential activation of second-order and third-order neurons within the brain stem, hypothalamus, and thalamus, leading to cortical spreading depression. The upper cervical sensory nerve roots that converge on the trigeminal nucleus caudalis may also contribute to the activation process, because inciting trauma results in forced flexion and extension of the cervical spine.[12]

Diagnosis

The patient in the case presented is experiencing persistent posttraumatic headache. Although a majority of patients with PTH have complete resolution of symptoms within 3 months from the time of injury, a small percentage of patients develop chronic headache (ie, persistent posttraumatic headache).[13] Multiple studies have documented recovery rates; however, the methodology of those studies varied greatly, providing for inconsistent results. The percentage of patients with headaches at 1 month varies from 31.3% to 90%, at 3 months from 47% to 78%, and at 1 year from 8.4% to 35%. Approximately 25% of patients report refractory headaches at 4 years.[14] The International Classification of Headache Disorders, 3rd edition (beta version) (ICHD-3), requires headache duration of greater than 3 months after traumatic injury to the head to fulfill the formal diagnosis of persistent headache attributed to traumatic brain injury to the head[15] (**Box 1**). When a new-onset headache occurs in close temporal

---

Box 1
Persistent headache attributed to traumatic injury to the head

A. Any headache fulfilling criteria C and D

B. Traumatic injury to the head has occurred

C. Headache is reported to have developed within 7 days after one of the following:
1. The injury to the head
2. Regaining consciousness after the injury to the head
3. Discontinuation of medication(s) that impair ability or sense or report headache after the injury to the head

D. Headache persists for greater than 3 months after the injury to the head

E. Not better accounted for by another ICHD-3 diagnosis

---

relation to trauma or injury to the head and/or neck, it is considered a secondary headache attributed to the trauma or injury. When a preexisting headache with the characteristics of a primary headache disorder becomes chronic after trauma or injury, both the initial headache diagnosis and an ICHD-3 diagnosis of headache attributed to trauma or injury to the head and/or neck (or 1 of its subtypes) is provided.[15]

Treatment

With regard to persistent posttraumatic headache, there is legitimate concern that duration of symptoms may have an impact on the efficacy of future treatment attempts. For this reason, some investigators have proposed an earlier and more aggressive treatment paradigm with regard to PTH; however, there is little evidence on its medical management.[16] Generally, treatment is approached as the primary headache disorder it most closely resembles in phenotype. A majority of PTHs exhibit migraine or probable migraine characteristics, although similarities to all primary headache types have been noted.[17]

A multidisciplinary approach is recommended in the management of PTH due to the spectrum of associated symptoms and presentations. For acute treatment, prophylactic nonsteroidal anti-inflammatory drugs, simple analgesics, and triptans are the usual first-line options depending on the symptomatology. Clinicians should be aware of potential medication overuse headaches with frequent use of these agents. Prescription drug formulations containing narcotics, butalbital, or benzodiazepines are generally not endorsed due to the risk of abuse and habituation. Prophylactic therapy typically includes an approach similar to migraine and/or tension-type headache treatment. This includes a standardized approach with β-blockers, antidepressants, or antiepileptic drugs. Propanolol, amitriptyline, and valproate have all shown statistically significant efficacy in the treatment of PTH.[18] Clinicians, however, should be mindful when using β-blockers in conditioned athletes, given the risk of exercise intolerance. Antiepileptics, such as topiramate, should also be used with caution given their propensity for perceived cognitive slowing – a common complaint in patients after concussion.

Other options in the treatment of PTH include trigger point injections and occipital nerve blocks. Loder and Biondi[19] reported effective treatment of chronic PTH with botulinum toxin injections. Although a valuable resource for the lay population, the concern that botulinum toxin may mask persistent headache could prevent a clinician from returning an asymptomatic athlete to play until the medication's 3-month duration of action has passed. Nonpharmacologic treatment methods also include physical therapy and manipulation, biofeedback and relaxation therapy, transcutaneous nerve stimulators, and behavioral therapies. Vestibular rehabilitation aids in the treatment of balance dysfunction due to migraine, cervicogenic dizziness, and other peripheral vestibular disorders.[20] Similar to cognitive rehabilitation, this remains a viable option in those athletes with prolonged symptoms postinjury.

Medical management of collegiate and professional athletes also requires strict adherence to various governing bodies and their respective regulations. Most organizations use the World Anti-Doping Association guidelines, which are the most regimented.[21] Others, including the National Football League, Major League Baseball, and the National Collegiate Athletic Association, have similar policies. Prohibited substances vary but in general include such drugs as anabolic steroids, amphetamines and other stimulants, glucocorticoids, β-agonists, β-blockers, peptide hormones and growth factors, hormone antagonists and modulators, diuretics and other masking agents, blood/oxygen transport enhancers, narcotics, and cannabinoids. Many of these medications are used in outpatient headache management, further increasing the demand for due diligence on the part of physicians treating such athletes.[22]

CASE 2: CHRONIC TRAUMATIC ENCEPHALOPATHY

A 51-year-old retired male boxer presented to an area neurologist at the urging of his wife. She reports a 3-year history of progressive mood swings, memory loss, emotional outbursts, and sleep disturbances. The patient had previously been reticent to seeking out formal medical evaluation due to an inherent distrust of medical professionals. He acknowledges feeling overwhelmed with an associated feeling of "loss of control." His boxing career encompassed a 20-year time period with his ultimate retirement from the sport occurring at age of 32. He reports being knocked unconscious 6 times during his amateur and professional career; however, he also reports other concussion-like episodes not involving loss of consciousness being "too numerous to count." Although endorsing definite elements of depression, he adamantly denies suicidal ideations – past or present. His past medical history is remarkable for opiate addiction in his late 20s but he denies active drug or alcohol use. His family history is remarkable for addiction and major depression in his mother. His father's medical history is unknown. The patient's spouse reports tremendous concern over recent media reports of former contact sport athletes suffering from chronic neurologic issues after retirement.

Discussion

CTE is a neurodegenerative disease associated with recurrent head trauma, including concussive and subconcussive injuries. It is thought to result in executive dysfunction, memory impairment, depression, apathy, poor impulse control, and eventually dementia. Since the description of CTE by Omalu and colleagues in a former professional football player, further cases of contact sports athletes have shown gross and microscopic pathology attributed to repeated exposure to concussive blows.[23–25] The disease has gained widespread public attention and has now been described postmortem in former hockey, baseball, rugby, and soccer players.[26] In these cases, tau protein deposition was proposed as the pathologic hallmark of the condition now known as CTE; however, tau deposition is a nonspecific marker of brain inflammation in response to many different stimuli, not all of which are traumatic.[26] McKee and colleagues[24,27,28] have reported findings consistent with CTE in the brains of approximately 80% to 100% of the former football players studied. This substantially high rate has led some to question a possible selection bias in the samples studied.[29] To date, the baseline rate of CTE in amateur and professional athletes is still unknown, and it remains uncertain how head trauma itself initiates disease pathology, acts to accelerate an underlying predisposition, or both.

More convincing evidence for the chronic sequelae of recurrent/cumulative head trauma has long been reported in the pathologic studies of combat sport athletes, such as boxers.[30] The syndrome of dementia pugilistica, or punch-drunk syndrome, was first described in the medical literature by Martland in 1928,[31] when he described a 38-year-old retired boxer with advanced parkinsonism, ataxia, behavioral changes, and pyramidal tract dysfunction. The clinical spectrum of dementia pugilistica is now known to be synonymous with the clinical phenotype of modern day CTE. The findings are typically delayed in onset and occur after an extended exposure to the sport, usually after a boxer retires or late in a boxer's career. Due to this delayed onset in clinical symptomatology, chronic neurologic dysfunction remains the most difficult safety challenge in combat sports. The true incidence and prevalence of chronic neurologic impairment in modern-day boxing remains unknown. The prevalence was approximately 17% among former professional boxers who were licensed by the British Boxing Board of Control from 1929 to 1955, with further increases seen as exposure to head trauma accumulated.[32] Despite this knowledge base within the professional boxing ranks, strong objective evidence of chronic neurologic pathology associated with amateur boxers remains elusive.[33]

Pathophysiology

The neurodegenerative pathophysiology of CTE is complex, and the neurologic sequelae are poorly understood. Areas of the cerebral cortex and limbic system seem most affected, with typical findings characterized by neurofibrillary tangles of TAR DNA-binding protein and phosphorylated tau.[34–36] Neurofibrillary tangles pathology in CTE is concentrated near the bottom of sulci, distinguishing it from Alzheimer disease (AD) pathology that is located primarily within the cerebral and entorhinal cortices.[37] Postmortem brain analysis also points to substantial brain atrophy, notably in the frontal cortex and medial temporal lobe in structures, such as the thalamus, hypothalamus, and mammillary glands.[34,38]

Diagnosis

Although the diagnosis of CTE in this patient should be included in the differential diagnosis, it can only be formally diagnosed postmortem. At the present time, the clinical diagnosis of CTE is difficult because there are no consensus diagnostic criteria or large-scale longitudinal clinicopathologic correlation studies. Although a history of remote head trauma may be suggestive of CTE, head trauma has been implicated as a risk factor for AD, Parkinson disease, amyotrophic lateral sclerosis, and other neurodegenerative diseases.[39–41] Multiple other clinical entities should also be ruled out in the setting of possible CTE, including primary psychiatric disorders, substance abuse, sleep disorders, and other subtypes of cognitive impairment. Therefore, without neuropathologic confirmation, at the present time, a clinical diagnosis of CTE cannot be made with a high degree of confidence. Some researchers are attempting to identify reliable screenings for CTE that can be used premortem. Ultimately, a range of neuropsychological tests, brain imaging, and biomarkers likely will be used to accurately diagnose CTE.

Comments

Lehman and colleagues[42] recently reported on the neurodegenerative causes of death among retired National Football League players. Although the overall mortality of the studied population was lower than predicted, the neurodegenerative mortality was li uuul :l liiries yreater than that of the general US pupululiun. Specifically, the rates of AD and amyotrophic lateral sclerosis were 4 times higher.

Despite the resurgence of interest in the long-term effects of sports concussion, it should be stressed that no empirical data yet exist regarding a dose-dependent threshold of developing chronic neurologic sequelae after head trauma (ie, How much head trauma is too much?). Furthermore, no level I evidence has demonstrated a causal link between concussion in sports and the development of CTE later in life. Some investigators have suggested a divergence of media accounts of sports-related concussion in relation to the existing scientific and medical findings.[43] Andrikopoulos[44] raised the question of whether individuals were creating a concussion crisis regarding CTE in a recent *JAMA Neurology* issue. The most recent version of the International Conference on Concussion in Sport consensus statement concluded, "It was further agreed that a cause and effect relationship has not yet been demonstrated between CTE and concussions or exposure to contact sports." At present, the interpretation of causation in the modern CTE case studies should proceed cautiously.[45] Prospective longitudinal studies are necessary to clarify the underlying biological mechanism of acute concussive injury and its influence in the evolution to chronic neuropathology.

CASE 3: SPORT-RELATED HEADACHE

An 18-year-old female swimmer presents with the complaint of recurrent headaches associated with each morning workout. Her past medical history is remarkable only for attention-deficit disorder, which has not required medical intervention. She has no prior history of headache or concussion. There is a strong family history of migraine in both mother and older sister. The headaches are described as migrainous in nature, with associated throbbing pain, photophobia, and phonophobia. They occur exclusively with onset of exercise and generally resolve within 30 minutes of physical activity cessation. She reports that use of over-the-counter analgesics provides some symptomatic relief, she but has not attempted preventative approaches.

Discussion

Sport-related and exercise-related headaches have received increased attention over the past 10 years, largely through increased awareness of concussive injury in sport and the military. Despite this renewed interest in postconcussive headache, other nontraumatic headaches occurring in sport are often misdiagnosed or overlooked altogether. These scenarios can complicate return-to-play decisions, because it is often unclear whether an athlete has an exacerbation of a primary headache disorder, has new-onset headache unrelated to trauma, or is in the recovery phase after concussion.[17] In the current case of the 18-year-old competitive swimmer, she reports a clear relationship of headache onset with exercise and was ultimately diagnosed with primary exercise headache (PEH).

Clinical Features

Previously known as benign exertional headache, it is now formally referred to as PEH in the ICHD-3[15] (**Box 2**). It was first described in 1968 by Rooke, who published a case series of 103 patients with exertional headache, concluding that this presentation may be a separate primary headache disorder.[46] Clinically, PEH often has migrainous features, such as throbbing pain, photophobia, phonophobia, nausea, and vomiting; however, this headache is described as a distinct entity, precipitated by any form of exercise in the absence of an intracranial disorder.[15] This self-limited disorder is prompted by exercise and becomes more severe with prolonged physical exertion,

---

Box 2
Primary exercise headache

A. At least 2 episodes fulfilling criteria B and C

B. Brought on by and occurring only during or after strenuous physical exercise

C. Lasting less than 48 hours

D. Not better accounted for by another ICHD-3 diagnosis

---

although short-duration isometric exertion alone can also serve as the sole precipitant. Initially termed, *weight lifter's headache*, there were early case reports of headaches occurring after maximal lifts, at times associated with arterial blood pressure readings of greater than 400/300 mm.[47]

A study 2008 by Pascual and colleagues[48] sought to clarify, among other factors, the prevalence and clinical features of PEH in patients presenting to a tertiary headache clinic. Of 6412 patients, only 11 reported headache provoked by prolonged physical exercise. This study remains the only prospective study to date in which neuroimaging was performed on all patients to exclude underlying secondary causes. Their study also substantiated previous findings that PEH is an uncommon, and most often self-limited, headache disorder that is frequently associated with comorbid migraine. In 2012, however, van der Ende-Kastelijn and colleagues[49] reported a PEH prevalence of 26% among a population of competitive cyclists, suggesting a higher prevalence of this headache type among athletes. Proposed risk factors in these patients included extreme exertion, decreased fluid intake, and warm weather. Although 54% of women (vs 44% of men) participating in this survey reported PEH, there is limited evidence identifying one gender as higher risk for the development of this disorder.[49] A family history of migraine has also been identified as an underlying risk factor for PEH.[50]

Pathophysiology

Although the exact pathophysiology of PEH remains unclear, some investigators have implicated internal jugular vein incompetence as a potential contributing source. Doepp and colleagues[51] found retrograde jugular flow via venous duplex ultrasound more frequently in patients with exertional headache versus control. These findings support the idea that dilated pain-sensitive venous sinuses as a result of venous congestion play a role in generating PEH. The presence of internal jugular vein incompetence does not fully explain the mechanism of PEH, however, because this finding is also seen in persons without the clinical complaint of headache.[52] Another theory involves the increase of cerebral arterial pressure and/or intrathoracic pressure resulting, similarly, in the dilation of pain-sensitive venous sinuses.[53,54] Other investigators posit that intracranial vascular anomalies, such as bilateral transverse sinus stenosis, can promote a paroxysmal and short-lasting increase of both cerebrospinal fluid pressure and venous pressure proximal to the stenosis, leading to the abrupt onset of short-lasting headaches with exertion.[55] Lastly, other mechanisms have been proposed, including the hypothesis that metabolic and myogenic factors may cause impaired cerebrovascular autoregulation.[56]

Differential Diagnosis

Other primary and secondary headaches can be precipitated by physical activity and subsequently mimic PEH. Secondary causes are present in up to one-third of exertional headaches: thus, it is mandatory in a first time occurrence to exclude other more ominous etiologies, such as arterial dissection, cardiac cephalalgia, or subarachnoid hemorrhage.[57]

Treatment

The prognosis for athletes with PEH is good; however, as discussed previously, this must be a diagnosis of exclusion. Treatment of PEH typically consists of indometh-acin, beginning at a dose of 25 mg to 50 mg prior to physical activity.[58] β-blockers, other prophylactic nonsteroidal anti-inflammatory drugs, and various migraine-specific preparations have also been reported, although firm evidence is lacking.[59–61] Lastly, there is good evidence that gradual warm-up prior to exertion and graded exercise programs can be beneficial in the prevention of the pain-inducing effects of moderate exercise.[62]

CASE 4: THE NEUROLOGIC BENEFIT OF EXERCISE

A 39-year-old healthy woman with a history of migraines without aura presented to her neurologist with an increased number of migraine attacks. Her headache frequency and severity had started to have a negative impact on her work and social functioning. She was concerned about what to do going forward and asked about the potential nonpharmacologic remedies as an alternative to the previous treatment attempts for her headaches. She had previously tried several prescription and herbal preventative measures without success, either because of lack of efficacy or the development of intolerable side effects. She was reluctant to consider botulinum toxin because a friend had a bad experience with the treatment. The patient inquires as to whether a regular exercise regimen is an option as an alternative to traditional headache prophylaxis.

Introduction

Understanding the influence of exercise on disease prevention and treatment is critical to the management of neurologic disorders. The general health benefits of exercise are widely accepted and encouraged in today's sedentary society. Routine exercise enhances the immune system and helps prevent cardiovascular disease, diabetes mellitus, obesity, and osteoporosis. Numerous age-related disorders are also known to benefit from exercise. In the general population, a physically active lifestyle during midlife is associated with longer survival rates in prospective studies. Increasing evidence shows that exercise also has significant benefits on cognition.[63,64] Unfortu-nately, routine physical activity is commonly neglected in both normal aging as well as neurologic disease states.[63] Effectively communicating the numerous benefits of physical exercise to the competitive athlete and layperson alike are key aspects to the practice of sports neurology.

Background

Physical activity is defined by the National Institutes of Health as bodily movement produced by skeletal muscles that results in energy expenditure.[65] In 2011, the American College of Sports Medicine issued its updated guidelines recommending at least 150 minutes of moderate-intensity physical exertion per week for most healthy adults[66] (**Box 3**). Despite these formal guidelines, fewer than 50% of Americans exer-cise on a regular basis.[67] A majority of studies on physical activity in various disease states involve dynamic exercise, which increases strength through active movement of muscles and joints. In contrast, static exercise exerts isometric contraction of a

---

Box 3
American College of Sports Medicine cardiorespiratory exercise guidelines

Adults should get at least 150 minutes of moderate-intensity exercise per week.

Exercise recommendations can be met through 30 to 60 minutes of moderate-intensity exercise (5 days per week) or 20 to 60 minutes of vigorous-intensity exercise (3 days per week).

One continuous session and multiple shorter sessions (of at least 10 minutes) are both acceptable to accumulate desired amount of daily exercise.

Gradual progression of exercise time, frequency, and intensity is recommended for best adherence and lowest injury risk.

People unable to meet these minimums can still benefit from some activity.

---

muscle without visible movement of the joint. Resistance in isometric exercise generally involves movement using the body's own resistance, structural objects, or weight lifting.[67] Rehabilitation methods used in neurologic disorders can involve both static and dynamic exercise.

Physiologic and Structural Changes

Despite ongoing interest in the effects of exercise on the CNS, it is still unclear how exercise alters the neurophysiologic activity of specific brain regions. Standardized low-resolution electromagnetic tomography has recently been used in combination with EEG to localize changes in cerebral activity with exercise. Acclimation to specific exercises and intensities resulted in unique cortical activation patterns with each stimulus, suggesting brain cortical activity variations induced by exercise depend on both exercise type and intensity.[68] These neurophysiologic data indicate that individualized exercise approaches may be necessary to achieve optimal outcomes.

A hallmark of the aging process is a progressive decrease in brain cortical volume. Several cross-sectional neuroimaging studies suggest that exercise may help slow this trend. Elderly people participating in regular aerobic exercise displayed less pronounced volume loss of the cortex and hippocampus.[69,70] In prospective studies, older people who engaged in up to 1 year of physical activity exhibited increased hippocampal or cortical gray matter volumes relative to more sedentary controls.[71] One study even found a direct relationship between walking distance as a measure of activity and stability of brain volume when studied prospectively.[72]

A 2013 study by Gons and colleagues,[73] using conventional MRI analysis, investigated the relationship between physical exercise and the structural integrity of cerebral white matter. Decreased levels of physical activity were associated with increased diffusivity measures in multiple white matter regions, reflecting impaired microstructural integrity. Multiple other studies using diffusion tensor imaging have supported the inverse relationship between impaired white matter integrity and cognitive status in subjects with radiographic small vessel disease.[74] Physical activity conceivably bestows a protective benefit on cerebral white matter integrity by modifying cardiovascular risk factors, which then results in improved cerebral perfusion.[73] A common mechanism between many of these vascular risk factors is inflammation, which exercise is known to ameliorate.[75] Prospective studies are necessary to confirm a causal relationship between sedentary habits and neuroimaging abnormalities.

In addition to its relationship with brain cytoarchitecture and electrophysiology, exercise may promote neuroprotection through systemic mechanisms. Cardiovascular modifications seen in aerobic exercise are influenced by central regions involved in autonomic nervous system regulation. This CNS plasticity involves several neuronal regions involved in sympathetic output, such as the caudal ventrolateral medulla, rostral ventrolateral medulla, and nucleus tractus solitarii. This suggests that some positive effects of exercise are partially because of reductions in sympathetic nervous system expression. It is also conceivable that increased sympathetic activity in sedentary people relate to their increased cardiovascular risks.[76]

Discussion

Regarding the case of the 39 year old seeking other treatment options for migraine prevention, several studies have confirmed that exercise therapy results in a reduction in frequency and duration of migraine attacks.[77,78] Darabaneanu and colleagues[78] reported a significant reduction in migraine frequency and duration after completing a 10-week program of aerobic exercise 3 times a week, although high-intensity training was required to reach clinically significant improvement. Assuming no contraindication to physical activity exists in this patient (and no history of exercise precipitating her headaches), this recommendation could be offered as an adjunct treatment. Furthermore, regular physical exercise may also prove beneficial to multiple neurologic disease states other than migraine. Credible evidence exists for its efficacy in Parkinson disease, AD, traumatic brain injury, epilepsy, and multiple sclerosis. The broad-reaching need for exercise therapy in neurologic disease is clear, and neurologists should address this with all patients encountered.

REFERENCES

1. Choe MC, Babikian T, DiFiori J, et al. A pediatric perspective on concussion pathophysiology. Curr Opin Pediatr 2012;24:689–95.
2. Barkhoudarian G, Hovda DA, Giza CC. The molecular pathophysiology of concussive brain injury. Clin Sports Med 2011;30:33–48.
3. Giza CC, Hovda DA. The new neurometabolic cascade of concussion. Neurosurgery 2014;75:524–33.
4. Guskiewicz KM, Weaver NL, Paudua DA, et al. Epidemiology of concussion in collegiate and high school football players. Am J Sports Med 2000;28:643–50.
5. Guskiewicz KM, McCrea M, Marshall SW, et al. Cumulative effects associated with recurrent concussion in collegiate football players: the NCAA concussion study. JAMA 2003;290(19):2549–55.
6. Eisenberg MA, Andrea J, Meehan W, et al. Time interval between concussions and symptom duration. Pediatrics 2013;132(1):8–17.
7. Mihalik JP, Stump JE, Collins MW, et al. Posttraumatic migraine characteristics in athletes following sports-related concussion. J Neurosurg 2005;102:850–5.
8. Kontos AP, Elbin RJ, Lau B, et al. Posttraumatic migraine as a predictor of recovery and cognitive impairment after sport-related concussion. Am J Sports Med 2013; 41(7):1497–504.
9. Gilkey SJ, Ramadan NM, Aurora TK, et al. Cerebral blood flow in chronic posttraumatic headache. Headache 1997;37:583–7.
10. Lauritzen M. Pathophysiology of the migraine aura: the spreading depression theory. Brain 1994;117:119–210.
11. Lucas S. Headache management in concussion and mild traumatic brain injury. PM R 2011;2(1 Suppl 2):S406–12.
12. Piovesan EJ, Kowacs PA, Oshinsky ML. Convergence of cervical and trigeminal sensory afferents. Curr Pain Headache Rep 2003;7(5):377–83.
13. Seifert TD, Evans RW. Posttraumatic headache: a review. Curr Pain Headache Rep 2010;14:292–8.

14. Evans RW. The postconcussion syndrome. In: Aminoff M, editor. Neurology and general medicine. 4th edition. Philadelphia: Elsevier; 2007. p. 593–603.

15. Headache Classification Subcommittee of the International Headache Society. The International Classification of Headache Disorders, 3rd ed. (beta version). Cephalalgia 2013;33(9):629–808.

16. Lucas S, Hoffman JM, Bell KR, et al. A prospective study of prevalence and characterization of headache following mild traumatic brain injury. Cephalalgia 2014; 34(2):93–102.

17. Meehan WP. Medical therapies for concussion. Clin Sports Med 2011;30:115–24.

18. Gladstone J. From psychoneurosis to ICHD-2: an overview of the state of the art in post-traumatic headache. Headache 2009;49:1097–111.

19. Loder E, Biondi D. Use of botulinum toxins for chronic headaches: a focused review. Clin J Pain 2002;18:169–76.

20. Vidal PG, Goodman AM, Colin A, et al. Rehabilitation strategies for prolonged recovery in pediatric and adolescent concussion. Pediatr Ann 2012;41(9):1–6.

21. World Anti-Doping Agency. The world anti-doping code: the 2016 prohibited list, international standard. 2016. Available at: https://www.usada.org/wp-content/uploads/wada-2016-prohibited-list-en.pdf. Accessed May 1, 2016.

22. Conidi FX. Sports-related concussion: the role of the headache specialist. Headache 2012;52(S1):15–21.

23. Omalu BI, DeKosky ST, Minster RL, et al. Chronic traumatic encephalopathy in a National Football League player. Neurosurgery 2005;57(1):128–34.

24. McKee AC, Stein TD, Nowinski CJ, et al. The spectrum of disease in chronic traumatic encephalopathy. Brain 2013;136(Pt 1):43–64.

25. Baugh CM, Stamm JM, Riley DO, et al. Chronic traumatic encephalopathy: neurodegeneration following repetitive concussive and subconcussive brain trauma. Brain Imaging Behav 2012;6(2):244–54.

26. Mietelska-Porowska A, Wasik U, Goras M, et al. Tau protein modifications and interactions: their role in function and dysfunction. Int J Mol Sci 2014;15:4671–713.

27. McKee AC, Cantu RC, Nowinski CJ, et al. Chronic traumatic encephalopathy in athletes: progressive tauopathy after repetitive head injury. J Neuropathol Exp Neurol 2009;68(7):709–35.

28. McKee AC, Stein TD, Kiernan P, et al. The neuropathology of chronic traumatic encephalopathy. Brain Pathology 2015;25(3):350–64.

29. Solomon GS, Sills A. Chronic traumatic encephalopathy and the availability cascade. Phys Sportsmed 2014;42(3):26–31.

30. Corsellis JA, Bruton CJ, Freeman-Browne D. The aftermath of boxing. Psychol Med 1973;3(3):270–303.

31. Martland HS. Punch drunk. JAMA 1928;91(15):1103–7.

32. Roberts AH. Brain damage in boxers. London: Pitman Publishing; 1969.

33. Loosemore M, Knowles CH, Whyte GP. Amateur boxing and risk of chronic traumatic brain injury: systemic review of observational studies. Br J Sports Med 2008;42:564–7.

34. McKee AC, Cantu RC, Nowinski CJ, et al. Chronic traumatic encephalopathy in athletes: progressive tauopathy after repetitive head injury. J Neuropathol Exp Neurol 2009;68(7):709–35.

35. Stern RA, Riley DO, Daneshvar DH, et al. Long-term consequences of repetitive brain trauma: chronic traumatic encephalopathy. PM R 2011;3(10 Suppl 2): S460–7.

36. Gavett DE, Stern RA, McKee AC. Chronic traumatic encephalopathy: a potential late effect of sport-related concussive and subconcussive head trauma. Clin Sports Med 2011;30(1):179–88.

37. Braak H, Braak E. Neuropathological stageing of Alzheimer-related changes. Acta Neuropathol 1991;82(4):239–59.

38. Carman A, Ferguson R, Cantu R, et al. "Mind the gaps": a multidisciplinary proposal to advance research in short-term and long term cognitive outcomes following youth sports-related concussions. Nat Rev Neurol 2014;11:230–44.

39. Mortimer JA, van Duijn CM, Chandra V, et al. Head trauma as a risk factor for Alzheimer's disease: a collaborative re-analysis of case-control studies. EURODEM Risk Factors Research Group. Int J Epidemiol 1991;20:S28–35.

40. Goldman SM, Tanner CM, Oakes D, et al. Head injury and Parkinson's disease risk in twins. Ann Neurol 2006;60:65–72.

41. Chen H, Richard M, Sandler DP, et al. Head injury and amyotrophic lateral sclerosis. Am J Epidemiol 2007;166:810–6.

42. Lehman EJ, Hein MJ, Baron SL, et al. Neurodegenerative causes of death among retired National Football League players. Neurology 2012;79:1970–4.

43. Barr WB. An evidence based approach to sports concussion: confronting the availability cascade. Neuropsychol Rev 2013;23:271–2.

44. Andrikopoulos J. Creating a concussion crisis and chronic traumatic encephalopathy. JAMA Neurol 2014;71:654.

45. McCrory P, Meeuwisse W, Aubrey M, et al. Consensus statement on concussion in sport: the 4th International Conference on Concussion in Sport held in Zurich. Br J Sports Med 2012;2013(47):250–8.

46. Rooke ED. Benign exertional headache. Med Clin North Am 1968;52:801–8.

47. MacDougall JD, Tuxen D, Sale DG, et al. Arterial blood pressure response to heavy resistance exercise. J Appl Physiol 1985;58(3):785–90.

48. Pascual J, Gonzalez-Mandly A, Martin R, et al. Headaches precipitated by cough, prolonged exercise or sexual activity: a prospective etiological and clinical study. J Headache Pain 2008;9:259–66.

49. van der Ende-Kastelijn K, Oerlemans W, Goedegebuure S. An online survey of exercise-related headaches among cyclists. Headache 2012;52:1566–73.

50. Silbert PL, Edis RH, Stewart-Wynne EG, et al. Benign vascular sexual headache and exertional headache: interrelationships and long term prognosis. J Neurol Neurosurg Psychiatry 1991;54(5):417–21.

51. Doepp F, Valdueza JM, Schreiber SJ. Incompetence of internal jugular valve in patients with primary exertional headache: a risk factor? Cephalalgia 2007;28:182–5.

52. Halker RB, Vargas BB. Primary exertional headache: updates in the literature. Curr Pain Headache Rep 2013;17:337.

53. Thomaides T, Karapanayiotides T, Spantideas A, et al. Are transient increases in blood pressure during the treadmill stress test associated with headache? Cephalalgia 2006;26(7):837–42.

54. Smith ED, Swartzon M, McGrew CA. Headaches in athletes. Curr Sports Med Rep 2014;13(1):27–32.

55. Donnet A, Valade D, Houdart E, et al. Primary cough headache, primary exertional headache, and primary headache associated with sexual activity: a clinical and radiological study. Neuroradiology 2013;55:297–305.

56. Heckman JG, Hilz MJ, Muck-Weymann M, et al. Benign exertional headache/benign sexual headache: a disorder of myogenic cerebrovascular autoregulation? Headache 1997;37:597–8.

57. MacGregor A, Frith A. ABC of headache. Oxford (United Kingdom): Blackwell Publishing Ltd; 2009. p. 46–50.
58. Diamond S, Medina JL. Benign exertional headache: successful treatment with indomethacin. Headache 1979;19:249.
59. McCrory P. Headaches and exercise. Sports Med 2000;30:221–9.
60. Allena M, Rossi P, Tassorelli C, et al. Focus on therapy of the chapter IV headaches: primary cough headache, primary exertional headache, and primary headache associated with sexual activity. J Headache Pain 2010;11:525–30.
61. Pascual J. Other primary headache disorders. Neurol Clin 2009;27:557–61.
62. Hindiyeh NA, Krusz JC, Cowan RP. Does exercise make migraines worse and tension type headaches better? Curr Pain Headache Rep 2013;17:380.
63. Sun Q, Townsend MK, Okereke OI, et al. Physical activity at midlife in relation to successful survival in women at age 70 years or older. Arch Intern Med 2010; 170(2):194–201.
64. Middleton LE, Barnes DE, Lui LY, et al. Physical activity over the life course and its association with cognitive performance and impairment in old age. J Am Geriatr Soc 2010;58(7):1322–6.
65. Caspersen CJ, Powell KE, Christenson GM. Physical activity, exercise, and physical fitness: definitions and distinctions for health-related research. Public Health Rep 1985;100(2):126–31.
66. Garber CE, Blissmer B, Deschenes MR, et al. American College of Sports Medicine position stand. Quantity and quality of exercise for developing and maintaining cardiorespiratory, musculoskeletal, and neuromotor fitness in apparently healthy adults: guidance for prescribing exercise. Med Sci Sports Exerc 2011;43(7):1334–59.
67. Diehl JJ, Choi H. Exercise: the data on its role in health, mental health, disease prevention, and productivity. Prim Care 2008;35(4):803–16.
68. Brummer V, Schneider S, Abel T, et al. Brain cortical activity is influenced by exercise mode and intensity. Med Sci Sports Exerc 2011;43(10):1863–72.
69. Gordon BA, Rykhlevskaia EI, Brumback CR, et al. Neuroanatomical correlates of aging, cardiopulmonary fitness level, and education. Psychophysiology 2008; 45(5):825–38.
70. Erickson KI, Prakash RS, Voss MW, et al. Aerobic fitness is associated with hippocampal volume in elderly humans. Hippocampus 2009;19(10):1030–9.
71. Erickson KI, Voss MW, Prakash RS, et al. Exercise training increases size of hippocampus and improves memory. Proc Natl Acad Sci U S A 2011;108(7): 3017Y3022.
72. Erickson KI, Raji CA, Lopez OL, et al. Physical activity predicts gray matter volume in late adulthood: the cardiovascular health study. Neurology 2010; 75(16):1415–22.
73. Gons RA, Tuladhar AM, de Laat KF, et al. Physical activity is related to the structural integrity of cerebral white matter. Neurology 2013;81(11):971–6.
74. van Norden AG, de Laat KF, van Dijk EJ, et al. Diffusion tensor imaging and cognition in cerebral small vessel disease: the RUN DMC study. Biochim Biophys Acta 2012;1822(3):401–7.
75. Alonso-Frech F, Sanahuja JJ, Rodriguez AM. Exercise and physical therapy in early management of Parkinson disease. Neurologist 2011;17(6 Suppl 1):S47–53.
76. Martins-Pinge MC. Cardiovascular and autonomic modulation by the central nervous system after aerobic exercise training. Braz J Med Biol Res 2011;44(9):848–54.

77. Varkey E, Cider A, Carlsson J, et al. Exercise as migraine prophylaxis: a randomized study using relaxation and topiramate as controls. Cephalalgia 2011;31(14): 1428–38.

78. Darabaneanu S, Overath CH, Rubin D, et al. Aerobic exercise as a therapy option for migraine: a pilot study. Int J Sports Med 2011;32(6):455–60.

Neurological Fallacies Leading to Malpractice

A Case Studies Approach

James C. Johnston, MD, JD[a],*, Knut Wester, MD, PhD[b,c],
Thomas P. Sartwelle, BBA, LLB[d]

KEYWORDS

- Medical malpractice • Neurologic malpractice • Intracranial arachnoid cyst
- Migraine headache • Stroke • Cerebral palsy • Electronic fetal monitoring

KEY POINTS

- Decompressive surgery should be considered for any symptomatic intracranial arachnoid cyst regardless of size or location.
- More aggressive neuroimaging is warranted in patients with headache and a normal examination until further studies refine the current guidelines.
- Litigation for failing to recommend or administer tissue plasminogen activator (tPA) to eligible patients will continue to increase; however, tPA should be avoided in patients with stroke on awakening until randomized controlled trials identify a subset of patients that may benefit from treatment.
- Cerebral palsy (CP) litigation continues despite uncontradicted evidence that birth events rarely cause CP and electronic fetal monitoring neither predicts nor prevents CP. The next litigation target is hypothermia for neonatal encephalopathy.

Wisdom in recognizing cases that are likely to involve you in suits for malpractice, and in foreseeing and forestalling the suits themselves, is a valuable power. Take care that this wisdom does not come too late or cost you too much.
—DW Cathell, MD, The Physician Himself, 1890[1]

Neurology has evolved to a high-risk specialty plagued by steep indemnity claims, with a high payment ratio, that are more costly to defend than claims in any other

Funding: The authors received no financial support for the research, authorship, or publication of this article.
Disclosures: The authors have nothing to disclose.
[a] Legal Medicine Consultants, 1130 N Loop 1604 West, Suite 108-623, San Antonio, TX 78248, USA; [b] Department of Clinical Medicine K1, University of Bergen, Bergen, Norway; [c] Department of Neurosurgery, Haukeland University Hospital, Bergen 5021, Norway; [d] Deans and Lyons, LLP, 1001 Fannin, Houston, TX 77002, USA
* Corresponding author.
E-mail address: johnston@GlobalNeurology.com

Neurol Clin 34 (2016) 747–773
http://dx.doi.org/10.1016/j.ncl.2016.04.011
0733-8619/16/$ – see front matter © 2016 Elsevier Inc. All rights reserved.

neurologic.theclinics.com

Specialty.[7] Although the literature is replete with risk management recommendations for practicing neurologists, that mostly generic advice is of limited use when confronted with an office full of real-world patients seeking answers and relief from ongoing symptoms that have altered their lives. Importantly, that generic advice rarely assists neurologists when clinical symptoms fail to follow the textbook presentations as is so often the case. Thus true risk management consist of 2 principles: first, becoming familiar with fundamental medical malpractice litigation concepts like negligence, standard of care, and understanding the role of evidence-based medicine as that concept is used in the clinic as well as the courtroom; second, heightened attention to those patients presenting with clinical entities that are known to engender common diagnostic errors leading to claims and litigation.

There are several instructive articles and books describing generic litigation principles and providing guidance for the treatment of common neurologic presentations,[2–5] but this article highlights fact-specific cases in everyday clinical practice in which medical decision making is overburdened and clouded by myths and misinformation that, unrecognized, could lead to malpractice liability. These real cases were selected because they encompass conditions that affect a large segment of the population, generate recurring claims, and have the potential for exceptionally high indemnity payments or judgments because of catastrophic injury and suffering.

The discussion of each case focuses on specific malpractice issues, which necessitates omitting many conditions, truncating differential diagnoses, oversimplifying the medical points, and disregarding some diagnostic and therapeutic options. This article is not a substitute for conventional medical writings, nor does it provide legal advice or even discuss black letter law or legal theories. It is designed to provide neurologists with a rudimentary understanding of how lawsuits may arise from some commonly accepted medical practice myths, and thereby focus discussion on adapting practice patterns to improve patient care and minimize liability risk.

CASE 1: MANAGEMENT OF THE INTRACRANIAL ARACHNOID CYST
Case Presentation

A previously healthy 30-year-old woman presented with a 2-year history of headaches increasing in frequency and intensity. The headaches were described as starting in the forehead, then generalizing but with a clear left-sided dominance, and varying in duration between hours and a few days. Visual analog scale (VAS) intensity ranged from 2.5 on good days to 8.5 during attacks. These attacks initially occurred weekly, progressing to several times a week.

The patient did not experience any relief with ibuprofen or ketobemidon hydrochloride, and her family physician prescribed Imigran for a presumptive diagnosis of migraine. Her headaches continued to escalate over the next year, prompting her physician to order an MRI scan, which revealed a Galassi type 1 arachnoid cyst in the left temporal fossa[6] (**Fig. 1**). The family doctor referred the patient to the local department of neurology. The neurologist advised the patient that the cyst was an incidental finding, unrelated to the headaches, and there was no indication for surgery. The headaches progressively worsened over another year, at times so severe that the patient was unable to work, prompting her family doctor to refer her to a regional department of neurosurgery. The neurosurgeon (KGW) performed an uneventful craniotomy with fenestration of the cyst to the basal subarachnoid space (**Fig. 2**). In the immediate postoperative period the patient had pronounced headache and nausea, which is common after cyst fenestration. Subsequently the headaches resolved with

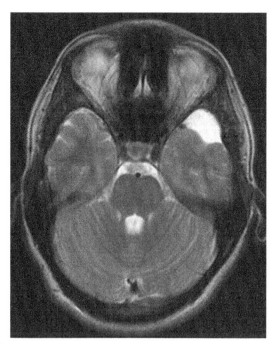

Fig. 1. Preoperative MRI.

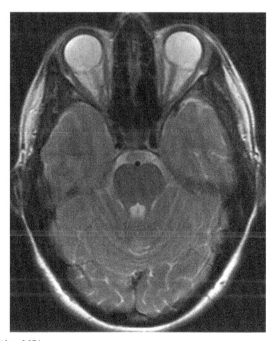

Fig. 2. Postoperative MRI.

a VAS of 1 to 2 at 3 months' follow-up and now, 5 years postoperatively, she remains without headache.

Questions

Do arachnoid cysts cause any symptoms? Does the size or location of the cyst matter? Should the neurologist have referred the patient for surgery?

Discussion

Comments

This story is fairly typical. Why? The intracranial arachnoid cyst remains the subject of outdated views and misconceptions, perpetuated by the neurosurgical training methodology. Initially, surgeons were craftsmen, trained outside universities through apprenticeships with a master of the trade. It was not until the Age of Enlightenment that the medical profession recognized the combination of science and surgery, and incorporated the trade as a formal discipline. Surgery evolved in tandem with the medical specialties, but remained a handicraft characterized by learning from more experienced colleagues. Even today, surgical training requires both an academic education as well as development of the necessary trade skills.

Although the ancient art of neurosurgery transitioned to a distinct specialty almost a century ago, modern neurosurgery evolved only during the last 40 to 50 years. In the 1950s intracranial surgery was a dangerous undertaking with extraordinarily high morbidity and mortality. At the time, masters of the trade wisely admonished their apprentices never to operate on benign intracranial cysts. The procedure was too risky, especially when the indication was not to save lives but improve the quality of life. These apprentices later became masters themselves, and conveyed this supposed wisdom to their apprentices without questioning the underlying truth, further entrenching the myth. This perpetuation of stale knowledge continues to influence neurosurgery, which affects neurology and remains an important reason for the current misunderstandings associated with arachnoid cysts.

What is an arachnoid cyst?

Arachnoid cysts are congenital space-occupying lesions formed by duplications of the arachnoid layer,[7] with an apparent cerebrospinal fluid (CSF)–like content,[8–10] and may present throughout the neuraxis but have a predilection for the temporal fossa, most often on the left side.[11,12] They are probably the most common intracranial expansive condition, with a reported prevalence of 0.2% to 1.7%.[13–17]

What symptoms are associated with arachnoid cysts?

Arachnoid cysts may present with specific sensorimotor findings or convulsions, but more commonly cause nondescript symptoms, including headache, nausea, dizziness, and impaired cognition.[18–35] Some patients have incidental cysts, are asymptomatic, and never warrant referral for further evaluation. However, the population-based data from patients with symptomatic arachnoid cysts who are referred to neurosurgery provides further insight regarding the clinical picture: 80% complain of headache; 25% of patients with temporal cysts and 60% of those with posterior fossa cysts patients report dizziness and nausea; and about 20% of patients with supratentorial cysts have epileptic seizures. These observations comport with other reports.[36,37] Only a small fraction approximating 10% of symptomatic patients complain of cognitive problems,[20] although systematic probing through neuropsychological testing shows both verbal and nonverbal dysfunction in patients with supratentorial cysts. The symptoms differ in children, in whom headache is less common (30%)

and a large proportion harbor cognitive or behavioral problems.[19] Arachnoid cysts rarely cause neurologic deficits.

The headache is generally nonspecific, of varying intensity, and may have symptom-free intervals followed by periods of incapacitating pain. It may be global or lateralized, albeit not necessarily to the side of the cyst. The dizziness may present as classic vertigo with well-defined spells or, more commonly, a nonspecific feeling of unsteadiness. Vertigo may occur with posterior fossa cysts as well as those in the temporal lobes.[29,30] Although few patients with intracranial arachnoid cysts present with subjective complaints of neurocognitive impairment, significant deficits are commonly uncovered through systematic neuropsychological testing. Several reports find these deficits spanning multiple cognitive spheres, including attention, memory, verbal, and visuospatial functions.[21,25,28,31,33,35,38] In addition, deficits in higher executive functions are evident.[23] Hitherto unpublished reports show that a large number of patients with supratentorial cysts have increased anxiety and depression scores. Several investigators have proposed that these types of cognitive deficits may be related to hypoperfusion of the cortical regions adjacent to the arachnoid cyst.[24,39–42]

One of the more common misconceptions regarding arachnoid cysts is that symptom intensity is related to cyst size, and it is often stated that small cysts do not cause major complaints. That statement does not seem to be true, because small and large cysts have the same capacity to elicit incapacitating complaints, at least for the most common symptoms of headache and dizziness. A recent study found no correlation between preoperative cyst volume and VAS scores for either of these symptoms.[43] What matters for the symptom intensity is the intracystic pressure, which seems to be independent of the cyst size.[18]

Decompressive surgery for arachnoid cysts

In principle, there are 4 different approaches for surgical cyst decompression: (1) craniotomy with fenestration of the cyst cavity to the basal cisterns; (2) endoscopic fenestration of the cyst cavity to the basal cisterns; (3) internal shunting of the cyst interior to another intracranial fluid compartment; and (4) shunting of the cyst interior to an extracranial compartment, such as the peritoneum.

Craniotomy seems to provide the best results. It requires general anesthesia and allows removal of the cyst wall, thus opening the closed cyst to the subarachnoid space and allowing drainage of the cyst fluid into the CSF. After opening the dura, the parietal cyst membrane covering the inside of the dura can be peeled off the dura, removed from its attachment to the surrounding cortex, and then excised. The arachnoid membrane attached to the brain surface (the visceral membrane) is not removed. The medial cyst wall covering the basal structures (the tentorial slit, the oculomotor nerve, the carotid artery, and the optic nerve) is fenestrated, thus creating communication from the previous cyst cavity to the basal cisterns and the posterior fossa. When accessible, the arachnoid covering the Sylvian fissure can also be opened, thus creating communication to the subarachnoid space surrounding the carotid and middle cerebral arteries. The goal of endoscopic fenestration is the same as for craniotomy: to achieve a communication between the cyst cavity and the subarachnoid space, but with a less invasive procedure.[44–46] Internal (cystosubdural) shunting is a minimally invasive procedure through a burr hole and can be performed under local anesthesia.[47,48] An ordinary ventricular drain is placed inside the cyst cavity, with the distal part of the drain sutured in place in the subdural compartment,[47,48] allowing drainage of the cyst fluid to this compartment. Alternatively, the distal drain may be placed in another intracranial fluid compartment (ventricle or CSF cistern). A cystoperitoneal shunt is similar to placement of a ventriculoperitonal uhunt and usually requires general anesthesia, but the proximal drain is placed in the cyst cavity and not in the ventricles.[49]

The advantage of the first 3 options is that they eliminate the pressure gradient between the cyst interior and the subarachnoid space. The cystoperitoneal shunt does not create such a balance between the intracystic and the intracranial pressure; to the contrary it may introduce a new pressure gradient, reducing the intracystic pressure to less than that of the intracranial pressure.

Does decompressive cyst surgery help?

Cyst decompression relieves the preoperative complaints in most patients, as in this case, and the risks associated with these procedures are limited.[19,20,47,48] About 80% of the patients with headache or dizziness experience an improvement of the preoperative complaints; the likelihood of improvement of epilepsy is lower. There is a reduction of fluid volume in approximately 80% of patients. However, there is no association between volume reduction and clinical improvement for adults.[18,20,47,48] In children, there is a correlation between volume reduction and clinical improvement.[18] More recently, other studies have shown similar results of surgical decompression.[36,37] Perfusion studies have shown that the preoperative cortical hypoperfusion adjacent to the cyst is normalized after decompression,[39–42] which seems to parallel the postoperative cognitive improvement.

What about the neurologist?

This case occurred in Norway, where the Norwegian System of Patient Injury Compensation precludes litigation. However, the neurologist, failing to recognize that intracranial arachnoid cysts may cause headaches, was admonished and provided with a copy of the records documenting proper patient care. In many nations, including the United States, it is possible that this case would have resulted in a malpractice suit against the neurologist.

Recommendations

In general, most patients with a symptomatic intracranial arachnoid cyst benefit from surgical decompression, which is a low-risk procedure. However, because improved quality of life is the main aim of surgical intervention for arachnoid cysts (except when the cyst has caused an intracystic and/or a subdural hematoma necessitating an emergency procedure),[50] it is of the utmost importance to provide the patient with all available information on the potential risks and benefits of surgery. Anything less constitutes a failure to provide informed consent.

CASE 2: NEUROIMAGING PATIENTS WITH ISOLATED HEADACHE
Case Presentation

A 28-year-old female architect described a 4-year history of episodic generalized headaches, sometimes more pronounced on one side or the other without predilection, occasionally throbbing and without any symptoms suggestive of an aura. Stress and lack of sleep were the only identifiable triggers. Initially the headaches occurred once or twice a month, lasting several hours, and sometimes improved with various nonprescription analgesics and nonsteroidal antiinflammatory medications. The headaches became more frequent over the past year, occurring once or twice a week, and she correspondingly increased the medication frequency without avail. Past medical history was unremarkable, family history revealed a maternal grandmother with headaches, and social history was notable for recent work absences attributed to the headaches. She presented to a family physician who diagnosed tension headaches and prescribed hydrocodone for the past 4 months, which the patient reports decreased the severity of pain. She returned for follow-up requesting another prescription and was referred to a neurologist.

The neurologist documented a normal neurologic examination, diagnosed common migraine headaches with possible medication overuse headaches, and advised the patient to discontinue all medications including over-the-counter drugs for 1 month. The patient returned after this drug holiday reporting that the headaches were worse. She was started on topiramate 100 mg twice a day. One month later the patient returned to clinic reporting no improvement. The neurologist advised her to give it more time and return in 2 months. At that time, she reported that the headaches were more frequent. Topiramate was increased to 200 mg twice a day, with follow-up in 2 months. She returned with no improvement and was advised to remain on topiramate, resume nonsteroidal antiinflammatory agents as needed but no more than 2 or 3 times a week, and return in 2 months. She called the neurologist's office 3 weeks later requesting an earlier follow-up because of the severity of the headaches and was advised by the nurse to stay on the prescribed medication, limit over-the-counter drugs as instructed, and keep her scheduled appointment.

Two weeks later the patient consulted her family physician who referred her to a second neurologist. That neurologist performed an MRI scan showing a convexity meningioma in the right frontal region necessitating surgical intervention. She experienced postoperative cognitive deficits precluding a return to work.

The patient filed a lawsuit against the family doctor and first neurologist. The neurologist stated in deposition that "[the patient] had a normal exam so there was no reason to order an MRI." The second neurologist and an independent third neurologist provided expert opinions on behalf of the patient. Another neurologist reviewed the case at the request of the first neurologist's malpractice insurer and recommended settlement. Ultimately the family doctor was dismissed from the suit, and the first neurologist's insurer settled for an undisclosed amount.

Questions

Should the first neurologist have performed an MRI? Did that neurologist breach the standard of care despite following practice guidelines?

Discussion

Background

Headaches are ubiquitous. The primary headache disorders like migraine and tension-type headache must be distinguished from myriad conditions causing secondary headaches. Accurate diagnosis of any patient with headache requires a detailed, complete, and accurate history coupled with general and neurologic examinations designed to exclude secondary headaches, diagnose the primary headache, and formulate a treatment plan.[2,4,5] This requirement mandates a de novo approach to each patient because secondary and primary headaches may be clinically indistinguishable, some secondary causes may trigger primary headache phenotypes, and the overall diagnostic differential is extraordinarily broad.[2,4,5] Neurologists are trained to focus on warning signs of a secondary headache as an indication for neuroimaging.[2,4,5] However, the subtleties of these warning signs demand the clinician's utmost attention.

Comments

This case is an example of the single most common diagnostic error in neurology, year after year, over the past 3 decades: labeling a patient with migraine or another headache disorder when subsequent evaluation uncovers a brain tumor or other structural disease.[2,4,5] These repeated errors are disconcerting, especially in light of the contemporaneous advances in neuroimaging and widespread availability of imaging centers.[2,4,51]

Why does this particular error recur so often? Perhaps some clinicians, overwhelmed by the sheer volume of patients with headache, adopt an apathetic approach,[2,4,51] or maybe the diagnostic errors are partially attributable to the insidious presentation of intracranial tumors and other structural diseases[2,4,51]: many patients with intracranial tumors have an unremarkable presentation[2,4,52]; a significant percentage of patients with brain tumor present with isolated headache[2,4,53]; certain tumors mimic particular headache syndromes[2,4,54,55]; tumor-related headaches often meet the International Headache Society criteria for migraine, tension, or mixed headaches[2,4,56]; headaches triggered by cough, exertion, and sexual activity are trivialized despite the high association with posterior fossa structural disease[2,4,57]; and supratentorial tumors may cause headache with psychological symptoms leading to psychiatric referral.[2,4,58] More commonly, poorly trained, inexperienced, or hurried neurologists overlook subtle warning signs of a secondary headache, such as the increasing frequency in this case.[2,4,5] Whatever the reasons, the malpractice data unquestionably support more aggressive imaging for the many patients with headache.

However, the neurologist in the case at hand will defend his failure to order neuroimaging by pointing to the guidelines promulgated by the American Academy of Neurology and 6 other professional organizations under the auspices of the United States Headache Consortium (USHC), which state that "neuroimaging is not usually warranted in patients with migraine and a normal neurological examination."[59] The USHC based their recommendations for migraine on a meta-analysis of 11 studies yielding a 0.2% summary prevalence of significant intracranial abnormalities in patients with migraine with a normal neurologic examination.[60] However, close scrutiny of these studies reveals serious methodological flaws: they consisted of small retrospective reports, devoid of relevant clinical detail, and were completed between 1976 and 1995 when imaging techniques underestimated intracranial abnormalities. Almost one-half of the limited studies antedated 1984, using first-generation computed tomography (CT); others used MRI without paramagnetic contrast or high-resolution studies, and not following any standardized protocol.

The USHC recommendations were seemingly supported by further reports suggesting that neuroimaging rarely yielded significant abnormalities in patients with chronic headache. A Spanish study of 1876 consecutive patients with nonacute headache and a normal neurologic examination reported significant intracranial abnormalities on neuroimaging in 1.2% of all patients, including 0.4%, 0.8%, and 3.7% of patients with migraine, tension, and indeterminate headache, respectively.[61] Similarly, a UK study reported imaging 530 of 3655 new patients presenting to a headache clinic over a 5-year period, yielding significant intracranial abnormalities in 2.1% of all patients and 1.2% of patients with migraine.[62] However, these studies are of questionable import. They were plagued by limitations underestimating the prevalence of intracranial disorders, including referral bias, limited demographics, patient selection variability, and inconsistent and suboptimal imaging practices. Neither study consistently defined insignificant but arbitrarily excluded select patients with abnormal imaging, including, for example, small arachnoid cysts, despite there being no correlations between preoperative cyst volume and VAS scores for headache and dizziness, or between postoperative volume reduction and clinical improvement.[43] Moreover, the UK findings were rendered meaningless by a lack of follow-up to determine whether the patients not imaged were subsequently found to have intracranial abnormalities.

The use of the guidelines and their supporting studies can be placed in proper perspective if viewed against the prism of the incidental findings on neuroimaging in asymptomatic people. Doing so compels the conclusion that the guidelines grossly underestimate the incidence of intracranial disorder in patients with headache. One study imaging healthy asymptomatic military recruits uncovered intracranial lesions in 6.5% of 2500 men with a mean age of 20.5 years.[17] A meta-analysis of 16 studies performed from 1989 to 2008 incorporating 19,559 people showed a 2.7% prevalence of intracranial abnormalities.[15] These studies used different MRI equipment with varying field strengths and inconsistent imaging protocols, most using low-resolution sequences, without paramagnetic contrast, and in the absence of multiplanar image reconstruction. Advanced imaging influences were plainly evident on subgroup analysis in which, for example, the prevalence increased to 4.3% when at least 1 high-resolution MRI sequence was performed. The population-based Rotterdam study showed intracranial abnormalities in 271 of 2000 people with a mean age of 63.3 years, including benign primary tumors in 1.6%, aneurysms in 1.8%, and infarction in 7.2%.[16] A Chinese report of 2164 asymptomatic individuals revealed incidental brain findings in 8.3%.[63] Subsequently, a UK research study of 525 healthy individuals yielded significant abnormalities in 8.8% of people.[64] It would be illogical to conclude that asymptomatic people have significantly more intracranial abnormalities than patients presenting with isolated headache, leaving no question that the guidelines are premised on outdated data.

Moreover, neither the guidelines' supporting studies nor subsequent reports provide sufficient evidence to determine whether there is any appreciable difference in the incidence of findings in asymptomatic people compared to patients with headache. Another weakness of the guidelines is the presumption that patients with brain tumors or other structural disease present with more than isolated headache. This presumption is inconsistent with the medical misadventure data, anecdotal reports, and shared experience of many neurologists and neurosurgeons treating these patients.[2,4,51,53] In a recent retrospective study, one-quarter of patients with biopsy-proven brain tumor presented with an incidental lesion (3.2%), nonspecific symptoms (9.5%), or isolated headaches (11.6%).[53] Following the guidelines would have denied neuroimaging for 3% to 7% of patients with a brain tumor, resulting in an unknown number of claims and possibly lawsuits.[53]

Unfortunately, these very same Guidelines were parroted by two American Board of Internal Medicine Foundation Choosing Wisely member societies,[65] the American Headache Society ("Don't perform neuroimaging studies in patients with stable headaches that meet criteria for migraine")[66] and the American College of Radiology ("Don't do imaging for uncomplicated headache").[67] The Guidelines and related statements have led some investigators to suggest restricting neuroimaging for the patient with headache and a normal exam, mistakenly presuming that intracranial pathology is uncommon, occurs at the same rate in patients without headache, and structural disease does not present with isolated headache. For example, a recent review documenting neuroimaging in 12% of outpatient headache visits considered the procedure "common, costly and likely substantially overused," and recommended that restricting utilization should be a "major national priority."[68] These types of recommendations focus on reducing health care expenditure, and contend that incidental findings may lead to additional diagnostic intervention with further costs. As shown, this misguided approach is likely to lead clinicians into high-stakes litigation.

It is naive to assume that limiting neuroimaging will translate to reduced health care spending for patients with headache without considering the enormous costs associated with misdiagnosis, including unnecessary medical expenses, loss of patient productivity, liability costs, and related factors balanced against the cost of an imaging study. Earlier imaging allows prompt treatment, with more surgical options and ultimately an improved outcome.[2,4,50] This principle is particularly true with benign tumors, such as in this case, in which the delay in diagnosis increased the operative risk, and may have contributed to the increased postoperative morbidity precluding the patient's ability to return to work. In addition, many patients with headache have health concerns that are effectively addressed by imaging, resulting in higher patient satisfaction.[69] Likewise, early neuroimaging significantly reduces costs to patients scoring higher on the Hospital Anxiety and Depression Scale because of lower use of health care resources.[70]

Arguments against imaging patients with headache because of the possibility of uncovering incidental findings are plainly untenable. The harm of missing a treatable brain tumor or other structural lesion far outweighs the concern of an incidental finding. Moreover, some of the findings mislabeled incidental warrant treatment (eg, arachnoid cyst), continued monitoring (eg, aneurysm), or further investigation (eg, stroke). At the least the patient should be given the option of imaging after a frank discussion of the facts, not a recitation of the myths. This approach is simply respectful of patient autonomy, which is a fundamental tenet of clinical ethics. It also opens a dialogue to address expectations, which strengthens the physician-patient relationship, thereby improving patient care and reducing liability risks. Blindly following outdated or poorly constructed guidelines eviscerates any meaningful informed consent. It is antithetical to the ethical mandate of acting in the best interests of the patient.

The overarching issue in this case is what obligation do neurologists have to follow guidelines issued by various professional organizations? The answer is that guidelines are double-edged swords that may be used for or against physicians in litigation depending on the facts and circumstances of a particular case.[3,5,71] The first fact to remember, however, is that guidelines are exactly that: guides to diagnosis and treatment, "applicable in narrow circumstances, and subject to continuous modification based on the patient's clinical picture, disease severity, symptom progression, coexistent diseases, complications, medication reactions, and a host of other variables,"[51] rather than the final arbiter of a standard of care (SOC).[3] The second fact to remember is that guidelines are not a substitute for informed consent judgment applied to careful histories and complete examinations. Guideline use in litigation varies from jurisdiction to jurisdiction.[3–5,71] However, even if accepted as SOC, each case and each patient must be viewed through the lens of clinical judgment based on individual histories and findings; otherwise the physician is practicing cookbook medicine. If sued for failing to follow guidelines that are accepted as SOC, the physician must justify any decision to deviate from the guidelines and must produce expert witnesses agreeing with the clinical reasoning. The same is true for following the guidelines, as in this case. Now the position is reversed. The physician is sued for slavishly following outdated and poorly constructed guidelines, and failing to use clinical judgment. The patient brings experts testifying that the guidelines are not SOC, whereas the defense testifies to the opposite. Ultimately the trier of fact decides who to believe.

These decision-making concerns are an ongoing problem in clinical medicine. There is a plethora of guidelines, statements, practice parameters, and commentaries; the US Department of Health and Human Services Agency for Healthcare Research and Quality publishes the National Guideline Clearinghouse, which lists 341 guidelines under the search term neurology.[72] Methods vary considerably among published guidelines, some of which, because of rapid advances, are outdated soon after publication. Updated guidelines are also affected and therefore determining validity and current usefulness is sometimes extremely difficult. Not all guidelines are created equal. Some are simply based on poor science and low levels of evidence. Others are biased. Distinguishing between them is the key to guideline use, but that is easier written than done. For practitioners following a guideline or choosing not to follow a guideline, the advice is to be prepared to justify either decision and consider how to defend that decision in court and what medical expert witness would support that decision.[3]

Recommendations

Continued adherence to the guidelines and statements discussed herein will ensure that the failure to diagnose brain tumor or other intracranial structural disease remains the most common diagnostic error in neurology. Outdated or poorly constructed guidelines are of no use and simply help set up unsuspecting clinicians for potential claims. The current guidelines and statements that advise against imaging patients with headache and a normal examination should be deleted and further research undertaken to correlate intracranial abnormalities with individual patient data, headache patterns, underlying diseases, associated conditions, imaging protocols, and related factors in order to provide practitioners with rational imaging guidelines. In the intervening time, it would be prudent to consider imaging all patients presenting with a new headache, or a headache with increasing frequency or changing pattern, or any other warning sign. It is hoped that most neurologists now agree that MRI is preferred to CT in this type of setting because of the higher sensitivity for detecting intracranial neoplasms, white matter abnormalities, meningeal diseases, and other structural features, as well as the ability to visualize the pituitary region, posterior fossa, and cervicomedullary junction, all while avoiding radiation exposure.[2,4,5,51]

CASE 3: THROMBOLYSIS FOR STROKE ON AWAKENING
Case Presentation

A neurologist is called to the emergency room shortly before 11 AM to consult on a 79-year-old man with aphasia and right-sided hemiparesis, scoring 20 on the National Institutes of Health Stroke Scale. Family members report that he was independent, active, and fine when he went to bed at 11 PM the previous night, and was found awake in bed at 9 AM, unable to speak or move his right side. The emergency physician suggested treatment with intravenous recombinant tissue plasminogen activator (tPA). The neurologist documented a discussion with the family and administered tPA. The patient had a massive intracerebral hemorrhage and died 2 weeks later from pulmonary complications. The family subsequently sued the neurologist, emergency physician, internist, and hospital, under several theories, including negligence and lack of informed consent, and the case settled for an undisclosed sum after protracted legal proceedings. The neurologist stated in deposition that "current studies show treating wake up strokes may be helpful."

Questions

Why are neurologists sued over tPA? What is the best way to manage patients presenting with a stroke on awakening or of unknown onset?

Discussion

Background
Stroke causes almost 7 million deaths globally every year, and represents a leading source of disability.[73] In the United States 800,000 people have a stroke each year (predominantly ischemic strokes).[74–76] Intravenous tPA was approved by the US Food and Drug Administration 2 decades ago for the treatment of acute ischemic stroke and remains the mainstay of therapy.[77] The drug must be rapidly administered

because therapeutic efficacy is time sensitive, and earlier treatment is associated with improved functional outcome.[77–81] Every 30-minute delay in acute reperfusion results in a 10% relative reduction in the likelihood of a good outcome.[82] The current guidelines provide specific inclusion and exclusion criteria, and advise that tPA should be administered within 4.5 hours after stroke onset, even when the patient is being considered for endovascular therapy.[83,84] The combination of a narrow therapeutic window, discord over data analysis, misinterpretation of practice guidelines, and fear of litigation have created an inordinate amount of confusion thwarting the widespread use of tPA.[2,4,5,85–88] In the United States, fewer than 10% of patients with acute ischemic stroke receive tPA.[87,89]

Comments

Most physicians are fearful of lawsuits over tPA-related hemorrhagic complications despite repeated studies showing these constitute a minority of claims.[90] The initial trials indicated that tPA therapy increased the percentage of patients who developed intracerebral hemorrhage from 0.6% in placebo-treated patients to 6.4%,[77] but independent reanalysis of the original data more favorably showed that tPA rarely caused meaningful clinical deterioration,[91] and further evaluation concluded that patients were at least 10 times more likely to be helped than harmed with tPA for acute stroke.[92]

A decade ago one author proposed that "the failure to recommend or use tPA in an eligible patient – whether due to fear of liability [for hemorrhagic complications] or not – is, in fact, malpractice and an area ripe for litigation."[93] It turned out to be true. This area is now the most frequent stroke-related malpractice claim, followed by or associated with the failure to properly diagnose an ischemic stroke.[88,94,95] Therefore, neurologists deciding not to use tPA in an acute ischemic stroke should clearly document the reasons for that decision in the medical records. In contrast, it is imperative to resist pressure from the emergency physician or family to use tPA unless the patient unequivocally satisfies all inclusion and exclusion criteria. Modification of the criteria, especially exceeding the time constraint, diminishes the benefit of tPA and increases the risk of intracerebral hemorrhage with the concomitant patient harm and liability risks.[83]

It is, therefore, crucial to determine the exact time of stroke onset, which becomes problematic in the 20% to 25% of patients with stroke who wake up with symptoms.[96–98] A common error is to label the onset as the time symptoms were first observed rather than the last time the patient was known to be well.[2,4,5] For example, when the patient wakens with deficits, the onset must be considered the time when the patient went to bed, not when the symptoms were noted on awakening. The same principle holds true when a patient has aphasia or a stroke-related neglect syndrome and cannot reliably communicate, and there are no available witnesses to describe the onset.

In this case, the neurologist recognized a wake-up stroke with an onset time far beyond the acceptable window, and elected to administer tPA. The neurologist stated in deposition that this decision was based on education, experience, and understanding of the literature, and cited 1 study suggesting that patients with wake-up stroke may benefit from tPA thrombolysis.[99] But the question is, was this reliance on background, experience, and limited literature within the SOC for reasonable prudent neurologists under the same or similar circumstances (a form of the usual negligence definition in a medical malpractice case)?

Probably not. There is a lack of definitive evidence regarding the efficacy and safety of tPA for wake-up stroke because these patients were excluded from the formative clinical trials that led to the guidelines. The available limited data for reperfusion therapy in wake-up stroke include multiple small, single-center observational reports on the off-label use of tPA,[100–112] a multicenter study,[113] and a phase II study,[114] all with marked heterogeneity of methodology, inclusion criteria, imaging protocols, and reported treatment outcomes, and none providing sufficient evidence to recommend tPA for wake-up stroke.[115] The only large, multicenter, randomized, placebo-controlled trial on perfusion therapy in wake-up strokes used a glycoprotein IIb/IIIa inhibitor, abciximab, and was terminated because of an unacceptably high rate of hemorrhagic complications.[116,117] There are several ongoing trials of thrombolysis in wake-up stroke or stroke of unclear onset, but it will probably take considerable time before any consequential results are available for implementation in clinical practice.[118–120] At present, there are no known clinical or radiographic features allowing selection of patients with wake-up stroke who may benefit from reperfusion therapy. Thus, neurologists should adhere to the national guidelines recommending administration of tPA in eligible patients within 4.5 hours of stroke onset. The answer to the SOC-negligence question and the neurologist's reliance on select literature rather than the national guidelines becomes very problematic.

Causation issues, which are separate from SOC-negligence issues, may favor neurologists, because the literature unequivocally states that only a minority of patients benefit from tPA.[121] This view seems to be changing with the increasing tPA-related litigation, because more jurisdictions are adopting a relaxed causation standard in the so-called loss-of-chance cases.[94,122,123] In these cases the failure to treat patients with stroke results in injury by depriving the patients of an opportunity for a good outcome, regardless of whether the likelihood was less than 50%.

Informed consent actions are common when the neurologist fails to document a frank discussion of the potential risks of tPA, including intracerebral hemorrhage, coma, and death.[2,4] In this case the patient's family alleged not only negligence but a lack of informed consent because they were not advised of the increased risk of intracerebral hemorrhage related to tPA administration beyond the recommended time frame. If the patient has cognitive impairment or communication deficits that preclude participation in the consent process, then the options should be discussed with a family member; however, it is important to recognize that only a legal representative can give proxy consent. If the patient is unable to give informed consent and no legal representative is available, then the neurologist has an ethical and legal obligation to proceed with thrombolysis when it is indicated.[2,4] Courts recognize the well-established legal doctrine of implied consent by assuming that competent individuals would agree to a procedure in their best interests.[124]

Although unrelated to this case, it is worth noting that other possible litigation concerns include whether the hospital is capable of performing thrombolysis in a timely fashion. If not, then the neurologist may be liable for failure to promptly transfer tPA-eligible patients to another institution for definitive treatment, which is likely to be an area of increasing litigation as stroke care evolves, and may similarly affect endovascular techniques in the future.

Recommendations

The refinement of prevention strategies and expansion of treatment options have created a heightened expectation of proper stroke management, which, combined with the catastrophic impact of stroke, heralds increasing litigation targeting the failure to properly evaluate patients and offer tPA in a timely manner. However, at this time, based on the current available evidence, tPA should generally not be administered to patients with stroke on awakening or of uncertain onset.

CASE 4: CEREBRAL PALSY, ELECTRONIC FETAL MONITORING, AND HYPOTHERMIA
Case Presentation

A child neurology colleague is being sued, and asks you to be a consulting expert witness to educate legal counsel on the medical issues, and perhaps serve as a trial expert witness. The lawsuit involves a child born at 38 weeks who is now 4 years old with severe spastic diplegia cerebral palsy (CP) and pronounced cognitive impairment. Your colleague has been sued along with the obstetrician, pediatrician, anesthesiologist, hospital, and the nurses attending the birth and those in the neonatal intensive care unit (NICU). The family is represented by a lawyer claiming that the child's lifetime care plan is $50 million. This amount represents the future medical damages but does not cover past medical, past and future lost wages, lost earning capacity, and past and future pain and suffering. The lawyer wants $75 million to settle out of court. You have never been an expert witness but have read some articles and understand the function of an expert as well as the SOC concept, and believe you could serve as an expert in the case.[3]

Question

Your colleague's lawyer sends the medical records and expert witness reports that the family's lawyer has filed with the court setting out the alleged negligent care, and asks you to write a report on the medical issues and reply, if possible, to the family's negligence allegations and provide citations to the medical literature.

Discussion

The records
One family expert is an obstetrician. He writes that the defendant obstetrician began the unfortunate chain of events leading to the child's CP and neurologic devastation by failing to heed the electronic fetal monitoring (EFM) showing a category II pattern for several hours and that the child should have been delivered by cesarean section (C-section) at least 2 hours earlier. If this had been done, it would have prevented the child's CP and cognitive deficits.

A second expert, a child neurologist, writes that the neurologist examining the child immediately after birth (your colleague) failed to reverse the child's neonatal encephalopathy with hypothermia, which, the expert writes, has been proved to successfully reverse most hypoxic ischemic encephalopathy (HIE), repair neural tissue, and prevent CP in almost all cases. The expert says that the failure of the neurologist to timely institute hypothermia and continue it for 120 hours at 32°C was a proximate cause of the child's CP and cognitive devastation. The expert opines that the predominant cause of CP and neonatal birth injury is an acute asphyxia insult, which was revealed in this child's EFM for the last hour before birth.

The medical records reveal a normal uncomplicated pregnancy. During labor the EFM showed varying degrees of category II patterns, with varying heart rate for the last hour before a vaginal birth. The APGAR (American Pediatric Gross Assessment Record) scores were 5 at 1 minute and 6 at 10 minutes, arterial cord blood gas at birth was pH 7.2, with a base deficit of 10 mEq/L at 1 hour after birth. After some initial breathing problems and 3 otherwise uneventful days in the NICU, the child was discharged in good health. Although the child was born at term (38 weeks), the pediatrician noted that the birth weight was greater than 2 standard deviations (SD) less than optimal.

You do extensive research and prepare a report to the lawyer on the 3 medical subjects within your expertise: CP, EFM, and hypothermia.

The report

I have reviewed the medical records, the reports from the family's doctors, and the medical literature. My CV setting forth my qualifications is attached.

In summary, it is my opinion that none of the allegations made by the family's doctors are viable allegations of negligence. In my opinion the physician caregivers all acted within the SOC and none of the acts or omissions of any physician caregiver proximately caused or contributed to cause the child's CP or cognitive deficits.

In my report the concept of negligence (malpractice) means that a physician has failed to do those things that a reasonable, prudent physician practicing the same specialty would do, taking into account the same or similar circumstances faced by the defendant physician.[3,125] In other words, the question is whether the physicians in this case breached the SOC as that concept is used in medical malpractice cases. The SOC concept does not require perfection.[3] Meeting the SOC simply means that a physician has not significantly deviated from what ordinary, reasonable practitioners do in similar situations.[3,125]

Cerebral palsy section

CP, the most common childhood disability, "a congenital motor disability of cerebral origin, is a group of lifelong movement disorders affecting about 2 out of every 1000 children."[126] CP has multiple causes, multiple subgroups and clinical presentations, is often accompanied by congenital anomalies both cerebral and noncerebral, and may be accompanied by multiple developmental disorders such as intellectual disability, autism, epilepsy, and visual impairments.[126–128]

From the middle of the 1850s, conventional wisdom taught that the exclusive cause of CP was birth trauma and/or asphyxia, hypoxia, and/or cerebral ischemia reflected by out-of-norm fetal heart rate; HIE.[125,127–131] HIE was thought to be benign as far as physicians were concerned until a revolutionary expansion of medical malpractice liability law occurred in the 1970s,[125–131] and trial lawyers began to successfully blame obstetricians for not recognizing HIE in time and intervening to save the fetus with a quick, simple C-section. Trial lawyers have since promoted HIE as the sole cause of CP, and HIE is now accepted as the true CP cause by the public and a large number of physicians. However, CP research beginning in the 1970s has proved that HIE as the primary cause of CP is a myth,[125–131] and that most CP has origins that are unrelated to events at birth but originate in causes occurring long before labor begins: preterm delivery, congenital malformations, infections, maternal fever, fetal growth restrictions (FGRs), multiple pregnancy, placental abnormalities, and genetic variants,[125–134] with 14% likely having single-gene mutations and up to 31% having a clinically relevant copy number variation.[127]

This child's CP and cognitive deficits, based on reasonable medical probability, were not caused by anything the physicians did or failed to do. There have been 3 consensus statements addressing CP causation and the criteria necessary to link CP to labor and birth.[127,135–137] Those essential criteria absent in this case are metabolic acidosis at birth shown by pH less than 7.0 and base deficit more than 12 mmol/L; early moderate to severe neonatal encephalopathy; CP of the spastic quadriplegic or dyskinetic type; exclusion of other identifiable causes like intrauterine growth restriction, prematurity, genetic disorders, and similar conditions; sentinel hypoxic events like ruptured uterus; sudden, sustained bradycardia from the event; APGAR score less than 4 after 5 minutes; signs of multisystem failure; and early neuroimaging signs of edema and intracranial hemorrhage.[127]

Current research has made the terms birth asphyxia and HIE outdated. These terms purposely imply an acute hypoxic/ischemic event related to labor or delivery as causative of a newborn's compromise, often, in the past, said to be reflected in nonspecific factors like meconium-stained amniotic fluid, low APGAR scores, and acidosis.[127,128] It is now well established that all of these clinical signs may be present at birth but are the result of long standing disorders beginning in pregnancy, such as infections, placental and umbilical vessel thrombosis, and many other factors not detectable or preventable.[127–131,135–138] The current more descriptive terminology for a child compromised at birth is neonatal encephalopathy, which accounts for most compromised newborns having no objective evidence of acute hypoxia or ischemia but who were compromised by long-standing factors present in pregnancy or genetics. Importantly, only 13% of term infants showing neonatal encephalopathy are later diagnosed with CP.[127]

Term-born infants represent the largest group of infants who go on to manifest morbidities such as CP and neurodevelopmental delay.[126,138,139] For many years umbilical arterial pH and base excess were thought to be objective measures of infants at risk for CP and neurodevelopmental complications[138] even though most term infants with low pH and increased base excess developed normally.[138,140] However, recent research has shown that pH or base excess values are highly questionable for identifying infants at risk for morbidity[138–141] and that most acidemic newborns, in the absence of neurologic symptoms, do not have an increased risk of developing neurologic or behavioral difficulties in the future.[138,140] Thus, in this case, the pH and base excess values are neither significant nor indicative of any labor or birth problem causing this child's CP or cognitive deficits.

FGR, defined as 2 SD less than optimal birth weight,[142] is associated with an increased risk of a wide range of neonatal adverse consequences: antenatal or neonatal death, neonatal encephalopathy, perinatal stroke, CP, epilepsy, autism, and schizophrenia. The association of FGR with CP has been especially robust.[142]

As noted, this child was 2 SD less than optimal birthweight. Although FGR has been thought to be related to pregnancy-induced hypertension (PIH), it is now clear from several studies that most FGR in singletons at or near term arises in pregnancies uncomplicated by PIH.[142] This study also confirmed prior studies finding that infants with FGR developing CP did not have asphyxial births more often than children with CP who had normal birth weights for gestational age.[142] Although half of infants with FGR developing CP had major birth defects, half did not.[142] The causes of FGR are many and varied and not well delineated, but the fact remains that normotensive FGR, as in this case, is a significant risk factor for CP.[142]

Electronic fetal monitoring section

The opinions expressed by the family's expert witnesses that a C-section in response to EFM patterns 2 hours before vaginal delivery would have prevented this child CP and cognitive deficits are unreliable opinions unsupported in whole or in part by any current medical evidence. Substantiated worldwide research and almost 50 years of EFM use has unequivocally proved that intervention in labor based on any single or combination EFM pattern interpretation does not predict or prevent CP, neonatal neurologic injury, stillbirth, neonatal acidemia, or neonatal encephalopathy, and that C-sections as an obstetric intervention to prevent CP or neonatal encephalopathy are a failure.[125–131,135–137,143–149]

EFM was introduced into clinical practice in 1970 without clinical trials.[125–131] The first clinical trial in 1976 found no EFM benefit compared with auscultation, as did 11 other trials up to 1995.[125–131,147,150,151] These trials did reveal that EFM's C-section rate was dramatically increased compared with auscultation because of EFM's 99% false-positive rate.[125–131,147,150,151] By the mid-2000s EFM research revealed that EFM had no effect on the rate of CP, perinatal mortality, or neurologic morbidity,[125–131,147,150,151] and a few contemporary observers were convinced that EFM did more harm than good for mothers and babies primarily because EFM caused huge numbers of unnecessary C-sections,[125,126,129–131,143,144,149] with the attendant morbidity and mortality associated with that major abdominal operation.[125,127,128,131,143,145,151–155]

Importantly, EFM research, past and contemporary, also reveals that EFM pattern interpretation by the so-called EFM experts is subjective, difficult to standardize, poorly reproducible, and often biased.[125,127,130,143,147,148,151,156–159] In addition, although 80% of EFM patterns of fetuses in labor are category II according to the National Institute of Child Health and Human Development (NICHD) 2008 uniform system of terminology, as was this child's EFM patterns, the American College of Obstetrics and Gynecology has never issued any management recommendations for how clinicians should respond to such patterns and, therefore, there is no SOC applicable to the response to these patterns, nor is there valid scientific evidence affirming the effectiveness of the various measures taken by clinicians to relieve these abnormal patterns.[144,160,161] The NICHD 3-tier EFM interpretation system has performed so poorly in clinical practice that contemporary observers question its physiologic foundation and call for radical changes in reliance on EFM interpretative guidelines.[125,127,143–145,149,160–164] The known bias and lack of objectivity in supposedly expert EFM interpretation in CP lawsuits has also spawned increasing demands for eliminating EFM junk science from the world's courtrooms.[125–128,130,131,143,151,156,165]

Hypothermia section

The family's neurologist's statements regarding hypothermia as a treatment of neonatal encephalopathy do not reflect the current research reported in the peer-reviewed literature and are simply wrong and misleading. The first neonate was enrolled in a clinical cooling therapy trial in 1999, after extensive animal and in vitro studies proved the concept.[166–168] Since then there have been major clinical trials, articles, workshops, and reviews updating methods and results.[166–169] The exact cellular and metabolic processes taking place in neonatal encephalopathy are complex and not fully understood, just as the mechanisms of hypothermia actions are unclear.[167,170] What is known is that therapeutic cooling decreases mortality and long-term neurologic morbidity in only a minority of neonates[126,170,171] (mortality and long-term morbidity reduced by 15%; CP risk reduced by 12%; number needed to treat, 8),[170] and the reason so many seemingly eligible neonates fail to benefit is unknown.[170]

The family's neurologist's opinions regarding hypothermia depth and duration as well as results that could be achieved are wrong. Hypothermia for 120 hours at 32°C as suggested has been reported as unsuccessful in a randomized clinical trial that was stopped early for safety and futility issues.[166,172] Hypothermia, as indicated earlier, does not reverse HIE as the neurologist has opined nor do EFM abnormalities in the hour before delivery identify neonates that qualify for hypothermia.[173] Importantly, this child does not meet the criteria for hypothermia specified in the current literature.[168]

Recommendations

The long-running CP-EFM myths have resulted in unjustified lawsuits against all health care providers involved in the birth process from labor and delivery to the NICU. These cases are time consuming, expensive, distressing, and often end in huge verdicts and settlements merely because of the emotional aspect involved with the enduring disability experienced by children with OP and their families. CP-EFM myths not only involve difficult and unresolved litigation issues but, perhaps more importantly, raise unaddressed ethical compromises by caregivers that have endured for decades in the way of defensive medicine. These ethical compromises may, in the near future, result in even more litigation if left unresolved.[174]

SUMMARY

As much as practitioners wish it, medical malpractice litigation will not disappear in the near or even distant future. However, efforts to reform the litigation system nationally, in most of the states, and even in other countries with like litigation systems, have met with total failure for the half century since the first insurance coverage crisis of the early 1970s. Despite efforts of medical societies, professional organizations, and individual physicians, trial lawyers have successfully blocked most reforms and watered down many of those that have passed. The reality is that physicians must adjust to the situation by focusing on risk management techniques that offer the most value for the effort. The most important is to remain cognizant of potential liability by thoroughly understanding the fundamentals of malpractice litigation and by keeping abreast of contemporary clinical scenarios that are becoming the malpractice case de jour, cases like those presented here, cases based on enduring medical myths.

REFERENCES

1. Cathell DW. The physician himself. 9th edition. Philadelphia: FA Davis Publishing; 1890. p. 62.
2. Johnston JC. Neurological malpractice and non-malpractice liability. Neurol Clin 2010;28(2):441–58.
3. Johnston JC, Sartwelle TP. The expert witness in medical malpractice litigation: Through the looking glass. J Child Neurol 2013;28:484–501.
4. Johnston JC. Legal issues in neurology: observations on American medical jurisprudence. In: Beran R, editor. Legal and forensic medicine. Berlin: Springer-Verlag Publishing; 2013. p. 1237–64.
5. Johnston JC. Neurology. In: Wecht C, editor. Preparing and winning medical negligence cases. 3rd edition. New York: Juris Publishing; 2009. p. 581–710.
6. Galassi E, Tognetti F, Gaist G, et al. CT scan and metrizamide CT cisternography in arachnoid cysts of the middle cranial fossa: classification and pathophysiological aspects. Surg Neurol 1982;17:363–9.
7. Bright R. Reports of medical cases selected with a view of illustrating the symptoms and cure of diseases by a reference to morbid anatomy. London: Longman, Rees, Orme, Brown and Green; 1827.
8. Berle M, Wester KG, Ulvik RJ, et al. Arachnoid cysts do not contain cerebrospinal fluid: a comparative chemical analysis of arachnoid cyst fluid and cerebrospinal fluid in adults. Cerebrospinal Fluid Res 2010;7:8.
9. Berle M, Kroksveen AC, Haaland OA, et al. Protein profiling reveals inter-individual protein homogeneity of arachnoid cyst fluid and high qualitative similarity to cerebrospinal fluid. Fluids Barriers CNS 2011;8:19.
10. Berle M, Kroksveen AC, Garberg H, et al. Quantitative proteomics comparison of arachnoid cyst fluid and cerebrospinal fluid collected perioperatively from arachnoid cyst patients. Fluids Barriers CNS 2013;10:17.
11. Helland CA, Lund-Johansen M, Wester K. Location, sidedness, and sex distribution of intracranial arachnoid cysts in a population-based sample. J Neurosurg 2010;113:934–9.

12. Wester K. Gender distribution and sidedness of middle fossa arachnoid cysts: a review of cases diagnosed with computed imaging. Neurosurg 1992;31:940–4.
13. Eskandary H, Sabba M, Khajehpour F, et al. Incidental findings in brain computed tomography scans of 3000 head trauma patients. Surg Neurol 2005;63:550–3.
14. Katzman GL, Dagher AP, Patronas NJ. Incidental findings on brain magnetic resonance imaging from 1000 asymptomatic volunteers. JAMA 1999;282:36–9.
15. Morris Z, Whiteley WN, Longstreth WT, et al. Incidental findings on brain magnetic resonance imaging: systematic review and meta-analysis. BMJ 2009; 339:b3016.
16. Vernooij MW, Ikram MA, Tanghe HL, et al. Incidental findings on brain MRI in the general population. N Engl J Med 2007;357:1821–8.
17. Weber F, Knopf H. Incidental findings in magnetic resonance imaging of the brains of healthy young men. J Neurol Sci 2006;24(1–2):81–4.
18. Helland CA, Wester K. Intracystic pressure in patients with temporal arachnoid cysts. A prospective study of pre-operative complaints and post-operative outcome. J Neurol Neurosurg Psychiatry 2007;78(6):620–3.
19. Helland CA, Wester K. A population-based study of intracranial arachnoid cysts: clinical and neuroimaging outcomes following surgical cyst decompression in children. J Neurosurg 2006;105:385–90.
20. Helland CA, Wester K. A population based study of intracranial arachnoid cysts: clinical and neuroimaging outcomes following surgical cyst decompression in adults. J Neurol Neurosurg Psychiatry 2007;78:1129–35.
21. Torgersen J, Helland C, Flaatten H, et al. Reversible dyscognition in patients with a unilateral, middle fossa arachnoid cyst revealed by using a laptop based neuropsychological test battery (CANTAB). J Neurol 2010;257:1909–16.
22. Bechter K, Wittek R, Seitz K, et al. Personality disorders improved after arachnoid cyst neurosurgery, then rediagnosed as 'minor' organic personality disorders. Psychiatry Res 2010;184:196–200.
23. Gjerde B, Schmid M, Hammar A, et al. Intracranial arachnoid cysts: impairment of higher cognitive functions and postoperative improvement. J Neurodev Disord 2013;5:21.
24. Horiguchi T, Takeshita K. Cognitive function and language of a child with an arachnoid cyst in the left frontal fossa. World J Biol Psychiatry 2000;1:159–63.
25. Isaksen E, Leet TH, Helland CA, et al. Maze learning in patients with intracranial arachnoid cysts. Acta Neurochir (Wien) 2013;155:841–8.
26. Lang W, Lang M, Kornhuber A, et al. Neuropsychological and neuroendocrinological disturbances associated with extracerebral cysts of the anterior and middle cranial fossa. Eur Arch Psychiatry Neurol Sci 1985;235:38–41.
27. Lebowitz BK, Schefft BK, Testa SM, et al. Neurocognitive sequelae of a giant arachnoid cyst: case study. Neurocase 2006;12:339–45.
28. Raeder MB, Helland CA, Hugdahl K, et al. Arachnoid cysts cause cognitive deficits that improve after surgery. Neurology 2005;64:160–2.
29. Tunes C, Flones I, Helland C, et al. Pre- and post-operative dizziness and postural instability in temporal arachnoid cyst patients. Acta Neurol Scand 2014;129(5):335–42.
30. Tunes C, Flones I, Helland C, et al. Disequilibrium in patients with posterior fossa arachnoid cysts. Acta Neurol Scand 2015;132(1):23–30.
31. Wester K, Hugdahl K. Arachnoid cysts of the left temporal fossa: impaired preoperative cognition and postoperative improvement. J Neurol Neurosurg Psychiatry 1995;59:293–8.

32. Wester K, Hugdahl K. Verbal laterality and handedness in patients with intracranial arachnoid cysts. J Neurol 2003;250:36–41.

33. Wester K. Intracranial arachnoid cysts–do they impair mental functions? J Neurol 2008;255(8):1113–20.

34. Zaatreh MM, Bates ER, Hooper SR, et al. Morphometric and neuropsychologic studies in children with arachnoid cysts. Pediatr Neurol 2002;26:134–8.

35. Gundersen H, Helland CA, Raeder MB, et al. Visual attention in patients with intracranial arachnoid cysts. J Neurol 2007;254:60–6.

36. Couvreur T, Hallaert G, Van Der Heggen T, et al. Endoscopic treatment of temporal arachnoid cysts in 34 patients. World Neurosurg 2015;84:734–40.

37. Wang Y, Wang F, Yu M, et al. Clinical and radiological outcomes of surgical treatment for symptomatic arachnoid cysts in adults. J Clin Neurosci 2015;22:1456–61.

38. Matsuda W, Akutsu H, Miyamoto S, et al. Apparently asymptomatic arachnoid cyst: postoperative improvement of subtle neuropsychological impediment - case report. Neurol Med Chir (Tokyo) 2010;50:430–3.

39. De Volder AG, Michel C, Thauvoy C, et al. Brain glucose utilisation in acquired childhood aphasia associated with a sylvian arachnoid cyst: recovery after shunting as demonstrated by PET. J Neurol Neurosurg Psychiatry 1994;57:296–300.

40. Martinez-Lage JF, Valenti JA, Piqueras C, et al. Functional assessment of intracranial arachnoid cysts with TC99 m-HMPAO SPECT: a preliminary report. Childs Nerv Syst 2006;22(9):1091–7.

41. Sgouros S, Chapman S. Congenital middle fossa arachnoid cysts may cause global brain ischaemia: a study with 99Tc-hexamethylpropyleneamineoxime single photon emission computerised tomography scans. Pediatr Neurosurg 2001; 35:188–94.

42. Tsurushima H, Harakuni T, Saito A, et al. Symptomatic arachnoid cyst of the left frontal convexity presenting with memory disturbance–case report. Neurol Med Chir (Tokyo) 2000;40:339–41.

43. Morkve SH, Helland CA, Amus J, et al. Surgical decompression of arachnoid cysts leads to improved quality of life: a prospective study. Neurosurg 2015. http://dx.doi.org/10.1227/NEU0000000000001100.

44. Choi JU, Kim DS, Huh R. Endoscopic approach to arachnoid cyst. Childs Nerv Syst 1999;15:285–91.

45. Hopf NJ, Perneczky A. Endoscopic neurosurgery and endoscope-assisted microneurosurgery for the treatment of intracranial cysts. Neurosurg 1998;43:1330–6.

46. Schroeder HW, Gaab MR, Niendorf WR. Neuroendoscopic approach to arachnoid cysts. J Neurosurg 1996;85:293–8.

47. Helland CA, Wester K. Arachnoid cysts in adults: long-term follow-up of patients treated with internal shunts to the subdural compartment. Surg Neurol 2006;66: 56–61.

48. Wester K. Arachnoid cysts in adults: experience with internal shunts to the subdural compartment. Surg Neurol 1996;45:15–24.

49. Ciricillo SF, Cogen PH, Harsh GR, et al. Intracranial arachnoid cysts in children. A comparison of the effects of fenestration and shunting. J Neurosurg 1991;74: 230–5.

50. Helland CA, Wester K. How often do extra-cerebral haematomas occur in patients with intracranial arachnoid cysts? J Neuro Neurosurg Psychiatry 2008; 79:72–5.

51. Evans RW, Johnston JC. Migraine and medical malpractice. Headache 2011;51: 434–40.

52. Purdy RA, Kirby S. Headaches and brain tumors. Neurol Clin 2004;22:39–53.

53. Hawasli AH, Chicoine MR, Dacey RG. Choosing wisely: a neurosurgical perspective on neuroimaging for headaches. Neurosurg 2015;76:1–6.

54. Levy MJ, Matharu MS, Meeran K, et al. The clinical characteristics of headache in patients with pituitary tumors. Brain 2005;128:1921–30.

55. Favier I, van Vliet JA, Roon KL, et al. Trigeminal autonomic cephalgias due to structural lesions. Arch Neurol 2007;64:25–31.

56. Schankin C, Rerrari U, Reinish V, et al. Characteristics of brain tumor associated headache. Cephalalgia 2007;27:904–11.

57. Chen PK, Fuh JL, Wang SJ. Cough headache: a study of 83 consecutive patients. Cephalalgia 2009;29(10):1079–85.

58. Price TR, Goetz KL, Lovell MR. Neuropsychiatric aspects of brain tumors. In: Yudofsky SC, Hales RE, editors. Textbook of neuropsychiatry and behavioral neurosciences. 5th edition. Washington, DC: American Psychiatric Publishing; 2008. p. 735–64.

59. Silberstein SD, for the United States Headache Consortium. Practice parameter: Evidence-based guidelines for migraine headache (an evidence-based review): Report of the Quality Standards Subcommittee of the American Academy of Neurology. Neurology 2000;55:754–62.

60. Frishberg B, Rosenberg J, Matchar D, et al. Evidence-based guidelines in the primary care setting: neuroimaging in patients with nonacute headache. USHC. Available at: http://tools.aan.com/professionals/practice/pdfs/gl0088.pdf. Accessed November 10, 2015.

61. Sempere AP, Porta-Etessam J, Medrano V, et al. Neuroimaging in the evaluation of patients with non-acute headache. Cephalalgia 2005;25:30–5.

62. Clarke CE, Edwards J, Nicholl DJ, et al. Imaging results in a consecutive series of 530 new patients in the Birmingham Headache Service. J Neurol 2010;257: 1274–8.

63. Lee WJ, Chang LB, Lee YC. Incidental findings on brain MRI [letter]. N Engl J Med 2008;358:853–4.

64. Hoggard M, Darwent G, Capener D, et al. The high incidence and bioethics of findings on magnetic resonance brain imaging of normal volunteers for neuroscience research. J Med Ethics 2009;35:194–9.

65. Available at: http://www.choosingwisely.org/. Accessed November 11, 2015.

66. American Headache Society. Choosing wisely: five things physicians and patients should question. Available at: http://www.americanheadachesociety.org/education/choosing_wisely/. Accessed November 11, 2015.

67. American College of Radiology. Choosing wisely: Five things physicians and patients should question. Available at: http://www.choosingwisely.org/societies/american-college-of-radiology/. Accessed November 11, 2015.

68. Callaghan BC, Kerber KA, Pace RJ, et al. Headaches and neuroimaging – high utilization and costs despite guidelines. JAMA Intern Med 2014;174(5):819–21.

69. Fenton JJ, Jerant AF, Berkakis KD, et al. The cost of satisfaction: a national study on patient satisfaction, health care utilization, expenditures and mortality. Arch Intern Med 2012;172(5):405–11.

70. Howard L, Wessely S, Leese M, et al. Are investigations anxiolytic or anxiogenic? A randomized controlled trial of neuroimaging to provide reassurance in chronic daily headache. J Neurol Neurosurg Psychiatry 2005;76(11):1558–64.

71. Taylor C. The use of clinical practice guidelines in determining the standard of care. J Leg Med 2014;35:273–90.

72. Available at: https://www.guideline.gov. Accessed December 2, 2015.

70. World Health Organization. Global health estimates: deaths by cause, age, sex and country, 2000-2012. Geneva (Switzerland): WHO; 2014.

74. Mozzaffarian D, Benjamin EJ, Go AS, et al. Heart disease and stroke statistics—2015 update: a report from the American Heart Association. Circulation 2015; 131(4):e29–322.

75. Available at: http://www.cdc.gov/stroke/facts.htm. Accessed November 16, 2015.

76. Allender S, Scarborough P, Viv P, et al. European cardiovascular disease statistics. European Heart Network; 2008.

77. The National Institute of Neurological Disorders and Stroke rt-PA Stroke Study Group. Tissue plasminogen activator for acute ischemic stroke. N Engl J Med 1995;333(24):1581–7.

78. Hacke W, Donnan G, Fieschi C, et al. Association of outcome with early stroke treatment: pooled analysis of ATLANTIS, ECASS and NINDS rt-PA stroke trials. Lancet 2004;363(9411):768–74.

79. Hacke W, Kaste M, Bluhmki E, et al. Thrombolysis with altepase 3 to 4.5 hours after acute ischemic stroke. N Engl J Med 2008;359(13):1317–29.

80. Saver JL, Fonarow GC, Smith EE, et al. Time to treatment with tissue plasminogen activator and outcome from acute ischemic stroke. JAMA 2013;309(23): 2480–8.

81. Lees KR, Bluhmki E, von Kummer R, et al. Time to treatment with intravenous alteplase and outcome in stroke: an updated pooled analysis of ECASS, ATLANTIS, NINDS and EPITHET trials. Lancet 2010;375(9727):1695–703.

82. Khatri P, Abruzzo T, Yeatts SD, et al. Good clinical outcome after ischemic stroke with successful revascularization is time-dependent. Neurology 2009;73(13): 1066–72.

83. Jauch EC, Saver JL, Adams HP, et al. Guidelines for the early management of patients with acute ischemic stroke: a guideline for healthcare professionals from the American Heart Association/American Stroke Association. Stroke 2013;44:870–947.

84. Powers WS, Derdeyn CP, Biller J, et al. 2015 American Heart Association/American Stroke Association focused update of the 2013 guidelines for the early management of patients with acute ischemic stroke regarding endovascular treatment: a guideline for healthcare professionals from the American Heart Association/American Stroke Association. Stroke 2015;46:3020–35.

85. Avitzur O. As public expectation for tPA grows, so too do lawsuits: how neurologists can reduce malpractice risks. Neuro Today 2006;6(9):31–2.

86. Johnston JC. On lawsuits regarding tissue plasminogen activator. Neuro Today 2006;6(13):4.

87. Asaithambi G, Tong X, George MG, et al. Acute stroke reperfusion therapy in the expanded treatment window era. J Stroke Cerebrovasc Dis 2014;23(9): 2316–21.

88. Liang BA, Lew R, Zivin JA. Review of tissue plasminogen activator, ischemic stroke and potential legal issues. Arch Neurol 2008;65(11):1429–33.

89. Schwamm LH, Ali SF, Reeves MJ, et al. Temporal trends in patient characteristics and treatment with intravenous thrombolysis among acute ischemic stroke patients at Get With the Guidelines – stroke hospitals. Circ Cardiovasc Qual Outcomes 2013;6:543–9.

90. Bruce NT, Neil WP, Zivin JA. Medico-legal aspects of using tissue plasminogen activator in acute ischemic stroke. Curr Treat Options Cardiovasc Med 2011;13: 233–9.

91. Saver JL. Hemorrhage after thrombolytic therapy for stroke: the clinically relevant number needed to harm. Stroke 2007;38(8):2279–83.
92. Demaerschalk BM. Thrombolytic therapy for acute stroke: the likelihood of being helped versus harmed. Stroke 2007;38(8):2215–6.
93. Johnston JC. To use tPA or not? The legal implications. Neurol Today 2005;5(3):4.
94. Liang BA, Zivin JA. Empirical characteristics of litigation involving tissue plasminogen activator and ischemic stroke. Ann Emerg Med 2008;52:160–4.
95. Bhatt A, Safdar A, Chaudhari D, et al. Medicolegal considerations with intravenous tissue plasminogen activator in stroke: a systematic review. Stroke Res Treat 2013. http://dx.doi.org/10.1155/2013/562564.
96. Mackey J, Kleindorfer D, Sucharew H, et al. Population-based study of wake-up strokes. Neurology 2011;76(19):1662–7.
97. Moradiya Y, Janjua N. Presentation and outcomes of "wake-up strokes" in a large randomized stroke trial: analysis of data from the international stroke trial. J Stroke Cerebrovasc Dis 2013;22(8):e286–92.
98. Fink JN, Kumar S, Horkan C, et al. The stroke patient who woke up: clinical and radiographical features, including diffusion and perfusion MRI. Stroke 2002;23:988–93.
99. Roveri L, La Gioia S, Ghidinelli C, et al. Wake-up stroke within 3 hours of symptom awareness: imaging and clinical features compared to standard recombinant tissue plasminogen activator treated stroke. J Stroke Cerebrovasc Dis 2013;22:703–8.
100. Cho AH, Sohn SI, Han MK, et al. Safety and efficacy of MRI-based thrombolysis in unclear-onset stroke. Cerebrovasc Dis 2008;25(6):572–9.
101. Iosif C, Oppenheim C, Trystram D, et al. MR imaging-based decision in thrombolytic therapy for stroke on awakening: report of 2 cases. AJNR Am J Neuroradiol 2008;29(7):1314–6.
102. Barreto AD, Martin-Schild S, Hallevi H, et al. Thrombolytic therapy for patients who wake up with stroke. Stroke 2009;40(3):827–32.
103. Natarajan SK, Snyder KV, Siddiqui AH, et al. Safety and effectiveness of endovascular therapy after 8 hours of acute ischemic stroke onset and wake-up strokes. Stroke 2009;40(10):3269–74.
104. Breuer L, Schellinger PD, Huttner HB, et al. Feasibility and safety of magnetic resonance imaging-based thrombolysis in patients with stroke on awakening: initial single-center experience. Int J Stroke 2010;5(2):68–73.
105. Kim JT, Park MS, Nam TS, et al. Thrombolysis as a factor associated with favorable outcomes in patients with unclear-onset stroke. Eur J Neurol 2011;18(7):988–94.
106. Aoki J, Kimura K, Iguchi Y, et al. Intravenous thrombolysis based on diffusion-weighted imaging and fluid-attenuated inversion recovery mismatch in acute stroke patients with unknown onset time. Cerebrovasc Dis 2011;31(5):435–41.
107. Natarajan SK, Karmon Y, Snyder KV, et al. Prospective acute ischemic stroke outcomes after endovascular therapy: a real-world experience. World Neurosurg 2010;74(4–5):455–64.
108. Manawadu D, Bodla S, Jarosz J, et al. A case-controlled comparison of thrombolysis outcomes between wake-up and known time of onset ischemic stroke patients. Stroke 2013;44(8):2226–31.
109. Bai Q, Zhao Z, Fu P, et al. Clinical outcomes of fast MRI-based thrombolysis in wake-up strokes compared to superacute ischemic strokes within 12 hours. Neurol Res 2013;35(5):492–7.
110. Manawadu D, Bodla S, Keep J, et al. Influence of age on thrombolysis outcome in wake-up stroke. Stroke 2013;44(10):2898–900.

111. Dhamoon D, Tassi R, Guerrini P, et al. Wake-ups (or wake up for) stroke a treatable stroke. Neuroradiol J 2013;26(5):573–8.

112. Jung S, Gralla J, Fischer U, et al. Safety of endovascular treatment beyond the 6 h time window in 205 patients. Eur J Neurol 2013;20(6):865–71.

113. Kang DW, Sohn SI, Hong KS, et al. Reperfusion therapy in unclear-onset stroke based on MRI evaluation (RESTORE): a prospective multi-center study. Stroke 2012;43(12):3278–83.

114. Hill MD, Kenney C, Dzialowski I, et al. Tissue Window in Stroke Thrombolysis study (TWIST): a safety study. Can J Neurol Sci 2013;40(1):17–20.

115. Buck D, Shaw LS, Price CI, et al. Reperfusion therapies for wake-up stroke: systematic review. Stroke 2014;45:1869–75.

116. Adams HP, Leira EC, Torner JC, et al. Emergency administration of abciximab for treatment of patients with acute ischemic stroke: results of an international phase III trial: abciximab in Emergency Treatment of Stroke Trial (abESTT-II). Stroke 2008;39(1):87–99.

117. Adams HP, Leira EC, Torner JC, et al. Treating patients with "wake-up" stroke: the experience of the abESTT-II trial. Stroke 2008;39(12):3277–82.

118. Ma H, Parsons MW, Christensen S, et al. A multicentre, randomized, double-blinded, placebo-controlled phase III study to investigate EXtending the time for Thrombolysis in Emergency Neurological Deficits (EXTEND). Int J Stroke 2012;7:74–80.

119. Thomalla G, Fiebach JB, Ostergaard L, et al. A multicenter, randomized, double-blind, placebo-controlled trial to test efficacy and safety of magnetic resonance imaging-based thrombolysis in wake-up stroke (WAKE-UP). Int J Stroke 2014;9:829–36.

120. Koga M, Toyoda K, Kimura K, et al. THAWS Investigators. THrombolysis in Acute Wake-up and unclear-onset strokes with alteplase at 0.6 mg/kg (THAWS) Trial. Int J Stroke 2014;9:1117–24.

121. Wardlaw JM, Muray V, Berge E, et al. Recombinant tissue plasminogen activator for acute ischaemic stroke: an updated systematic review and meta-analysis. Lancet 2012;379:2364–72.

122. Bambauer KZ, Johnston SC, Bambauer DE, et al. Reasons why few patients with acute stroke receive tissue plasminogen activator. Arch Neurol 2006;63: 661–4.

123. Fisher M, Schneider P. Stroke and the law. Stroke 2014;45:3141–6.

124. Canterbury v. Spence, 464 F.2d 772 (D.C. Cir 1972), cert. denied, 408 U.S. 1064 (1974) and its progeny.

125. Sartwelle TP, Johnston JC. Cerebral palsy litigation: change course or abandon ship. J Child Neurol 2015;30(7):828–41.

126. Nelson KB, Blair E. Prenatal factors in singletons with cerebral palsy born at or near term. N Engl J Med 2015;373(10):946–53.

127. MacLennan AH, Thompson SC, Gecz J. Cerebral palsy – causes, pathways, and the role of genetic variants. Am J Obstet Gynecol 2015;213(6):779–88.

128. Badawi N, Keogh JM. Causal pathways in cerebral palsy. J Paediatr Child Health 2013;49(1):5–8.

129. Donn SM, Chiswick ML, Fanaroff JM. Medico-legal implications of hypoxic-ischemic birth injury. Semin Fetal Neonatal Med 2014;19(5):317–21.

130. MacLennan A, Hankins G, Speer N. Only an expert witness can prevent cerebral palsy. Obstet Gynecol 2006;8(1):28–30.

131. Sartwelle TP. Defending a neurologic birth injury: asphyxia neonatorum redux. J Leg Med 2009;30(2):181–247.

132. Tollanes MC, Wilcox AJ, Lie RT, et al. Familial risk of cerebral palsy: population based cohort study. BMJ 2014;349:g4294–302.

133. Schnekenberg RP, Perkins EM, Miller JW, et al. De novo point mutations in patients diagnosed with ataxic cerebral palsy. Brain 2015;138(7):1817–32.

134. Moreno-DeLuca A, Ledbetter DH, Martin CL. Genomic insights into the causes and classifications of the cerebral palsies. Lancet Neurol 2012;11:383–92.

135. Am Coll Obstet & Gynecol and Am Acad Pediatrics. Neonatal encephalopathy and neurologic outcome. 2nd edition. 2014.

136. Am Coll Obstet & Gynecol and Am Acad Pediatricians. Neonatal encephalopathy and cerebral palsy: defining the pathogenesis and pathophysiology. 2003.

137. MacLennan AH. A template for defining a causal relationship between acute intrapartum events and cerebral palsy: international consensus statement. Br Med J 1999;319:1054–9.

138. Cahill AG. Umbilical artery pH and base deficit in obstetrics. Am J Obstet Gynecol 2015;2013(3):257–8.

139. Moster D, Wilcox AJ, Vollset SE, et al. Cerebral palsy among term and past term births. JAMA 2010;304:976–82.

140. Olofsson P. Determination of base excess in umbilical cord blood at birth: accessory or excess? Am J Obstet Gynecol 2015;213(3):259–61.

141. Tuuli MG, Stout MJ, Shanks A, et al. Umbilical cord arterial lactate compared with pH for predicting neonatal morbidity at term. Obstet Gynecol 2014;124: 756–61.

142. Blair E, Nelson KB. Fetal growth restrictions and risk of cerebral palsy in singletons born after at least 35 weeks gestation. Am J Obstet Gynecol 2015;212: 520.e1–7.

143. Sartwelle TP, Johnston JC. Neonatal encephalopathy 2015: opportunity lost and words unspoken. J Maternal Fetal Neonatal Med 2016;29(9):1372–5.

144. Constantine MM, Saade GR. The first cesarean: role of "fetal distress" diagnosis. Semin Perinatol 2012;36:379–83.

145. Grimes DA, Peipert JF. Electronic fetal monitoring as a public health screening program: the arithmetic of failure. Obstet Gynecol 2010;116(6):1397–400.

146. Khalil A, O'Brien P. Fetal heart rate monitoring – is it a waste of time? J Obstet Gynaecol India 2006;56(6):481–5.

147. Greene MF. Obstetricians still await a *deus ex machine*. N Engl J Med 2006; 355(21):2247–8.

148. MacLennan A, Nelson KB, Hankins G, et al. Who will deliver our grandchildren? JAMA 2005;294(13):1688–90.

149. Clarke S, Hankins G. Temporal and demographic trends in cerebral palsy – facts and fiction. Am J Obstet Gynecol 2003;188:628–33.

150. Graham EM, Petersen SM, Christo DK, et al. Intra-partum electronic fetal heart rate monitoring and prevention of perinatal brain injury. Obstet Gynecol 2006; 108(3):656–66.

151. Sartwelle TP. Electronic fetal monitoring: a bridge too far. J Leg Med 2012;33: 313–79.

152. Creanga AA, Bateman BT, Butwick AJ, et al. Morbidity associated with cesarean delivery in the United States: is placenta accrete an increasingly important contributor? Am J Obstet Gynecol 2015;213(3):384–6.

153. Silver RM, Fox KA, Barton JR, et al. Center for excellence for placenta accrete. Am J Obstet Gynecol 2015;212(5):561–8.

154. Spong CY, Berghella V, Wenstrom KD, et al. Preventing the first cesarean delivery: summary of a joint Eunice Kennedy Shriver National Institute of Child

Health and Human Development, Society for Maternal Fetal Medicine, and American College of Obstetrics and Gynecology Workshop. Obstet Gynecol 2012;120:1181–93.

155. American College of Obstetricians & Gynecologists and Society for Maternal Fetal Medicine. Safe prevention of the primary cesarean delivery. Am J Obstet Gynecol 2014;210(3):179–93.

156. Sabiani L, LeDu R, Loundou CA, et al. Intra and interobserver agreement among obstetric experts in court regarding the review of abnormal fetal heart rate tracings and obstetrical management. Am J Obstet Gynecol 2015;213(6): 856.e 1-8.

157. Sholapurkar SL. Interpretation of British experts' illustrations of fetal heart rate decelerations by consultant obstetricians, registrars and midwives: a prospective study – reasons for major disagreements with the experts and implications for clinical practice. Open J Obstet Gynecol 2013;3:454–65.

158. Hruban L, Spilka J, Chudacek V, et al. Agreement on intrapartum cardiotocogram recordings between expert obstetricians. J Eval Clin Pract 2015;21(4): 694–702.

159. Spilka J, Chudacek V, Janku P, et al. Analysis of obstetricians' decision making on CTG recordings. J Biomed Inform 2014;51:72–9.

160. Clark SL, Nageotte MP, Garite TJ, et al. Intrapartum management of category II fetal heart rate tracings: toward standardization of care. Am J Obstet Gynecol 2013;209(2):89–97.

161. Nageotte MP. Fetal heart rate monitoring. Semin Fetal Neonatal Med 2015;20(3): 144–8.

162. Sholapurkar SL. Categorization of fetal heart rate decelerations in American and European practice: importance and imperative of avoiding framing and confirmation biases. J Clin Med Res 2015;7(9):672–80.

163. Ugwumadu A. Are we (mis)guided by current guidelines on intrapartum fetal heart rate monitoring? Case for a more physiological approach to interpretation. BJOG 2014;121:1063–70.

164. Parer JT. Standardization of fetal heart rate pattern management: is international consensus possible? Hypertension Res Pregnancy 2014;2:51–8.

165. Maso G, Piccoli M, Deseta F, et al. Intrapartum fetal heart monitoring interpretation in labour: a critical appraisal. Minvera Ginecol 2015;67:65–79.

166. Robertson NJ, Marlow DM. Depth and duration of cooling for perinatal asphyxia encephalopathy. JAMA 2014;312(24):2623–39.

167. Perez JM, Feldman DO, Alpan G. Treating hypoxic ischemic encephalopathy with hypothermia. Neoreviews 2015;16(7):e413–9.

168. American Academy of Pediatrics. Hypothermia and neonatal encephalopathy, CLINICAL Report. Pediatrics 2014;133(6):1146–50.

169. Jacobs SE, Berg M, Hunt R, et al. Cooling for newborns with hypoxic ischemic encephalopathy. Cochrane Database Syst Rev 2013;(1):CD003311.

170. McIntyre S, Badawi N, Blair E, et al. Does aetiology of neonatal encephalopathy influence the outcome of treatment? Dev Med Child Neurol 2015;57(Suppl 3): 2–7.

171. Berg MT. Prevention of cerebral palsy: which infants will benefit from therapeutic hypothermia? J Pediatr 2015;167(1):8–10.

172. Shankaran S, Laptook AR, Pappas A. Effect of depth and duration of cooling on death in the NICU among neonates with hypoxic ischemic encephalopathy. JAMA 2014;312(24):2629–39.

173. Graham EM, Adami RR, McKenney SL, et al. Diagnostic accuracy of fetal heart rate monitoring in the identification of neonatal encephalopathy. Obstet Gynecol 2014;124(3):507–13.

174. Sartwelle TP, Johnston JC, Arda B. Perpetuating myths, fables and fairy tales: a half century of electronic fetal monitoring. Surg J 2015;01(01):e28–34.

Index

Note: Page numbers of article titles are in **boldface** type.

Neurol Clin 34 (2016) 775–814
http://dx.doi.org/10.1016/S0733-8619(16)30046-9
0733-8619/16/$ – see front matter

neurologic.theclinics.com

Moving?

Make sure your subscription moves with you!

To notify us of your new address, find your **Clinics Account Number** (located on your mailing label above your name), and contact customer service at:

Email: journalscustomerservice-usa@elsevier.com

800-654-2452 (subscribers in the U.S. & Canada)
314-447-8871 (subscribers outside of the U.S. & Canada)

Fax number: 314-447-8029

Elsevier Health Sciences Division
Subscription Customer Service
3251 Riverport Lane
Maryland Heights, MO 63043

*To ensure uninterrupted delivery of your subscription, please notify us at least 4 weeks in advance of move.

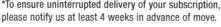